INTRODUCTION TO SONOGRAPHY AND PATIENT CARE

Steven M. Penny, MA, RT (R), RDMS (AB, PS, OB/GYN)
Medical Sonography Lead Instructor
Johnston Community College
Smithfield, North Carolina

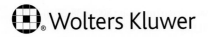. Wolters Kluwer

Philadelphia • Baltimore • New York • London
Buenos Aires • Hong Kong • Sydney • Tokyo

Acquisitions Editor: Jay Campbell
Product Development Editor: Staci Wolfson
Editorial Assistant: Tish Rogers
Marketing Manager: Shauna Kelley
Production Product Manager: Priscilla Crater
Design Coordinator: Teresa Mallon
Art Director: Jennifer Clements
Manufacturing Coordinator: Margie Orzech
Production Service: SPi Global

Library of Congress Cataloging-in-Publication Data
Penny, Steven M., author.
    Introduction to sonography and patient care / Steven M. Penny.
        p. ; cm.
    Includes bibliographical references.
    ISBN 978-1-4511-9259-9
    I. Title.
    [DNLM: 1. Ultrasonography—methods. 2. Career Choice. 3. Patient Care. WN 208]
    RC78.7.U4
    616.07'543—dc23

2015024250

RRS1809

INTRODUCTION TO SONOGRAPHY AND PATIENT CARE

To Him, the Ultimate Physician—Thank you for providing me with everything that I have or will have. Thank you for knowledge and the ability to share it with others. But most of all, thank you for your sacrifice for me. I know that this book would not be possible without your inspiration and your soft voice reminding me of my potential, a potential that I could obtain only through the strength that you can supply. I am grateful—but undeserving—of your everlasting, faultless love.

To Lisa—Thank you for everything you do for me and our children, for your compassionate spirit, your personal sacrifices for my career, and for being my best friend. I know that I could not have done any of this without you surrendering some of our shared valuable time together over the past few years. I love you. You have been, and will always be, the only one for me.

To Devin and Reagan—Thank you for being my kids. I can't imagine my life without you. I am so proud of both of you. I love both of you equally, exceptionally, and eternally. There is nothing that I would not sacrifice for you.
—Steven M. Penny

Contributors

Traci B. Fox, EdD, RT(R), RDMS, RVT
Assistant Professor and Clinical Coordinator
Diagnostic Medical and Vascular Sonography
  Program
Department of Radiologic Sciences
Research Assistant Professor, Radiology, Sidney
  Kimmel Medical College
Thomas Jefferson University
Philadelphia, Pennsylvania

Maureen McDonald, MBA, RDMS, RDCS, FASE
Assistant Professor/Cardiovascular Clinical
  Coordinator
Thomas Jefferson University, School of Health
  Professions
Philadelphia, Pennsylvania

Reviewers

Michael Beauford, RDMS, RVT
Instructor
Diagnostic Medical Sonography
Baton Rouge Community College
Baton Rouge, Louisiana

Patty Braga, RT, RDMS, RVT, RDCS
Associate Professor
Diagnostic Medical Sonography
Palm Beach Community College
Lake Worth, Florida

Erin Burns, BS, RT, RDMS, RVT
Coordinator of Clinical Education
Sonography Department
St. Catherine College
Springfield, Kentucky

Keith Farwell, MS, BS, BA
Program Director
Allied Health, School of Applied Studies
Washburn University
Topeka, Kansas

Leonardo Faundez, MA, BS
Professor
Ultrasound Program
The Michener Institute
Toronto, Ontario, Canada

Elena Guyer, MEd, RT, RDMS, RVT
Program Coordinator
Diagnostic Medical Sonography
Delaware Technical Community College
Dover, Delaware

Tiffany Johnson, MBA, RDMS, RVT, RT
Program Director
Saint Luke's Hospital
Kansas City, Missouri

Jo Ann Lamb, BS, RDMS, RVT, RT
Assistant Professor
School of Diagnostic Medical
  Sonography
Cuyahoga Community College
Parma, Ohio

Diana Martin, BS, AAS
Assistant Professor
Diagnostic Sonography
Cuyahoga Community College
Parma, Ohio

Jessica Murphy, BS, RRT-NPS, RDCS, RCS, RVT
Department Chair
Diagnostic Cardiovascular Sonography
Alvin Community College
Alvin, Texas

Kathleen Murphy, MBA, RDMS, RT
Director
Diagnostic Sonography
Central Arizona College
Apache Junction, Arizona

Ryan Parnell, ARRT, ARDMS
Term Instructor
Diagnostic Medical Sonography
University of Alaska Anchorage
Anchorage, Alaska

Sonia Rodriguez, RDMS
Ultrasound Instructor
Diagnostic Medical Sonography
National Polytechnic College
South Gate, California

Donna Rubosky, RDMS, RDCS, RVT
Program Director
Allied Health
Spokane Community College
Nine Mile Falls, Washington

Kitty Sheets, BA, RDMS
Director
Diagnostic Medical Sonography Program
East Coast Polytechnic Institute University
Newport News, Virginia

Angela Smith, RDMS
Instructor
Medical Sonography
Parker University
Dallas, Texas

Felicia Toreno, PhD, RDMS, RDCS, RVT
Program Director
Diagnostic Medical Sonography
Tidewater Community College
Virginia Beach, Virginia

Cara Vickery, RDMS, RT
Program Director
Diagnostic Medical Sonography
Bowling Green State University
Bowling Green, Ohio

Kerry Weinberg, MA, MPA, RDMS, RDCS, RT
Program Director
School of Health Professions
Diagnostic Medical Sonography
Long Island University
Brookville, New York
Sonography Specialty Advisors/Contributors

Preface

Patient care is the keystone of sonography. And although the sonographer is ultimately fashioned through the trials and tribulations of clinical practice, fundamental patient care exists as the basis of all that we do. Before a sonographer has the ability to distinguish a subtle renal malignancy, a small ventricular septal defect, or slight intimal thickening in a tortuous carotid artery, he or she must be capable of providing superior patient care. Regardless of your motive behind the selection of sonography as a profession, whether it is the result of intellectual curiosity or monetary gain, you must accept that patient well-being is the primary obligation of the sonographer. And for that reason, you are intrinsically required not only to provide healthcare for each patient but to truly care for the health of each patient.

The primary purpose of *Introduction to Sonography and Patient Care* is to provide the sonography student with an overview of the sonography profession and basic patient care. However, ultimately the book provides further evidence of the essential role that sonography and the sonographer play in medicine. Part I, Introduction to Sonography, offers a fundamental approach to learning more about the profession and about the practitioner.

One of the primary struggles for beginning sonography students is the initial shock experienced when he or she must combine the stresses of didactic and clinical sonography education with the strains of everyday life. In Chapter 1, helpful tips regarding specific classroom and clinical survival skills are provided, and an explanation of the importance of involving your support system in your studies. In Chapter 2, the focus is on the sonographer and the workplace obligations of those in the profession. Chapters 3 and 4 combine to provide a historical analysis of the use of ultrasound in medicine, specialties in sonography, and professional organizations. Chapter 4 ends with leadership roles in sonography and career establishment.

The use of proper ergonomics has gradually become more valued over the years for sonographers, and it is encouraging to see how much research has been conducted not only to highlight the risks for work-related musculoskeletal disorders for sonographers but to attempt to mediate this potential personal and professional calamity. Thanks to those involved in bringing the issue to the forefront, the sonography profession is now much more safe and sound. However, one must at the outset recognize the risks, know the consequences of flawed mechanics, and strive to use best practices every day. For this reason, Chapter 5 focuses on the prevention of work-related musculoskeletal disorders.

Permeated through every chapter in the book are direct references to the importance of being a professional and why demonstrating ethical behavior consistently is vital to the sonographer. However, Chapter 6 provides more facts regarding ethics and personal values. The chapter ends with a brief warning for students, asserting that every interaction should be viewed as a job interview and that first impressions are vital to future success.

Chapter 7 provides a brief analysis of legal essentials for the sonography student, including patient rights and the responsibility of the sonographer regarding confidentiality. Finally, basic principles and common knobology are offered in Chapter 8. This is a unique chapter for an introductory book, and though this chapter is not expansive, it will hopefully provide the reader with a succinct overview of transducer manipulation, scanning planes, and transducer care.

Part II, Introduction to Patient Care, begins with Chapter 9. Communication elements and a 10-step process for the sonographic examination are offered, from the assessment of relevant documents to the final release of the patient. Chapters 10 and 11 offer information regarding basic patient care and vital emergency care, respectively. One of the most important roles in patient care for the sonographer is to prevent the spread of infection among our patients. Consequently, in Chapter 12, infection control objectives abound. In Chapter 13, the primary focus is surgical asepsis technique and the role of the sonographer in invasive procedures. Lastly, Chapter 14 offers guidelines, patient preparation, and a brief synopsis of some suggested exam specifications for abdominal, small parts, musculoskeletal, gynecologic, obstetric, vascular, and echocardiography specialties.

FOR STUDENTS

Undoubtedly, the most distinctive quality of this textbook is that it is readable. It is written in a manner that is overtly conversational. Accordingly, the user should find this patient care book unique, understandable, and most importantly, applicable. Each chapter begins with chapter objectives and a brief introduction. Next, key terms, which are highlighted in the text in bold, are briefly defined for the reader. At the end of each chapter, following a brief summary, there is a critical thinking section. It is provided to advance the reader's acquaintance with the information and to allow for further illumination regarding the chapter content. Lastly, this book offers chapter review questions. The questions help the student evaluate comprehension of key chapter components. For students, the online components of this book include online cases studies and a quiz bank. To access the online resources, please visit thePoint.lww.com/PennyIntro1e.

FOR INSTRUCTORS

For the instructor, *Introduction to Sonography and Patient Care* provides you with a comprehensive text and a vast supply of textbook and ancillary resources. Within the chapters, important images and diagrams, "Sound Off" boxes, and carefully constructed tables are dispersed. "Sound Off" boxes highlight key points within the text. The procedures section for patient care is in the back of the book. This section provides bullet point instructions for important clinical competencies such as how to don sterile gloves, how to open a sterile pack, and how to take a blood pressure. These procedures can be practiced in the classroom, laboratory, or the clinical setting. Online, you will find a robust test generator, PowerPoint presentations, lesson plans, and a complete image bank (with color images), as well as course cartridges for learning management systems. To access the online resources, please visit thePoint.lww.com/PennyIntro1e.

FINAL NOTE

National certification in sonography is vital to confirm competency and to ensure a high standard of care. However, perhaps even more vital for the individual patient is the personal interaction, compassion, and respect received from the sonographer. It is my strong belief that while didactic testing is invaluable for assessing comprehension, knowledge, and retention, clinical practice is the most vital component of becoming a sonographer, and clinical is where the most tangible testing occurs. It is my hope that this book will outline the need to always place the patient's welfare first.

Steven M. Penny

Acknowledgments

I would first like to thank Pete Sabatini, the primary person who created the spark, which eventually lit the fire to begin this project. Next, I would like to thank Mike Nobel at Lippincott Williams & Wilkins (LWW) for his guidance in the process and for providing the fuel to a nearly faltering small flame. Thanks also to my remarkably bright product development editor Staci Wolfson at LWW for offering her invaluable insight and editing abilities to the project. Thanks to marketing manager Shauna Kelley, other editors, product specialists, and special minions who worked behind the scenes at LWW to get this book to the marketplace.

To my parents, Ted and Linda Penny, thank you for providing me with a home that was strict but forgiving, honest, and loving. You instilled in me the work ethic to take on a task as large as this. Thanks for believing in me.

To my brother Jeff and his family, Tammy, Nick, and Mackenzie—thank you for being in my life and for your support.

To Dr. Traci B. Fox and Maureen McDonald, thank you for offering your knowledge concerning vascular technology and echocardiography, respectively.

Thank you to Angela Hansen for your help as well.

Thank you to my coworkers at Johnston Community College for your support. I enjoy working with you daily and greatly value our alliance as we partner together in education.

Thanks to all of my students, past, present, and future. You are the reason why I stay in education.

To all of my past patients—I pray that I helped you in some way. I pray that my concern for your well-being was overtly demonstrated through my actions, even when my patience and time were strained. I pray that if and when I faltered to make you feel special or irreplaceable, that you forgive me. Playing a small role in your care was a privilege.

Steven M. Penny

Contents

PART I

Introduction to Sonography

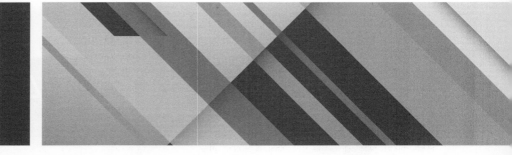

1

Foundations for the Sonography Student

CHAPTER OBJECTIVES

- Briefly explore vital concepts related to student success in sonography.
- Offer insight into classroom and clinical survival skills for sonography students.
- Understand workflow in the hospital setting.
- Appreciate the different imaging modalities that a sonography student will encounter while in the hospital or office setting.
- Recognize how vital critical thinking skills are in the sonography profession.

KEY TERMS

Acoustic windows (sonographic window) – the optimal location on the body for placement of the ultrasound transducer to demonstrate both normal anatomy and pathology; the best image acquired by manipulating and placing the ultrasound transducer in the most favorable position; some organs can provide a better acoustic window for improved viewing adjacent anatomy

American Registry for Diagnostic Medical Sonography – an organization that offers national certification exams for all sonography specialties

American Registry of Radiologic Technologists – an organization that offers national certification exams for radiographers and some sonography specialties

Anxiety – the general state of feeling worry and fear before confronting something emotionally or physically challenging

Arthrography – an x-ray procedure that utilizes contrast agent to examine a joint, such as the shoulder, knee, or hip

Assumptions – reasoning based on guesses or opinion

Audible sound – sound range that can be detected by the human ear

Brain dumping – a test preparation technique in which a large amount of information is memorized by a test taker, and when the test commences, the test taker "dumps" the information on a scrap piece of paper or the test

Cardiolite – a pharmaceutical agent used in nuclear medicine imaging to examine the blood flow of the heart

Cardiologist – a physician who diagnoses and treats cardiac and blood vessels disorders

Cardiovascular interventional technologist – a specialized radiographer that assists physicians in the treatment and diagnosis of cardiac and blood vessel disorders under fluoroscopy

Clinical competencies – unassisted sonographic examinations which are graded to determine fundamental proficiency

Clinical findings – the information gathered by obtaining a clinical history

Clinical history – includes signs and symptoms, pertinent illnesses, past surgeries, laboratory findings, and the results of other diagnostic testing of a patient

Clinical journal – a book used by students for personal and professional reflection

Computed tomography – an imaging modality that uses x-ray to obtain cross-sectional images of the body in multiple planes; also referred to as CT or CAT scan

Contrast agent – a substance that is either ingested or injected into the body to enhance the visualization of specific anatomy; disease contrast agents may also be used to treat disease; also referred to as a contrast medium

Coupling gel – a medium placed on the skin to allow ultrasound waves to enter the body also referred to as ultrasound gel

Critical thinking skills – resourceful actions, judgments, and decisions based on the combination of professional knowledge, experience, integrity, and ethical standards

Cross-training – when radiographers or other imaging specialists are training to perform another imaging modality in the clinical setting without specific classroom training

CT technologist – typically a registered radiographer who has undergone specific classroom and clinical training to perform computed tomography examinations

Diagnostic mammogram – a targeted mammogram, typically performed after a screening mammogram to further analyze the characteristics of a breast lesion

Diagnostician – an interpreting physician who provides a diagnosis

Differential diagnosis – a diagnostic method used to create a short list of possible diseases based on signs and symptoms

Fight-or-flight response – the body's physiologic reaction to a real or imagined threat that arises from situations that cause fear or anger

Fluoroscopy – an x-ray procedure that allows direct or realtime imaging of structures within the body

Gadolinium – a contrast agent used in MRI

Gold standard – the leading tool to diagnose certain diseases; for example, mammography is the gold standard for breast imaging, and sonography is the gold standard for gallbladder disease

Heart catheterization – a fluoroscopic procedure that involves the passing of a catheter into the right or left side of the heart, typically from the groin or arm, in order to evaluate and treat disorders related to the blood flow of the heart

Hippocratic Oath – a pledge observed by physicians and occasionally other healthcare professionals containing some basic guidelines for ethical standards and conduct between the healthcare provider and the patient

Indication – a basis for an examination; a valid reason to perform a certain test

Inference – reasoning that is based on gained factual knowledge using critical thinking.

Infrasound – the sound range below the normal hearing range of humans

International Classification of Disease, Ninth Edition (ICD9) code – a healthcare classification system that provides a system of diagnostic codes for classifying diseases

Interventional radiology – a branch of radiology that uses various imaging modalities to treat or further characterize disease by means of biopsy or minimally invasive procedures

Invasive procedures – procedures that include an imaging modality to treat disease; typically involves the use of catheters, needles, and surgical asepsis techniques (sterile techniques)

Investigative imaging – technique used by sonographers by which they obtain sonographic protocol images while simultaneously searching for and identifying abnormalities

Magnetic resonance angiogram – MRI technique used to visualize blood vessels

Magnetic resonance imaging – imaging modality that utilizes magnetic waves to obtain images of the human body in various planes

Mammography – Breast imaging technique that utilizes x-rays

Maternal-fetal medicine specialist – a physician who has specialized training that focuses on the medical and surgical management of high-risk pregnancies

Megahertz – 1 million hertz

Mnemonics – memorization technique; an acronym is an example of a mnemonic; an abbreviation is formed from the initial components in a phrase or a word in order to aid in quick recall

MRI technologist – imaging specialist trained in magnetic resonance imaging procedures

Myelography – an x-ray procedure that utilizes a contrast agent to identify abnormalities of the spinal cord

Nuclear medicine – imaging modality that employs the use of radioactive material for the diagnosis and treatment of various diseases

Nuclear medicine technologist – imaging specialist trained in nuclear medicine procedures

Nuclear stress test – a nuclear medicine test that requires the patient to exercise or be injected with a medication that stresses the heart for imaging purposes

Nurse practitioner – an advanced practice registered nurse who provides patient care and has the ability to order diagnostic tests under the supervision of a physician

Objective – something that is not influenced by personal feeling or opinion in regard to facts

Obstetrician – a physician trained in the care of pregnant patients

Pathology – a disease process; also could be referring to the profession of pathology, which is the precise study and diagnosis of disease by a pathologist

Physician assistant – a healthcare professional who practices medicine on a team under the supervision of a physician or surgeon and who has the ability to order diagnostic tests

Picture Archiving and Communication System – medical imaging technology that allows for the storage of digital studies for quick access and easy storage

Positron emission tomography – a technique that utilizes both the radionuclide imaging principles of nuclear medicine and the imaging techniques of computed tomography

Protocol (sonographic) – an inclusive order of necessary images acquired during a sonographic examination

Pulse-echo technique – ultrasound waves are pulsed into the body by a transducer; the sonographic image is produced when the pulsed wave returns to the transducer

Radiograph – an x-ray image

Radiographer – an imaging professional trained to obtain x-ray images and assist the radiologist in x-ray procedures

Radiography – the imaging specialty that utilizes x-rays to obtain images of the body

Radiologist – a physician that interprets radiologic procedures and also uses imaging modalities to treat disease

Radiopharmaceutical – a nuclear medicine radioactive material that the patient inhales, ingests, or is injected with for a nuclear medicine test that is capable of concentrating on specific organs or systems in order to evaluate organ function

Realtime imaging – instant viewing of internal structures

Scan (ultrasound) – to perform a sonographic examination

Scan lab – a practice room with ultrasound machines for students to use to gain scanning experience

Scintigraphy – a test in nuclear medicine in which the radiopharmaceutical is taken internally and the emitted radiation is captured by a gamma camera

Screening mammogram – the initial mammographic images of the breast

Signs – objective evidence of a disease

Society of Diagnostic Medical Sonography – the national membership society for all specialties in sonography; offers membership benefits and helps set standards for the sonography profession

Sonographer report – typically a written or typed document that provides basic descriptive information of the sonographic examination, including measurements of normal and abnormal structures, the sonographic appearance of organs and structures, and the manifestation of any sonographically identifiable abnormalities noted during the examination

Sonographic findings – information gathered by performing the sonographic examination

Sonography phantom – a simulation object that provides tissue similar to the human body that can be used to practice sonographic examination

Stress – the body's typical reaction to challenging situations that are perceived as demands on time, energy, or resources with the threat that not enough time, energy, or resources exist to fulfill an obligation

Stressors – individual events or perceived challenges placed upon time, energy, or resources that increase stress

Subjective – something that is potentially influenced by personal feeling or opinion in regard to facts

Surgical asepsis – the absence of viable pathogenic organisms; also referred to as sterile technique

Symptoms – any subjective indication of disease, like nausea, weakness, or numbness

Transducer – an instrument that emits ultrasound waves that is used by the sonographer to acquire sonographic images

Ultrasound – the sound range above the normal hearing range of humans

Vascular interventional radiographers – radiographers specialized in vascular intervention

Work ethic – effort consisting of perseverance and diligence

INTRODUCTION

Welcome to the sonography profession! If you are reading this text, you have most likely already started pursuing a career in sonography. The sonographer is a critical part of the healthcare team (Fig. 1-1). Before we recognize the unique function of the sonographer within the medical profession, we must first investigate where you as a student fit in and how you can plan for success now and in your future studies. Students can perform at varying levels of competency within a sonography department, from simple observations to completing unassisted but supervised sonographic examinations. This chapter will serve as a guide for student success by providing you with some insight into your educational pursuit and recommended skills to master as you progress through both your didactic and clinical training. Therefore, this chapter will offer an overview of the workflow and the layout of an imaging department, including an overview of the different imaging modalities that you

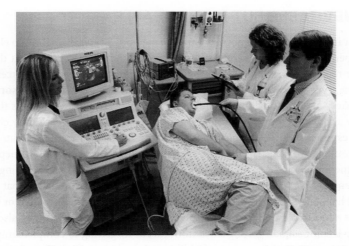

Figure 1-1. As a vital healthcare team member, the sonographer (*left*) must be capable of working with other professionals, including physicians and nurses, as demonstrated here during a transesophageal echocardiogram.

may encounter during your clinical rotations. The overarching objectives that you establish now as you begin your training should be aimed at becoming the best sonographer that you can be. Many of the concepts in this chapter will be returned to again later in this book. However, by initially understanding what is going on around you and how your environment impacts your role as a student, your responsibilities will hopefully be more clearly defined, and your objective toward becoming a registered sonographer will not just be a far-off dream, but a rewarding journey that has only just begun.

GOING BACK TO SCHOOL

Prior to endeavoring to comprehend the life-altering obstacles that sonography school entails, we must first recognize the blended group of students that you will refer to as classmates. For some of you, pursuing a career in sonography is a continuation of a career in radiology, cardiology, nursing, vascular technology, or some other medical specialty. Without a sabbatical between academic programs, you have chosen to pursue advanced studies in sonography. Your study skills may be highly developed, and your goals may be clearly established. However, there are two other groups of individuals who may find unique challenges. Some of you may have been unemployed for several years, or some of you could possibly be previous stay-at-home moms or dads.

First, for some students, sonography has become a secondary profession. This means that this person may have worked in a non-medical profession before deciding to pursue a career in sonography. These individuals may have limited patient care experience, though they find that they have a passion for helping others. Secondly, there may be some individuals who have chosen to obtain a degree in sonography, having recently graduated from high school. Though you may not fall into one of these categories specifically, you all share the same goal of becoming a registered sonographer. In preparation for a patient care environment where compassion should persist, offer support to those you recognize as struggling in their studies, and work together to help each other succeed.

Sound Off

In preparation for a patient care environment where compassion should persist, offer support to those you recognize as struggling in their studies, and work together to help each other succeed.

STRESS: INEVITABLE BUT MANAGEABLE

Stress is not just inevitable, but it is normal. Stress is the body's typical reaction to challenging situations that are perceived as demands on time, energy, or resources with the threat that not enough time, energy, or resources exist to fulfill an obligation.[1] Individual events or perceived challenges placed upon time, energy, or resources that increase stress are referred to as **stressors**. These stressors increase **anxiety** and do so with consequent physiologic responses. Anxiety is the general state of feeling worry and fear before confronting something emotionally or physically challenging. The **fight-or-flight response** is the body's physiologic reaction to real or imagined threats that arise from situations that cause fear or anger.[1] Hormones released by the adrenal glands, epinephrine (adrenaline) and norepinephrine, cause an increase in heart rate, shallow and rapid breathing, sweaty palms, and a surge in energy. We have all experienced the sudden rush of adrenaline that occurs when a surprising event happens, such as nearly being involved in an automobile accident or being suddenly awakened in the middle of the night by a telephone call during sleep. Stress can also build up over time. Waking up late for school, getting stuck in traffic, or forgetting to complete important assignments contribute to stress and cause us to feel like we have lost control. Therefore, it is important to recognize the causes of stress in our lives, be prepared in advance, and develop intervention techniques (Table 1-1).

TABLE 1-1	Dealing with stress and anxiety
Dealing with Stress and Anxiety	**Explanation**
Anticipate stress, and be prepared.	You can do this by being financially prepared, having a good support system made up of friends and family, maintaining a healthy lifestyle, and managing your time wisely (further details provided in this chapter).
Recognize the symptoms.	Symptoms may include feeling overwhelmed, suffocated, behind on daily tasks, and physical symptoms like sweaty palms, racing heart, abdominal discomfort, and shortness of breath. Try to identify and remove negative thoughts that contribute to anxiety and increase stress.
Use positive language.	Oftentimes, if you think more positively and use positive language with self-acknowledging statements like "I can do this," you will be successful. Maintain a positive outlook, and watch yourself meet goals.
Practice stress-reducing activities.	Walking, running, breathing exercises, playing a sport, practicing relaxation techniques, sleep, listening to music, and starting a new hobby are all good ways to reduce stress and distract your mind from the stressor.

Anxiety, according to the authors of *Under Pressure and Overwhelmed: Coping with Anxiety in College*,[2] is fueled by three mechanisms: cognitive component, physical component, and behavioral component. The cognitive components relate to how we interpret our circumstances. People who experience increased anxiety characteristically expect the worst out of situations. These individuals are generally pessimistic and constantly worry. It is important to note that less than 5% of events that we worry about actually come to fruition.[1] The second component of anxiety is the physical component, the aforementioned physical manifestation or symptoms of anxiety. The last component of anxiety is behavior. Of course, we all perform differently when faced with anxiety caused by stress. Destructive behavior resulting from anxiety includes removing yourself from a situation to avoid potential negative outcomes, dealing with stress with excessive alcohol use or reckless behavior, or procrastinating.[1] Some individuals may overcompensate to avoid anxiety and ultimately overprepare for tests, resulting in poor scores. For test anxiety tips, refer to the section in this chapter titled "Preparing for Tests."

Stress can be used as a motivator for some people. Studying harder for a difficult exam so that you are prepared is a means to compensate for and combat against anxiety. Feeling prepared and rising to the occasion makes you feel successful and boosts self-esteem. We have all had to face the stresses of school. The following sections will assist you in your quest to resolve stressful situations, but also keep in mind that your college or academic institution has resources for students and your professors should also be able to assist you in finding help.

Financial Preparedness

Annual salaries vary per specialty within the sonography profession. In 2012, the **Society of Diagnostic Medical Sonography** (SDMS) reported that the median annual income for sonographers was $78,520 (Table 1-2).[3] Although you have chosen to pursue a career that is in demand, you must be financially prepared to survive college. One of the most vital steps in the arduous process of pursuing a new career is to consider the possible financial ramifications. This means that you must contemplate the consequences of your educational pursuit for not only yourself but for your family

TABLE 1-2	Median annual compensation for sonographers in 2012
Registered Sonographer	**Median Annual Income**
RDMS	$77,000
RDCS	$85,644
RVT	$80,509

By credentials for registered diagnostic medical sonographers (RDMS), registered diagnostic cardiac sonographers (RDCS), and registered vascular technologists (RVT) according to the SDMS annual salary survey.
From SDMS News Wave, January 2013. Retrieved from http://www.sdms.org/members/news/NewsWave/NW-January-2013.pdf.

and others. Furthermore, economic woes can greatly inhibit your ability to focus on your studies, resulting in anxiety, academic issues, and emotional instability. Developing a financial budget and agreeing upon this budget with your significant other if you have one can greatly reduce the likelihood of financial tension in the future. Along with all of the other expenses of life, you must consider the ramification of the costs associated with child care, tuition, activities, technology, books, and travel related to school when you attempt to develop a working budget (Table 1-3).

Sound Off

Developing a financial budget and agreeing upon this budget with your significant other if you have one can greatly reduce the likelihood of financial tension in the future.

For many, working during school to pay bills is the only option. In fact, more than half of students attending college have a job.[4] Sonography programs are highly demanding fulltime programs, meaning your didactic workload is much like having a fulltime job. The requirements

TABLE 1-3	Money-saving tips for the sonography student	
Five Tips for Saving Money in School	**Explanation**
Buy e-books.	E-book versions of texts can be purchased, and these are typically slightly cheaper than traditional textbooks.
Carpool.	Carpooling with a fellow classmate can save everyone involved some money, and it is better for the environment.
Bring your lunch.	Making your lunch at home and bringing it to school or clinical can save you money every week that you might otherwise be spending on eating out.
Take online courses.	Though online courses may not be cheaper than traditional courses, you will typically save some money in travel expenses, as much of the coursework can be completed at home.
Seek employer reimbursement.	Some healthcare employers may assist you financially while in school and even offer you a position when you graduate.

of studying for many hours each night combined with clinical and laboratory rotations can be physically draining. Physical exhaustion can then lead to a lack of focus, and your academic goals could be derailed. Therefore, it may be best to work on weekends and avoid night shifts when possible.

Though additional debt is not always the appropriate solution, many students choose to take advantage of financial assistance. Financial stability throughout school can be maintained with support from employers and the state or federal government through low-interest loans, gifts, grants, and scholarships. Federal student aid applications are available online at www.fafsa.ed.gov. Also, secondary forms of savings that some may be eligible to receive include tax credits for both tuition and fees. It would be wise to consult your tax advisor while in school to determine what tax incentives exist for fulltime students, as these may vary from year to year. Seek help when needed, and take advantage of student support services, your academic advisor, and student counseling when you encounter financial strain.

Emotional Stability and Support

One of the most significant and ongoing struggles for many students is the challenge of maintaining emotional stability. In preparation for time away from family to study, it is best to preemptively share with loved ones the demands that will impact your individual relationship. Children and spouses need time to adjust to your busy schedule just like you do. But those same individuals can also provide encouragement during difficult times. Therefore, a solid support system made up of friends and family can provide one with the emotional sustenance needed to be successful. For some, the spiritual nourishment found in a place of worship strengthens determination and offers a respite from the stresses of life also.

Involving your family or friends in your studies can be both beneficial and work to strengthen relationships. Explain to them your assignments, and utilize them while studying for tests, practicing transducer manipulation, patient positioning, or practicing new procedures. Students can also find assistance from other students, sonographers, and faculty members. Sonography program administrators may develop a student mentoring program between first- and second-level students to encourage relationship development and provide additional distinctive student support.

Sound Off

A solid support system made up of friends and family can provide one with the emotional sustenance needed to be successful.

Physical Well-Being

Before beginning most sonography educational programs, students must undergo a physical examination, which includes immunizations, laboratory tests, and a drug screen. A drug screen tests for various chemical in the bloodstream, including alcohol and illegal drugs. If alcohol or illegal drugs are discovered on a drug screen, you may be dismissed from your educational program or prohibited from your clinical assignment. If a positive drug screen is discovered when you are employed as a sonographer, you will most likely lose your job.

Maintaining your physical well-being is strongly associated with your overall success. Your physical wellness can be maintained with regular exercise, eating a well-balanced diet, and getting adequate sleep. Taking breaks while studying to take a walk outside or to play some basketball can provide a quick stress release and some exercise at the same time.

Sound Off

If alcohol or illegal drugs are discovered on a drug screen, you may be dismissed from your educational program or prohibited from your clinical assignment. If a positive drug screen is discovered when you are employed as a sonographer, you will most likely lose your job.

TIME MANAGEMENT

Time management is crucial while in school. For those with immediate families, finding a balance between spending time with family and working on schoolwork consists of developing good time management skills (Table 1-4). Many external forces attempt to take up our time. Limit your extracurricular activities until your schoolwork is complete in order to reach deadlines and plan your day wisely. If you are not using electronic devices for school, put the device down and walk away! Instead, open your textbooks and read. Delay watching television as well. Instead, if you have the ability, record your favorite shows and use watching them as a reward after your studies are complete.

Sound Off

If you are not using electronic devices for school, put the device down and walk away! Instead, open your textbooks and read.

ESTABLISHING EDUCATIONAL GOALS

Educational requirements for acceptance into sonography programs vary. Creating educational goals starts with research into one's chosen profession and obtaining the foundation needed to have a successful, long-lasting career. Gregory Gottesman, author of *College Survival: A Crash Course for Students by Students*,[5] suggests five basic steps of goal setting (Table 1-5). Involving family members

TABLE 1-4	Time management tips for sonography students
Time Management Tip	**Explanation**
Use watching television or a movie as a reward, not as time-wasters.	This may sound impossible for some people. Many of us are addicted to television, but it takes us away from schoolwork.
Put the devices down, and walk away.	Our day is full of seemingly innocent distractions from our electronic devices (tablets, computers, smartphones, etc.). Most of what is accomplished may seem important, but most likely it is not.
Plan your day and week.	Your academic studies should rank high on your list of priorities. Afford time for reading, writing, and studying. Include adequate time in your day planning for eating, relaxing, sleeping, exercising, and family time.
Create your own academic calendar.	When you are provided assignments via a lesson plan from your instructors at the beginning of courses, organize your test, assignments and projects by writing them on a calendar.
Set your own deadlines for assignments early.	Use the deadlines provided by your professors for assignments as being late. Instead, set your own deadlines early so that you are prepared in advance.

TABLE 1-5	Five basic steps of goal setting
Five Basic Steps of Goal Setting	**Explanation**
Make a list of priorities, and rank them.	For the sonography student, your academic studies should rank high on this list. School should be a main priority. Be dedicated, and strive for achievement.
Set measurable and realistic long-term goals.	Establish a realistic GPA to achieve each semester and by the end of your academic studies.
Set short-term goals for classroom and clinical.	Long-term goals are not accomplished without meeting short-term goals along the way. Completing all lab assignments, homework, meeting attendance requirements, and mastering specific scanning skills are all short-term goals to establish from week to week.
Make social and personal goals.	Set aside some time for family and friends, and strive to reach personal fitness, financial, and spiritual goals.
Strive to meet those goals.	Write your goals down and mark them off when you complete them. If you do not achieve them at first, don't stop trying.

From Gottesman G, et al. *College Survival: A Crash Course for Students by Students.* 4th ed. New York, NY: Macmillan Company; 1996.

and fellow students in the establishment and implementation of these goals will undoubtedly help you achieve them. Keep in mind that your achievements in school will influence your likelihood for employment and your ability to provide sufficient patient care.

CLASSROOM SURVIVAL SKILLS

There are numerous common skills that successful students have, according to Susan Roubidoux, author of *101 Ways to Make Studying Easier and Faster for College Students*. Roubidoux claims that among the items on the list, successful students sit near the front of the classroom, have healthy snacks before lectures begin, take good notes, ask questions when clarity is needed, and prepare for tests efficiently.[6] The didactic or classroom portion of your training can take place before, after, or during your clinical rotations. That is, sonography programs vary as to the time during which didactic training occurs. However, when one encounters a large amount of complicated information, as found in a sonography educational program, it is easy to become overwhelmed. The following classroom survival skills will provide you with some insight and tips to help you prepare for the challenges of a sonography didactic education.

Pertinent Coursework

Courses relevant to your studies can strengthen your understanding of sonography. Sonographers must have a thorough understanding of anatomy, physiology, and pathophysiology. Therefore, these classes can provide both a foundation for your studies and reinforce information that you will encounter in your sonography program. Public speaking or communications, writing, fine arts, math, and basic physics courses will enhance your likelihood for success as well. Medical terminology courses are crucial in understanding the vocabulary of the medical world. Appendix 1 provides a list of common medical abbreviations, prefixes, and suffixes commonly used by sonographers.

With the growing Spanish-speaking population in North America, one could certainly benefit from taking a Spanish medical communication course. Some clinical facilities employ interpreters or use technology to communicate with patients who do not speak English. Appendix 2 provides some basic Spanish phrases that may be utilized. However, utilizing a trained medical interpreter is always the proper decision for ensuring accurate communication and providing optimal patient care.

Sound Off

Utilizing a trained medical interpreter is always the proper decision for ensuring accurate communication and providing optimal patient care.

There may be sonography programs that require applicants to be registered healthcare professionals, like a radiographer or nurse, before acceptance. Conversely, there are also programs with minimum entrance requirements, and these are available to individuals with very little medical background. One health occupation one can pursue to encourage the development of patient care skills is that of certified nursing assistant (CNA). Accordingly, obtaining a CNA certification and working in a patient care setting, even in a part-time or casual position, can provide you with some valuable patient care experience and practice with interacting with ill patients. The following chapters will further provide insight into how sonographers must interact with patients and how effective communication helps us gather useful information before performing an examination.

Within some sonography programs, online coursework consists of testing, course lecture retrieval, video sharing, and discussion board postings. Occasionally, online modules are provided with textbooks, and assignments are conducted by means of an online administration through Blackboard or Moodle. For some individuals returning to school, or those accustomed to a traditional education, maneuvering through online resources can be daunting. You should take advantage of introductory computer training programs offered by your institution to familiarize yourself with online classroom navigation. Purchasing a personal desktop or laptop computer would be wise as well, as online research at home may be encouraged by your instructors. When pricing items for school, especially higher-priced items like computers or tablets, ask the retailer about unique discounts for college students. At some institutions, laptop computers can be checked out from the school library as well.

Sound Off

When pricing items for school, especially higher-priced items like computers or tablets, ask the retailer about unique discounts for college students.

Preparing for Tests

We all prepare for tests differently. Some of us prepare well in advance for tests by studying some every night, while others prepare only the night before. Your institution typically has study resources for students, and Table 1-6 provides additional helpful tips for preparing for tests. Regardless of how you study, your aim should be to learn the information, not just to memorize it. You should genuinely understand the concepts because the information that is covered in your didactic classes is applicable to clinical practice and consequently directly impacts patient care.

Sound Off

Regardless of how you study, your aim should be to learn the information, not just to memorize it. You should genuinely understand the concepts because the information that is covered in your didactic classes is applicable to clinical practice and consequently directly impacts patient care.

Test anxiety is a common educational issue that all students have encountered at times. However, for some students, test anxiety can affect them to the point where their test results are dramatically altered, despite having prepared and grasped the information prior to the test.[7] In fact, studies have

TABLE 1-6	Test preparation tips
Test Preparation Tips	**Specific Goal**
Read your textbooks for comprehension.	• Read often: Though medical literature is dissimilar, reading fiction and nonfiction books can also strengthen your reading skills. • Take notes as you read: Highlight specific points, and write notes in the margins. • Take breaks: With a long reading assignment, take intermittent breaks to relax your brain and eyes. • Be prepared for lectures by reading the information in advance.
Take quality lecture notes.	• Be organized and prepared with pencils for note taking. If utilizing an e-book, have your computer ready to insert notes. • Use highlighters, but remember that simply highlighting information on a PowerPoint presentation or in the textbook is not necessarily adequate note taking. • Make notes of key points made by your instructor. • If classroom drawings or sketches are utilized by your instructor, draw them yourself in your notes. • If allowed, make audio recordings of lectures.
Create study cards and **mnemonics**.	• Developing a study method that incorporates note cards with questions on one side and answers on the other is a great way to study. • Create mnemonics for lists of materials in order for quick recall.
Form a study group, or find a study partner.	• Exchange e-mail addresses and phone numbers with fellow students, and form a study group. • You and your study partner(s) can meet early before tests to quiz each other.
Develop a study schedule, and take breaks.	• Study several times a week or some each night to prevent cramming and information overload. This may help you retain information. • Take breaks between studying, and sometimes use music to help you focus better while you are studying.

shown the scores of students suffering from test anxiety reduce by more than 12% compared to the non-anxious student.[7]

Essentially, overcoming severe test anxiety can result in an increase in test scores by a whole letter grade. Some colleges offer resources and counseling for students suffering from test anxiety, and special testing situations for students may be offered by some instructors for those with extreme testing issues. For example, study skills courses and one-on-one behavioral counseling have been shown to be the most effective at reducing test anxiety.[7] Table 1-7 provides some test-taking tips for all students, not just those suffering from anxiety.

Though some instructors may encourage a technique called **brain dumping**, it is not necessarily the best way to approach a test. Brain dumping is a test preparation technique whereby a large amount of information is memorized by a test taker, and when the test commences, the test taker "dumps" the information on a scrap piece of paper or the test. Therefore, if allowed before a test, students write down information on the test that one will most likely encounter. Some students may even be allowed to draw quick sketches of anatomy. Brain dumping is something that should be a last resort, however, as you should strive to learn and not memorize. And though your classroom instructors may allow this practice, the **American Registry for Diagnostic Medical Sonography** (ARDMS), the organization that offers national certification exams for sonographers, absolutely prohibits brain dumping on

TABLE 1-7	Test-taking tips

- Examine the length of the test.
- Estimate the time for different parts.
- Answer one item at a time.
- Look for keywords in the questions.
- Eliminate obviously erroneous answers.
- Return to harder questions.
- Hesitate before changing an answer.
- Make a quick outline of your thoughts before answering essay questions.

From Motevalli S, et al. New study skills training intervention for students who suffer from test anxiety. *Asian Soc Sci* 2013;9(7):85–96.

national certification exams.[8] Regarding this concept, sonographic information is cumulative. Your goal should be retaining and comprehending the information, not approaching each test in hopes of dumping the information just to obtain a good grade. Learning the material is better for developing your skills, and ultimately it is better for your patients.

Following the test, return to your notes and books, and highlight information that you recognized on the test. As many final examinations are cumulative, this technique will certainly help you prepare for a large amount of information. It is best to continually review information throughout the program. Go back to previous materials, and look over your notes when you have an opportunity. If allowed, take your books or notes to clinical to review during times that are slow.

Maintaining Motivation in the Classroom

Motivation is an additional key to educational success. Students can become easily overloaded with the amount of work that must be completed in a sonography program. Striving to do your best on every exam can be overwhelming, but it should always be your aim. Although you should be prepared, looking too far ahead can also increase anxiety. Approach one examination at a time, and put full effort into focused, dedicated study time for that one exam, and then move on to the next. Learn to reward your efforts after you do well on a test or examination, and try to avoid feeling depressed over tests on which you think you could have done better. Simply strive to do better on the next one, and make notes of information with which you struggled. Ask your instructors questions regarding specific concepts to gain a better understanding. Lastly, you should utilize your breaks from school to relax your mind and to do enjoyable activities, like gardening, exercising, traveling, or even catching up on sleep. Also, maintain motivation by setting individual academic goals so that the foundations of understanding established concepts in the classroom impact your clinical practice in a positive manner.

CLINICAL SURVIVAL SKILLS

The following sections will provide a brief overview of the role of sonographer, how important professionalism is in clinical settings, an explanation of workflow in an imaging department, and a concise explanation of several imaging modalities. As a student, in preparation for clinical, you should utilize a **scan lab** if your program provides one for students. As you progress into clinical, you should initially observe how sonographers interact with patients, the interpreting physician, and others on the healthcare team. It is also imperative for you to recognize the role of the sonographer within the healthcare team and workplace. The following sections will provide some clinical survival skills that may help you even before your first clinical experience.

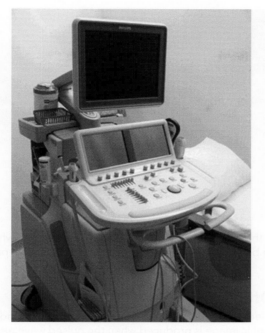

Figure 1-2. A Philips ie33 ultrasound machine.

The Sonographer: A Brief Overview

Though Chapters 2 and 4 provide further information regarding the sonographer and the sonography profession, respectively, it is vital at this time to provide a short synopsis of the obligations of a sonographer before delving into the clinical survival skills themselves. Sonography can be literally interpreted to mean "to draw with sound." A sonographer is a highly skilled medical professional who utilizes special equipment that emits **ultrasound** waves to create a diagnostic image of the human body (Fig. 1-2). These images are interpreted by a physician. **Audible sound** ranges are typically between 2 and 20,000 Hz. While **infrasound** is less than 2 Hz, ultrasound is greater than 20,000 Hz (Table 1-8). However, sonographers, when performing diagnostic ultrasound, utilize a much higher frequency range, typically between 2 **megahertz** (MHz) and 15 MHz, though some transducers may incorporate higher frequencies. Essentially, ultrasound waves are pulsed into the body by a **transducer** with the help of a **coupling gel** (Fig. 1-3). The sonographic image is produced when the pulse strikes an object within the body and returns again to the transducer, a process referred to as the **pulse-echo technique** (Fig. 1-4). Therefore, sonography offers a **realtime imaging** analysis of dynamic internal structures.

TABLE 1-8	Ranges of sound
Sound	**Ranges**
Infrasound	Less than 2 Hz
Audible sound	Between 2 and 20,000 Hz
Ultrasound	Greater than 20,000 Hz
Diagnostic ultrasound	Between 2 MHz and 15 MHz

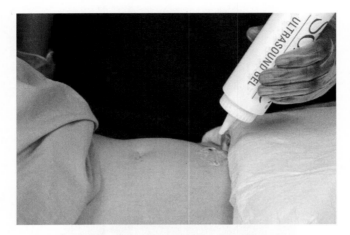

Figure 1-3. To image the body, sonographers utilize ultrasound gel, which may be dispensed in a bottle, as seen here, or contained in individual packets.

 Sound Off

In the pulse-echo technique, a transducer pulses ultrasound waves into the body. The sonographic image is produced when the pulsed wave returns to the transducer.

Before the examination, the sonographer obtains a **clinical history**, ultimately acquiring **clinical findings**, which are used to form a basis for the examination. After the examination, the sonographer offers a **sonographer report**, which provides basic descriptive information of the study, including measurement, the **sonographic findings** (such as appearance of organs and structures), and the manifestation of any sonographically identifiable abnormalities noted during the examination (Fig. 1-5). Interpreting physicians utilize this information along with viewing the sonographic images to develop a diagnosis. Therefore, it is the obligation of the sonographer to locate, measure, and describe **pathology** within the body.

Although you may witness it at times, sonographers should not be **diagnosticians**. A diagnostician is someone who produces a diagnosis from images and oftentimes shares the diagnosis with the patient. Physicians are diagnosticians. Furthermore, though the **investigative imaging** that we

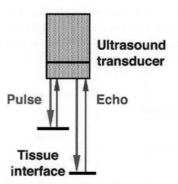

Figure 1-4. Pulse-echo technique. The transducer transmits a brief pulse of sound energy into tissue. The transmitted pulse encounters tissue interfaces, or boundaries, that reflect a portion of the sound beam back to the transducer. The depth of the tissue interface is determined by the round-trip time of flight for the transmitted pulse and the returning echo. The echo is then demonstrated on the monitor as a single dot.

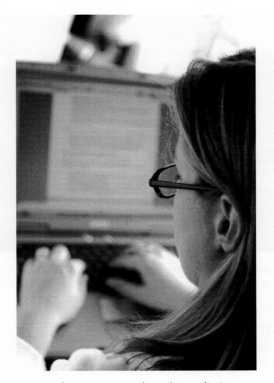

Figure 1-5. The sonographer must complete the preliminary report immediately after the procedure.

perform helps the interpreting physician to create a diagnosis, sonographers do not officially diagnose images. Sonographers who provide diagnostic information to patients may be held legally liable. Ask questions, and become familiar with sonographic dialogue. Specific sonographic descriptive terminology will be provided throughout this book, and you will encounter this unique form of analysis in the clinical setting daily. This book will further guide you in interacting with patients, sonographers, and physicians in clinical settings in upcoming chapters and offer some insight into the legal implications that exist in the medical profession.

Sound Off

Sonographers who provide diagnostic information to patients may be held legally liable.

Utilizing the Scan Lab

As you can easily deduce from the above brief description of the sonographer, the ability to accurately **scan** is essential. However, scanning experience is cumulative. In essence, the more you scan, the better scanner you will be and the more confidence you gain in your abilities. Your instructors cannot teach confidence. Confidence is something you acquire with time. If your sonography program provides a place where students can practice basic sonographic procedures on each other, often referred to as a scan lab, you should utilize it as much as possible (Fig. 1-6). And since the act of scanning takes much practice whether an instructor is available to provide assistance or not, being in the scan lab offers more exposure to sonography equipment, more scan time, and more experience with normal anatomy.

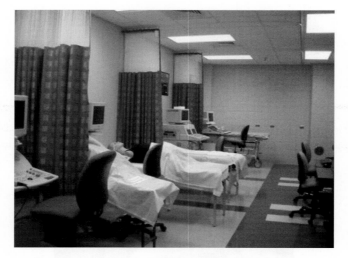

Figure 1-6. Image of an ultrasound scanning laboratory where students practice sonographic imaging. Image provided by Johnston Community College with permission.

Sound Off

Confidence cannot be taught by your instructors. The more you scan, the better scanner you will be and the more confidence you will gain in your abilities.

Your program most likely contains **clinical competencies**. These are unassisted sonographic examinations for which you are graded to determine fundamental proficiency. The scan lab can provide the student sonographer with much needed scanning practice in preparation for competencies. If scan lab instructors are not available, one can utilize his or her textbooks and other students for assistance. Furthermore, if a fellow student is not available, some sonography programs provide **sonography phantoms**, which offer simulation for practice (Fig. 1-7). When creating your time management for the week, include time for scan lab practice, as routine scanning practice is critical for success as a sonographer. You should also be in the scan lab to observe other students scanning.

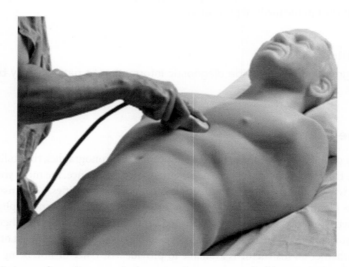

Figure 1-7. Image of an ultrasound phantom. Image provided by CAE Blue Phantom with permission.

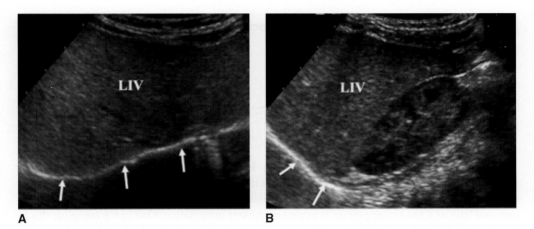

Figure 1-8. Transverse (**A**) and longitudinal subcostal (**B**) sonographic image using the liver (LIV) as an acoustic window demonstrates the echotexture of the diaphragm (*arrows*) and right kidney.

One study of sonography students claimed that the majority of first-year students prefer to scan after the sonographer in the clinical setting.[9] The research claimed that the students preferred this method of observation because they were more capable of finding organs in the specific patient by recognizing how the sonographer demonstrates the organs; they were more able to mimic the transducer manipulation and techniques after they watched the sonographers; they were more likely to discover **acoustic windows**, also referred to as sonographic windows; and they were able to learn protocols more easily (Fig. 1-8).[9] However, more advanced students may choose to scan before the sonographer. Whether you choose to scan before or after the sonographer, you should always strive to scan as much as possible.

Essentials of Professionalism in Clinical

How you perform in clinical settings is equally if not more important than how you perform in the classroom. Though obtaining good grades in the classroom is critical, the sonographer is ultimately defined by clinical competence and the ability to provide skilled patient care. Sonography is a profession. It was officially identified as such in 2002 when the Bureau of Labor and Statistics classified diagnostic medical sonographer as a distinct occupation. Consequently, there are specific requirements that a professional is expected to meet. For example, a professional must achieve certain educational criteria, they must meet minimum standards to practice within the profession, they are often required to obtain certification, and the profession in which they practice typically has professional associations with established codes of ethics and competency standards.[10] Sonographers are thus professionals and should therefore conduct themselves as such.

 Sound Off
Though obtaining good grades in the classroom is critical, the sonographer is ultimately defined by clinical competence and the ability to provide skilled patient care.

Closely associated with professionalism is the concept of medical ethics. Although Chapter 5 will provide greater detail concerning patient confidentiality and ethical standards that sonographers must appreciate and practice, one must recognize the importance of the **Hippocratic Oath**. The Hippocratic Oath, observed by physicians and occasionally other healthcare professionals, contains some basic guidelines for ethical standards and conduct between the healthcare provider and the patient. Table 1-9 provides a summary of concepts found in the Hippocratic Oath.

TABLE 1-9	Key concepts of the Hippocratic Oath

- Place the patient's interests before your own.
- Protect your patients from harm or injustice.
- Treat all patients equally.
- Respect the patient's rights.
- Protect patient confidentiality.

Regarding patient confidentiality, the Health Insurance Portability and Accountability Act (HIPAA) of 1996 included provisions that required the safeguarding of patient information, thereby establishing strict rules for maintaining patient confidentiality. Your obligation as a student in healthcare and later as a healthcare worker is to protect patient information. One can accomplish this by not sharing diagnostic information with those who are not directly involved in the patient's care, including the patient's family members, your family members, and strangers. One should never speak about a patient's sonographic exam or confidential medical information in front of another person, in an elevator, at the lunch table, or anywhere information could be overheard by bystanders, even if unintentionally. There are confidential locations in clinical that have been designated by clinical instructors where case discussions can take place.

Maintaining patient privacy is another continual objective for healthcare workers. Keeping our patients content and unexposed to maintain their dignity is of utmost significance. Sonography involves examining personal areas, including the chest, breast, and genital organs. You must attempt to maintain a patient's dignity by keeping him or her covered, especially when the examination is not in process.

Essentials of Work Ethic in Clinical Settings

There is always some task that needs to be performed in the department, and your role as a sonography student is to be supportive. Table 1-10 provides some minor tasks that you can perform in clinical that assist sonographers in their daily responsibilities. Maintaining professional conduct is critical to clinical achievement. Whether you recognize it or not, every clinical rotation is a job interview. Your clinical preceptors and instructors evaluate your successes and deficits in clinical, and consequently, you should view them as a prospective employer. In regard to treating your clinical assignment as a job, attendance and punctuality are essential. Make the commitment early in your training to be at clinical and to be there on time.

Employers not only recognize employees and students who are on time, they also appreciate someone on whom they can count. Being reliable and accountable can prove to be invaluable components

TABLE 1-10	Daily tasks for the sonography student

- Assist in completing paperwork.
- Assist in patient care and transporting patients.
- Clean stretchers, chairs, and ultrasound machines.
- Clean ultrasound transducers.
- Inform sonographers of needed supplies.
- Replace dirty linens after exams.
- Review protocols.
- Stock coupling gel.
- Stock rooms with linens and supplies.

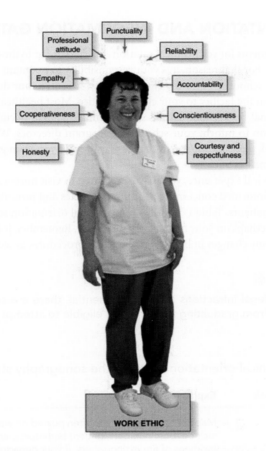

Figure 1-9. Professionalism and a strong work ethic are vital in healthcare. Many qualities contribute to a strong work ethic, including reliability, honesty, and empathy.

of **work ethic** (Fig. 1-9). Everyone appreciates someone on whom they can rely. And everyone has been frustrated by broken promises from those who have offered assistance but not delivered. Being accountable means upholding your obligations in clinical and admitting when you have made mistakes. Sonographers are responsible for patients' lives, and mistakes should be identified and remediated as quickly as possible. Therefore, honesty is always the best policy in patient care. Chapter 2 will provide greater detail regarding work ethic and professionalism.

Sonography departments are centered on a common theme—patient service. Consequently, daily schedules are constructed to accommodate a certain amount of allotted time for each examination. As a sonography student, your ultimate goal should be to increase your scanning speed without sacrificing accuracy. But how does one gain more scan time? Getting work done on time and accurately helps sustain a work environment with reduced stress and thus one that is more conducive to learning.

 ## Sound Off

Whether you recognize it or not, every clinical rotation is a job interview. Your clinical preceptors and instructors evaluate your successes and deficits in clinical, and consequently, you should view them as prospective employers.

As a student, your attitude and amount of enthusiasm that you bring to clinical are constantly examined. If you consistently have a negative attitude about learning your chosen profession, you may possibly want to review the reasons why you chose this profession to pursue.

CLINICAL ORIENTATION AND INFORMATION GATHERING

As a student, the requirements for your clinical rotations may be similar to those for another employee of the healthcare facility. For that reason, it is your responsibility to maintain professionalism, as you represent not only your school but also the clinical facility. It is also your duty to apply up-to-date changes that occur within the facility to your clinical practice. Most healthcare facilities require that students undergo criminal background checks. If a criminal incident occurs during your years of study, it is your obligation to inform your school and program directors. While many legal infractions are inconsequential, there are some crimes that may prevent you from graduating and/or being eligible to attempt national certification.

Throughout your clinical experience, you may be required to visit numerous healthcare facilities. Therefore, you must be informed concerning the unique policies and procedures of each institution before interacting with patients. Table 1-11 offers some clinical orientation recommended tasks that you should undertake, perhaps on your first day of attendance. Remember, it is your responsibility to recognize and adjust to any changes in hospital policies and procedures as well.

Sound Off

While many legal infractions are inconsequential, there are some crimes that may prevent you from graduating and/or being eligible to attempt national certification.

TABLE 1-11	Clinical orientation tasks for the sonography student
Clinical Orientation Task	**Explanation**
Obtain a map of the department.	Maps of departments are often posted on walls. These maps include room numbers, patient bathrooms, emergency exits, and locations of fire extinguishers. If your department does not have one, you can draw one for yourself.
Locate emergency crash carts (Fig. 1-10).	It is vital that you know the exact location of emergency crash carts. Some departments may have separate pediatric and adult crash carts, so know the difference.
Make copies of sono-graphic protocols.	Have protocols available in your pocket or in a notebook. Memorize the protocols, and ask questions concerning any variations in protocols.
Familiarize yourself with ultrasound machines.	Study the keyboards of each ultrasound machine in the department. Especially, find vital keys such as freeze, depth, overall gain, color Doppler, pulsed-wave Doppler, M-mode, and focus. Learn how to power on the machines and change transducers.
Locate supplies.	Masks, gowns, coupling gel, towels, sheets, invasive procedure supplies, and other patient care items should be located.
Locate material safety data sheets (MSDS) and policies and procedure manuals.	Ask your clinical supervisor where you can locate the MSDS material concerning chemicals used within the sonography department as well as the location of the policy and procedure manuals.
Obtain a list of emergency codes.	You should know the emergency codes for the department as well as how and when you should make an emergency call. For example, "code red" often refers to a fire. You should know what to do when a code red is announced.

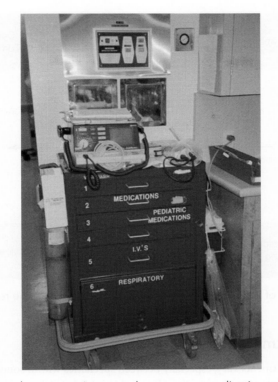

Figure 1-10. The crash cart contains several emergency medications and vital equipment used to perform emergency resuscitation. Always be aware of where the closest crash cart is in the clinical setting. (Photo by M. Kowalski.)

Understanding Workflow

Gaining an appreciation on a systemic level of an organization by viewing the entire process of how a patient moves through the organization can help you see just where you fit in. Consequently, it is vital for a sonographer and sonography student to not only understand his or her role in the imaging department but also appreciate how sonographic studies work to serve the goal of providing ordering physicians a definitive diagnosis. A patient would need to visit an imaging department when a licensed medical practitioner has ordered an imaging examination. The ordering physician targets the examination clinically based on clinical history, physical examination, and laboratory reports, and he or she develops a **differential diagnosis** with the information gathered.

All patients must have an order, similar to a prescription, from a licensed physician, **physician assistant**, or **nurse practitioner**. These healthcare practitioners may be employed within private practices or hospitals. For instance, an obstetrician can order an obstetric sonogram to be completed in the hospital setting. Also, an emergency room physician can order a lower venous sonogram to be completed within the vascular sonography department of the same hospital. A patient may have to undergo multiple imaging tests during his or her visit. It is important to recognize when multiple examinations are requested, because some imaging studies should be performed before others.

Ordering physicians must clearly offer an **indication**, or reason, for a diagnostic examination. An example of an indication for an abdominal sonogram is right upper quadrant pain. An indication serves to provide the sonographers and interpreting physician with a limited clinical history with the goal of establishing the correct diagnosis. There is also an **International Classification of Disease, Ninth Edition (ICD9) code**, which is a healthcare classification system that provides a system of diagnostic codes for classifying diseases. It is important to note that the ICD10 will soon be in use.

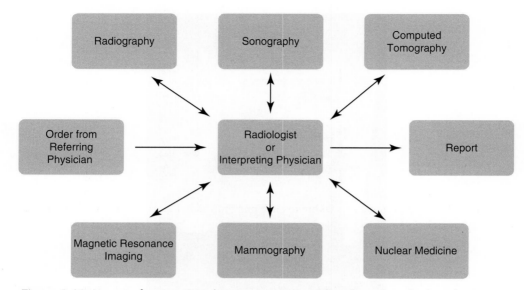

Figure 1-11. Layout of an imaging department and workflow from the referring physician to the final report.

Imaging Departments and Modalities

Though imaging departments vary, especially between specialties within sonography, most imaging facilities center on the interpreting physician (Figs. 1-11 and 1-12). All imaging studies must have an interpreting physician. For most general imaging, exams are interpreted or read by a **radiologist**. A radiologist is a physician who specializes in reading diagnostic imaging exams, and in some cases, he or she may utilize imaging modalities to assist in the treatment of disease. Furthermore, vascular surgeons may interpret vascular exams, and **cardiologists** may interpret echocardiograms. For obstetric and gynecologic studies, a radiologist, **obstetrician**, or **maternal-fetal medicine specialist** may be

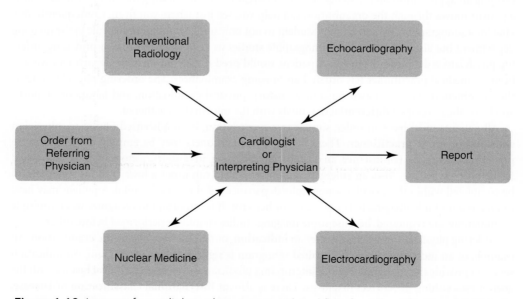

Figure 1-12. Layout of a cardiology department and workflow from the referring physician to the final report.

involved in proposing a diagnosis. Other physicians may be trained to interpret diagnostic imaging exams, though extensive training is frequently required.

Sonography departments differ in location and responsibility. In the hospital, echocardiography and vascular sonography may be located near or within the cardiology department, while general abdominal, gynecology, and obstetrics is often located in radiology. Vascular sonography may be performed in radiology as well. Separate physicians' offices that utilize sonography may require sonographers to perform a wide range of sonographic studies including several specialties. Regardless of the location, the sonography department will almost certainly consist of individuals with varying years of clinical and didactic training experience. The certifications of these individuals may vary as well. You may encounter lead sonographers, sonography department managers, and staff sonographers during your rotations. No matter what the role, each team member works to accomplish the goal of providing adequate and accurate patient care. The following sections will provide you with a brief overview of the different modalities within the imaging profession that you will most likely encounter during your clinical studies.

Radiography

Radiography is the oldest of the diagnostic modalities within the imaging department. On November 8, 1895, Wilhelm Conrad Röntgen accidentally discovered an invisible ray that produced an image of the bones within his hand.[1] He eventually created the first **radiograph**, when he imaged his wife's hand. His discovery ultimately led to what he termed "x-rays." Since then, the radiography field has been crucial in the diagnosis of not only broken bones but many other diseases within the human body. **Radiographers**, also referred to as radiologic technologists, are trained medical professionals that utilize x-ray or ionizing radiation to obtain images of the body. Radiographers not only image bones, they also use x-ray to evaluate the chest and gastrointestinal and genitourinary systems. Common gastrointestinal studies performed in radiography include barium enema examinations, upper gastrointestinal series, and pyloric stenosis examinations, while genitourinary examinations include intravenous pyelograms (IVPs) and voiding cystourethrograms (VCUGs) (Fig. 1-13). Most radiographic examinations require the radiographer to position an x-ray tube near the patient to obtain an exposure. However, radiographers may also assist the radiologist during **fluoroscopy**, **myelography**, and **arthrography**. Furthermore, portable radiography is often employed in patient rooms, within the emergency department, and during surgical procedures within the operating room. Since potential occupational exposure to radiation exists, radiographers must wear a radiation monitoring badge. These badges provide information regarding radiation exposure. Though x-ray films were once used, most departments now utilize digital radiography. Radiographers and other technologists use digital technology to store and view images on a computer within a **picture archiving and communication system** (PACS) (Fig. 1-14). These images are interpreted by a radiologist.

Many radiography educational programs in the United States now offer associated degrees, though some offer diplomas or baccalaureate degrees. The **American Registry of Radiologic Technologists** (ARRT) offers a national certification examination for radiography student candidates who meet certain didactic and clinical criteria. Once certified by the ARRT, a radiographer achieves the title of *registered technologist* (radiography) or *RT(R)*. There are also several sub-specialty modalities that a radiographer can further pursue within the field of radiology, like **computed tomography** and **mammography**.

Sound Off

The "ALARA" principle is practiced by imaging professionals, including sonographers. This mnemonic reminds professionals to keep patient exposure "as low as reasonably achievable." Though ultrasound does not involve ionizing radiation, sonographers should practice ALARA.

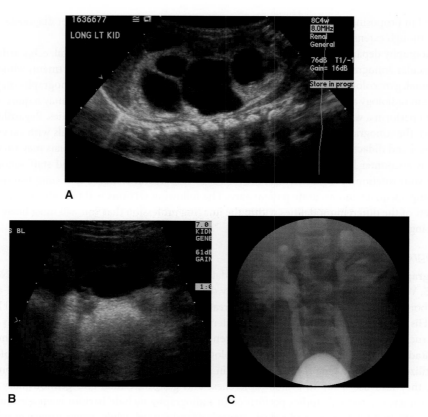

Figure 1-13. Sonogram of the left kidney (A) and urinary bladder (B) reveals a ureterocele. A voiding cystourethrogram (VCUG) is an x-ray procedure that helps to confirm the diagnosis (C).

Computed Tomography

Computed tomography (CT) also uses x-ray, like radiography, to obtain images of the body. For that reason, some radiographers have utilized **cross-training** to specialize in the field of CT, though dedicated didactic training is currently available. CT provides high-resolution sectional viewing of the body in multiple planes (Fig. 1-15). Instead of a stationary x-ray tube, as utilized in radiography, CT

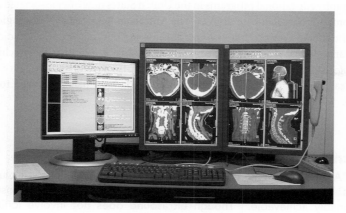

Figure 1-14. PACS reading consoles.

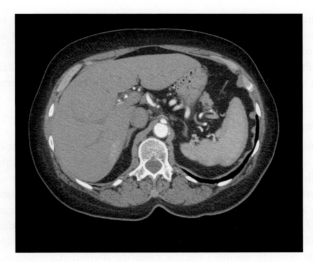

Figure 1-15. A CT image of the abdomen is excellent at delineating various soft tissue densities. In this CT image, fat, the liver, and bone all demonstrate different densities.

employs an x-ray tube that rotates around the patient, thereby offering the ability to obtain imaging slices of the patient (Fig. 1-16).

CT is often utilized in trauma, during **invasive procedures**, and routine outpatient procedures. Occasionally, **CT technologists** perform examinations that require the patient to ingest or be injected with a **contrast agent**. For example, for some gastrointestinal CT examinations, patients must drink barium or other ingestible contrast agents. Other CT examinations require an injection of iodine-based contrast into the venous system, thereby facilitating evaluation of the vascular system and improved characterization of certain masses.

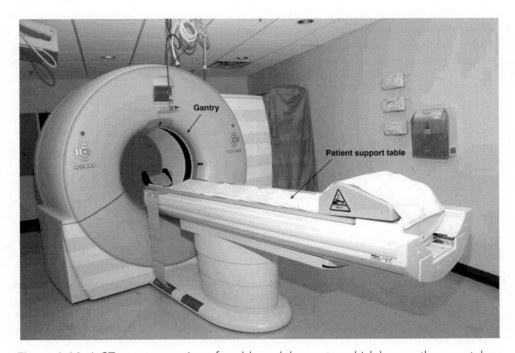

Figure 1-16. A CT scanner consists of a table and the gantry, which houses the x-ray tubes.

Sonographers should work to establish an understanding of CT, as many sonographic procedures are often correlated with CT studies. Also, it is important to note that some CT and radiography examinations should be completed after sonographic examinations, as contrast agents may inhibit the ability to obtain optimal sonographic images, especially if barium is employed. Radiographers may specialize in CT through the ARRT by obtaining post-primary education and clinical training.

Nuclear Medicine Technology

Nuclear medicine utilizes radioactive material for the diagnosis and treatment of various diseases. A nuclear medicine test requires that the patient inhale, ingest, or be injected with radioactive material known as a **radiopharmaceutical**. These radiopharmaceuticals are capable of concentrating on specific organs or systems in order to evaluate organ function, like the thyroid gland, kidneys, skeletal system, and urinary system. **Nuclear medicine technologists** operate a gamma camera strategically placed near the patient to detect the radiation emitted by the radiopharmaceutical, thus creating an image. The radiopharmaceutical may also be used to differentiate normal and abnormal structures within the body. For example, during a nuclear medicine thyroid examination, the radiopharmaceuticals can accumulate in an area of pathology that may be referred to as a "hot spot." Conversely, a "cold spot" indicates an area of decreased absorption of the radiopharmaceutical and could also indicate the presence of various diseases (Fig. 1-17). This two-dimensional imaging of various organs in nuclear medicine may be referred to as **scintigraphy**, and a special camera called a gamma camera acquires the images of the emitted radiation from inside the patient. Furthermore, some radiopharmaceuticals are utilized to treat disease or evaluate the function of organs. For example, a hepatobiliary iminodiacetic acid (HIDA) scan is another nuclear medicine test that can be used to evaluate the liver and biliary system, including the gallbladder, for appropriate function.

Technetium (Tc99m) sestamibi, often designated under the trade name **Cardiolite**, is a pharmaceutical agent used in nuclear medicine imaging to examine the blood flow of the heart. This test, often referred to as a **nuclear stress test**, requires that the patient exercise, often by way of a treadmill, though some patients require a special drug that artificially stresses the heart, thus simulating active exercise. Echocardiography may be utilized to further analyze the heart and surrounding anatomy before or following nuclear medicine tests.

Positron emission tomography (PET) is a technique that utilizes both the radionuclide imaging principles of nuclear medicine and the imaging techniques of CT. Some facilities may purchase

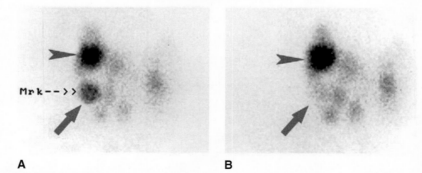

A   **B**

Figure 1-17. Nuclear medicine images of thyroid nodules. **A.** A radioactive marker (Mrk) was placed over a 2-cm palpable nodule (*arrow*) in the right thyroid lobe. **B.** The image on the right, without the marker, demonstrates the palpable nodule (*arrow*) to be cold. The second palpable nodule in the right upper lobe (*arrowhead*) is shown to be hot. A biopsy of the cold, palpable nodule demonstrated in **(B)** confirmed that the nodule was papillary thyroid cancer.

a CT scanner that includes PET technology. Nuclear medicine technologists may also acquire images with a single-photon emission tomography (SPECT) imaging machine, which adds further physiologic analysis of organs and specific diagnosis of pathology in order to develop a specialized treatment plan.

There exists several dedicated nuclear medicine training programs throughout the United States, and the ARRT and the Nuclear Medicine Technology Certification Board offer certification for technologists. A nuclear medicine technologist must undergo specific training dedicated to radiation safety, as exposure to both them and the patient is inevitable. Furthermore, some radiation exposure to sonographers during sonographic examination may occur following nuclear medicine injections or studies when patients are required to have further testing. For example, a patient who has recently undergone a thyroid nuclear medicine examination may still have some active radiation emitted from the thyroid. Though exposure is minimal to bystanders in most cases, student sonographers who are pregnant may be required to wear a fetal radiation monitoring badge to screen for possible exposure.

Sound Off

In some facilities, radiologists have the ability to overlay CT and nuclear medicine imaging examination, such as SPECT/CT or PET/CT, a process referred to as hybrid imaging.

Mammography

Mammography, the **gold standard** in breast imaging, employs x-rays to obtain an image of the breast. Like CT technologists, mammographers are specialized radiographers who pursue continuing education and specific on-the-job clinical training, with the ARRT offering a national certification examination. Currently, the American Medical Association and the American Cancer Society recommend that all women have an annual **screening mammogram** starting at the age of 40.[11] Patients may also present to the imaging department with a palpable nodule or lump within the breast. Mammography is not recommended in some cases of palpable disease, especially in younger patients, and thus, sonography may be used as the initial screening tool.

Women suspected to have disease on screening mammograms may require further breast imaging, including a **diagnostic mammogram**, breast sonogram, or an MRI of the breast. For this reason, sonographers should familiarize themselves with mammographic views of the breast in order to understand the location of breast pathology and the mammographic appearance of disease. Screening examinations typically involve two projections of the breast: cranial caudal (CC) and mediolateral oblique (MLO) (Fig. 1-18). Diagnostic mammograms include special compression views and focal imaging for specific lesions.

Magnetic Resonance Imaging

Unlike radiography and CT, **magnetic resonance imaging** (MRI) uses a powerful magnetic field, radio waves, and a devoted computer system to create sectional images of the human body (Fig. 1-19). MRI provides excellent resolution of internal structures, and the images can be obtained in numerous sectional planes. To better visualize structures, patients may be injected with a contrast agent, most likely **gadolinium**. MRI is used to evaluate disease all over the body, including the extremities, brain, spine, breast, and abdominal structures. Occasionally, MRI is even utilized during pregnancy. A **magnetic resonance angiogram** (MRA) is a special MRI procedure that is used to evaluate vascular structures more closely. An **MRI technologist** is often a specialized radiographer who has been trained both in didactic information and clinical preparation to work in MRI. The MRI machine is essentially a large magnet, and therefore, special precautions must be taken in MRI to prevent metallic structures from entering the MRI room where the machine is located. Be aware of caution signs placed near an MRI machine, and always ask for help before transporting patients near the MRI room.

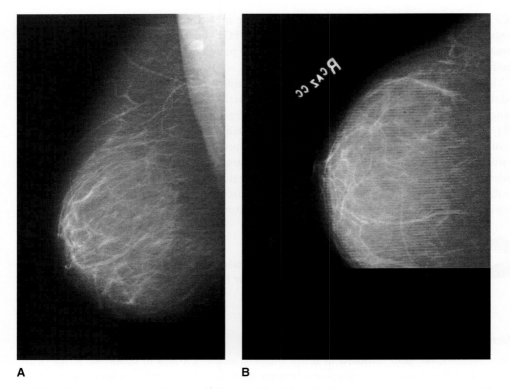

A   **B**

Figure 1-18. Mammogram images of the breast in medial lateral oblique projection (**A**) and cranial caudal projection (**B**).

Cardiovascular Interventional Technology and Vascular Interventional Technology

A **heart catheterization**, often referred to as heart caths or cardiac angiogram, is performed with the assistance of a **cardiovascular interventional technologist**. Specialized radiographers assist radiologists and other physicians in **interventional radiology** to complete these and other vascular studies

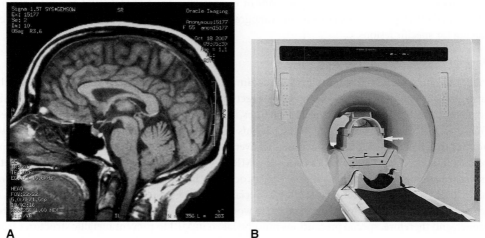

A   **B**

Figure 1-19. MRI image of the brain (**A**) and the MRI scanner (**B**).

under the assistance of fluoroscopy. During a heart catheterization, x-ray dye is utilized to image the vessels of the heart for signs of occlusion. The access point for the catheters used during the procedure is through either an upper extremity or leg. **Vascular interventional radiographers** also assist radiologists in stent placement for organs like the liver. Many of these procedures are performed under **surgical asepsis**, and treatment of certain diseases can be performed during the examination. The ARRT offers certification for both cardiovascular technology and vascular interventional technology.

APPRECIATING CRITICAL THINKING

A significant component of performing adequate patient care is both acquiring and utilizing **critical thinking skills**. Critical thinking skills are resourceful actions, judgments, and decisions based on the combination of professional knowledge, experience, integrity, and ethical standards.[1] Critical thinking has been described as the disciplined art of ensuring that you use the best thinking of which you are capable in any set of circumstances.[12] Furthermore, a critical thinker in sonography would utilize broad in-depth analysis of evidence to make decisions and communicate his or her beliefs clearly and accurately.[13] An important aspect of critical thinking in sonography is the application of a code of ethics to our decision-making process. Throughout this book, both ethical and legal issues related to sonography and health professions will be provided.

The function of problem solving and critical thinking skills is especially unique in the imaging profession for practicing sonographers. Whereas some imaging professionals utilize technical skills to acquire routine images for interpreting physicians, sonographers must have the ability to correlate clinical history with sonographic findings in order to guide the sonographic examination. The clinical history of a patient includes **symptoms** and **signs**, pertinent illnesses, past surgeries, laboratory findings, and the results of other diagnostic testing, including the results of the other aforementioned imaging studies in this chapter. It is important to note the difference between a sign and a symptom. A symptom is the **subjective** physical manifestation of a disease that a patient experiences. For example, abdominal pain, headaches, and nausea are all clinical symptoms. A sign is **objective** evidence of a disease. For example, a sign could be hematuria or high blood sugar, as both of these involve a specific test that can prove the presence of blood in the urine and high levels of sugar in the blood, respectively.

An example of clinical history information could be a patient who has persistent right upper quadrant pain, elevated laboratory values, and a recent cholecystectomy. Sonographic findings comprise the information gathered by completing the sonographic examination. An example of a sonographic finding includes the visualization of an enlarged common bile duct that contains gallstones in the same patient; these findings may lead to the diagnosis of retained gallstones in the common bile duct—choledocholithiasis.

Essentially, sonographers perform investigative imaging as previously discussed. This means that we obtain sonographic protocol images while simultaneously searching for and identifying abnormalities. That is to say, with the use of a standard sonographic **protocol**, the sonographer explores the relevant anatomy identifying normal structures and abnormalities with the goal of assisting the interpreting physician in establishing an accurate diagnosis. This task placed on the sonographer is a unique and vital responsibility. Placing this much responsibility on the sonographer can seem rather daunting, especially for students, but it is a duty that you, with much practice, can someday embrace. The more one observes and participates in sonographic examinations, the more one gains an appreciation for how vital critical thinking is to patient care. Table 1-12 provides some qualities of those who use critical thinking effectively.

Sound Off

With the use of a standard protocol, the information that we gather from the patient and from the medical history helps to guide our examinations with the goal of assisting the interpreting physician in establishing an accurate diagnosis.

TABLE 1-12	Qualities of well-cultivated critical thinkers

- Asks vital questions and recognizes problems
- Gathers and assesses relevant information
- Comes to well-reasoned conclusions and solutions
- Tests conclusions and solutions against relevant criteria
- Thinks with an open mind
- Communicates effectively with others in order to figure out solutions to complex problems

The development and utilization of critical thinking skills in sonography is an ongoing career-long undertaking that involves reasoning. There are many elements of reasoning, including information, **inferences**, and **assumptions**. In order to make optimal decisions in life, obtaining accurate information regarding the problem at hand is vital. Information includes observations, data, facts, and experiences.[12]

Obtaining reliable information is the most significant component of critical thinking and decision making. Furthermore, critical thinkers continually strive to learn not only the correct information but what portion of the information is imperative to understand. Medical books are full of important data, facts, and observations obtained through clinical studies and trials. A critical thinker should be able to take a large amount of information and break it down into understandable and usable facts. For example, a cardiac student who has been asked to read a journal article on the topic of tetralogy of Fallot can practice critical thinking by reading the article and then asking him or herself, "How does this article apply to patient care, and how can it improve my understanding about the disorder?" That is to say, one should determine through reasoning exactly how each assignment, whether didactic or clinical, applies to the ultimate goal of becoming a clinically minded sonographer. Once the aforementioned cardiac sonography student encounters a patient with tetralogy of Fallot in the clinical setting, the student should be capable of recalling the essential information needed to provide specific patient care for that individual with a more targeted sonographic examination.

Once the correct information is gathered, a sonographer can make certain inferences in which reasoning is based on gained factual knowledge using critical thinking. In the medical profession, our inferences must be based on facts. For example, a sonographer is asked to perform an abdominal sonogram. During the sonogram, the sonographer recognizes that the liver appears to have multiple liver masses. An inference made by the sonographer is that the patient has metastatic liver disease. This inference, or conclusion, can be further analyzed and essentially proven by correlating further sonographic findings with the patient's medical and laboratory history. Though the sonographer is not required to make a diagnosis, the sonographer must still understand the medical and sonographic implications of metastasis to the liver in order to evaluate the patient effectively with ultrasound, as other organs and systems may be involved. A skilled sonographer uses critical thinking skills to improve patient care. One author applied scientific methodology and specific steps to the art of critical thinking in sonography (Table 1-13).[14]

There is a vast difference between making inferences and making assumptions. Critical thinkers can distinguish between fact and opinion.[14] While inferences are based on fact, assumptions can be based on guesses or opinion. Making assumptions concerning patient care and safety is never appropriate. For example, assuming that a patient who has been sleeping on the stretcher throughout a sonogram can be left alone after a sonographic examination can be disastrous. The patient could fall off the stretcher and injure him or herself. A critical thinker will not only talk to the patient before leaving the room but put up the side rails of the stretcher and also inform a coworker that the patient is in the room or ask for someone to stay with the patient. Another example may be that a young patient presents to the sonography department with pelvic pain for a pelvic sonogram. The sonographer performs the pelvic sonogram without obtaining any medical history and does not visualize the uterus or ovaries during the sonogram. While presenting the sonogram to the interpreting physician, the

TABLE 1-13	Steps for successful critical thinking in sonography
Observation	Patient complaints, clinical symptoms, patient input and cues
Hypothesis	Reason for referral, tentative diagnosis, indications for examination, ICD9 code
Data collection	Subjective patient information, laboratory information, physical findings, sonographic findings, past medical history
Data analysis	Correlation of lab findings, clinical data, interpretation of sonographic images and other pertinent findings
Conclusion	Sonographer's description and impression of findings, sonographic diagnosis, final report

From Baun J. Scientific thinking as a framework for critical thinking in diagnostic medical sonography. *JDMS* 2004; 20:202–207.

sonographer is asked if the patient has had a hysterectomy. The sonographer claims "I assume she has. I could not find the uterus or ovaries." Making an assumption in this situation negatively affects patient care. A sonographer applying critical thinking skills will consistently delve deeper into patient history to discover the most essential facts and establish inferences or conclusions based only on those facts.

Student Application of Critical Thinking

There is a clear, positive correlation between the amount of clinical experience one has and diagnostic accuracy. Essentially, the more experience you gain in clinical, the higher the probability that your interpretation or suspected diagnosis will be correct.[14] As you progress through your education, you will naturally gain critical thinking skills by observing seasoned sonographers in practice. In fact, observation is crucial to critical thinking. We gain much knowledge from watching others. Student sonographers should evaluate the way in which sonographers interact with patients, other healthcare workers, and interpreting physicians. Students should take note of relevant clinical history for specific studies.

Observation in clinical includes making both mental and physical notes. The construction of a **clinical journal** (or clinical diary) for institutional information and professional reflection is a priceless practice for some students. Writing in a journal can be therapeutic, and returning to the journal weekly can help develop critical thinking skills, especially when writing down new pieces of information learned every day. Instructors may develop online discussion boards for students to confer about clinical experiences and candidly share thoughts. Table 1-14 provides some information to include in your clinical journal. Remember, everyone experiences bad days in clinical, but hopefully, the good days will ultimately outnumber the bad.

Sound Off
It is important to remember that everyone experiences bad days in clinical, but hopefully, the good days will ultimately outnumber the bad.

SUMMARY

Going back to school can be complicated, especially when it's sonography school. Stress is inevitable. However, with the help of some of the tips in this chapter, hopefully you will be better financially prepared, have better emotional stability and physical well-being, and understand the importance of time management. Classroom survival skills, such as test-taking preparation tips and maintaining motivation throughout your education, should facilitate a more conducive learning experience.

TABLE 1-14	Personal clinical journal components

Note: Clinical journals should never include patient identifiers like names and medical record numbers.

- Institutional components
  - Map of the department
  - Location of fire exits
  - List of codes
  - Location of crash carts
- Personal components
  - Goals for the day
  - Daily observations
  - Daily personal reflection
  - Interesting pathology
  - Interesting cases
  - New facts learned

Sonographers are created in clinical. This chapter provided insight into workflow and the various imaging modalities and professionals that sonographers encounter in clinical. The sonographer was briefly described with the hope that you can gain a basic understanding of the profession before greater details are offered in the upcoming chapters. The manner in which critical thinking skills permeate the sonographer's decision-making process was clearly established as well.

You have chosen a noble profession to pursue. Sonography school is demanding but rewarding. It is stressful but manageable. Make the decision now to develop classroom and clinical skills that are geared toward providing all patients with adequate care. Your ultimate goal should be to treat all patients with respect, protecting their dignity and serving them equally. This is something our patients both expect and deserve.

REFERENCES

1. Adler AM, Carlton RR. *Introduction to Radiologic Sciences and Patient Care*. 4th ed. St. Louis, MO: Saunders Elsevier; 2007.
2. Vye C, et al. *Under Pressure & Overwhelmed: Coping with Anxiety in College*. Westport, CT: Praeger; 2007.
3. SDMS. *News Wave*, January 2013. Retrieved from http://www.sdms.org/members/news/NewsWave/NW-January-2013.pdf
4. Siebert A, Karr M. *The Adult Student's Guide to Survival & Success*. 6th ed. Portland, OR: Practical Psychology Press; 2008.
5. Gottesman G, et al. *College Survival: a Crash Course for Students by Students*. 4th ed. New York, NY: Macmillan Company; 1996.
6. Roubidoux SM. *101 Ways to Make Studying Easier and Faster for College Students: What Every Students Needs to Know Explained Simply*. Ocala, FL: Atlantic Publishing Group; 2008.
7. Motevalli S, et al. New study skills training intervention for students who suffer from test anxiety. *Asian Soc Science* 2013;9(7):85–96.
8. ARDMS Registry Reports, Summer 2008. Retrieved from http://www.ardms.org/files/downloads/RegistryReports/RRSummer08PrintFINAL.pdf
9. Sonnagera T. Sonography clinical education: a student's perspective. *JDMS* 2004;20:356–359.
10. Makely S. *Professionalism in Healthcare*. 3rd ed. Upper Saddle River, NJ: Pearson Prentice Hall; 2009.
11. Breastcancer.org. (June 21, 2012). AMA updates mammogram policy, says screening should start at 40. Retrieved from http://www.breastcancer.org/research-news/20120621
12. Paul R, Edler L. *Critical Thinking: Learn the Tools the Best Thinkers Use*. Upper Saddle River, NJ: Pearson Prentice Hall; 2006.
13. Wilson M, et al. Critical thinking for sonographic breast imaging. *JDMS* 2010;26(5):226–237.
14. Baun J. Scientific thinking as a framework for critical thinking in diagnostic medical sonography. *JDMS* 2004;20:202–207.

Thinking Critically

1. Choose a pathology from another sonography class or one you have noted in clinical. Read your textbook concerning that pathology. On a piece of paper, write down the clinical findings of the pathology and sonographic findings. What would a sonographer need to know about this pathology in clinical?
2. It is Friday. You have three tests next week: one on Monday, one on Wednesday, and one on Friday. How would you manage your time wisely so that you can be successful on all three tests? Would you study just the night before each test? Would you study some each night for all three tests? Why?
3. What types of techniques would you use to prepare for the tests mentioned above? Would you make note cards? Would you study with a classmate?
4. Today is your first day at clinical. What tasks can you perform to assist the sonographer? What questions should you ask on your first day? What supplies should you locate?

Chapter 1
Review Questions

1. **What are resourceful actions, judgments, and decisions based on the combination of professional knowledge, experience, integrity, and ethical standards?**
   a. Critical thinking skills
   b. Investigative imaging skills
   c. Time management skills
   d. Clinical history skills

2. **What is the body's typical reaction to challenging situations that are perceived as demands on time, energy, or resources?**
   a. Subjective concerns
   b. Objective concerns
   c. Stress
   d. Anxiety

3. **Which of the following is the general state of feeling worry and fear before confronting something emotionally or physically challenging?**
   a. Subjective concerns
   b. Objective concerns
   c. Stress
   d. Anxiety

4. **What imaging modality utilizes both features of nuclear medicine and computed tomography?**
   a. PET
   b. CT
   c. MRI
   d. MRA

5. **Which of the following is not a quality of a well-cultivated critical thinker?**
   a. Gathers and assesses relevant information
   b. Asks vital questions and recognizes problems
   c. Thinks with a closed mind
   d. Tests conclusion and solutions against relevant criteria

6. All of the following are suggested daily tasks for the sonography student in clinical except:
   a. replaces dirty linens after exams.
   b. completes preliminary reports unassisted.
   c. informs sonographers of needed supplies.
   d. reviews protocols.

7. What is the normal range of human hearing?
   a. 2 to 4 kHz
   b. Less than 2 Hz
   c. Between 2 Hz and 20,000 Hz
   d. Above 20,000 Hz

8. What term is described as reasoning based on gained factual knowledge using critical thinking?
   a. Assumptions
   b. Inferences
   c. Brain dumping
   d. Work ethic

9. Which of the following would be a contrast agent used in MRI?
   a. Iodine
   b. Gas bubbles
   c. Gadolinium
   d. Technetium

10. Which of the following is not provided by the sonographer on a sonographer report?
    a. Diagnosis
    b. Descriptive sonographic terminology
    c. Location of pathology
    d. Measurements of normal and abnormal structures

11. Which of the following would be best described as a symptom?
    a. Positive urine pregnancy test
    b. Chest radiography report
    c. Biopsy results
    d. Nausea

12. Which of the following best describes the pulse-echo technique?
    a. The ultrasound transducer sends an ultrasound wave into the body.
    b. The ultrasound transducer listens to sound waves that are emitted naturally by the body.
    c. The ultrasound transducer sends an ultrasound wave into the body and then listens for the returning echo.
    d. The ultrasound transducer is a camera that utilizes pulsed magnetic waves and echoes to acquire images.

13. What term may be used to describe the optimal location on the body for placement of the ultrasound transducer to demonstrate both normal anatomy and pathology?
    a. Contrast window
    b. Protocol
    c. Realtime imaging
    d. Acoustic window

14. Which of the following would not be a valid time management tool for the sonography student?
    a. Plan your week.
    b. Set your own early deadlines.
    c. Create your own academic calendar.
    d. Check during class if any assignments are due for the day.

15. Which imaging modality technologist injects patients with radioactive material in order to acquire images?
    a. Nuclear medicine
    b. CT
    c. MRI
    d. Radiography

16. Which of the following should not be included in a personal clinical journal?
    a. Medical record numbers
    b. Interesting cases
    c. Personal thoughts
    d. Scanning tips learned

17. Which of the following would not be considered clinical history information?
    a. Headaches
    b. Gallbladder wall thickening demonstrated during the sonogram
    c. Microscopic hematuria
    d. Diarrhea

18. Which of the following would not be considered sonographic findings?
    a. A palpable breast mass noted during an examination
    b. A mass noted on the kidney during a sonogram
    c. Pericardial effusion noted during echocardiography
    d. Vascular stenosis noted during a sonogram of the renal arteries

19. Which of the following techniques does not employ ionizing radiation to acquire images?
    a. Fluoroscopy
    b. Radiography
    c. MRI
    d. CT

20. What are the typical ranges of diagnostic ultrasound?
    a. 2 to 4 kHz
    b. Less than 2 Hz
    c. Between 2 MHz and 15 MHz
    d. Above 20,000 Hz

The Sonographer: A Closer Look

CHAPTER OBJECTIVES

- Examine personality typewatching and emotional intelligence and how they relate to sonography.
- Appreciate work ethic in sonography.
- Recognize how vital character is to the sonographer.
- Understand the responsibilities and challenges of the clinical sonographer.
- Comprehend the need to effectively communicate with sonographers and interpreting physicians.

KEY TERMS

Accountability – responsibility for one's actions

Acute – sudden onset

Anechoic – without echoes

Assertiveness – being self-confident without being aggressive

Burnout – work-related condition during which one experiences physical and emotional exhaustion

Callback pay – additional monies earned because one is asked to return to work after normal business hours, results from taking call

Character – the way a person thinks, feels, and acts

Chronic – gradual onset or an ongoing condition

Clinical correlation – the process of obtaining clinical history and contrasting that information with sonographic findings

Clinical correlation ambiguity – lacking the ability to obtain a thorough clinical history and relate the information with the sonographic findings of the examination

Clinical hypotheses – educated guesses based on clinical history findings

Cognition – the act or process of knowing

Commission on Accreditation of Allied Health Education Programs – the national accreditation granting body for sonography education (CAAHEP)

Compassion – the ability to feel for others and for their well-being

Compassion fatigue – a complication often discovered in people who work in helping professions like sonography; results from the combination of traumatic stress and burnout

Compassion satisfaction – the pleasure one gains from being able to help others and the feeling that one has the ability to make a positive difference in patients' lives

Competence – the ability to complete a job successfully

Complex – a structure that has both fluid-filled and solid components

Constructive criticism – courteous manner of offering well-reasoned positive and negative opinions about the work of others

Continuing medical education – education required to maintain certification or licensure in a healthcare profession

Courtesy – demonstrating polite behavior

Echogenic – a structure that produces echoes; often used synonymously with hyperechoic

Echogenicity – the number of echoes within a structure

Emotional intelligence – the enhanced ability to recognize emotions in oneself and others and the capacity to use those emotions to improve emotional and intellectual growth and decision making

Empathy – a trait that demonstrates that one understands, to the point of feeling, how another person feels

Enthusiasm – eagerness or excitement for what one is doing

Fortitude – strength of mind that allows someone to face difficult circumstances with courage

Health Insurance Portability and Accountability Act of 1996 – law that is aimed at protecting the patient's rights and reducing waste, fraud, and abuse in the healthcare industry

Heterogeneous – of differing composition

Homogeneous – of uniform composition

Honesty – fairness and truthfulness in behavior

Humility – meekness in dealing with others

Hyperechoic – describes a structure that produces echoes; often used synonymously with echogenic

Hypoechoic – having few echoes within a structure

Inductive reasoning – form of reasoning whereby one makes an educated guess based on facts

Integrity – thinking with honesty and choosing the best paths to follow based on high standards

Isoechoic – having the same echogenicity

Joint Review Committee on Education in Diagnostic Medical Sonography – organization that establishes standards, reviews, and recommends education accreditation for sonography programs

Kinesthetic learning – hands-on learning

Occupational stress – stress related to job duties in the workplace; results in negative psychologic and physiologic effects

Personal values – things that someone holds in high regard and that are highly desirable and worthy of esteem

Physiology – the study of the function of the human body

Recertification – the process of completing tests following initial certification in sonography to maintain qualifications

Reputation – the way in which others view us

Respect – to demonstrate polite regard for others

Role ambiguity – the frustration that arises when job expectations differ between employer and employee

Self-confidence – belief in oneself and one's abilities

Self-motivation – the perception to recognize a goal and the courage and strength to reach that goal

Shadowing – failure of the sound beam to pass through a structure

Sincerity – genuineness

Sonographic anatomy – normal anatomy as it is demonstrated on a sonogram

Sonographic reasoning – a reasoning process for the sonographer by which he or she integrates the data obtained through clinical history gathering to the study at hand in order to facilitate optimum diagnostic results

Standards – the basis for one's conduct

Strength – the potential for effective action

Tact – always being aware of and considerate of the feelings of others

Taking call – the process by which a sonographer is paid a small amount of money to be on standby via telephone for emergency cases after regular department hours, including nights and weekends

Through transmission – the amount of sound passing through a structure; also known as acoustic enhancement

Traumatic stress – the consequence of wanting to help a traumatized or suffering person

Typewatching – the process of identifying personality types

INTRODUCTION

In Chapter 1, we briefly examined the role of the student in the clinical setting, including a brief overview of the sonographer. In this chapter, we will take a closer look at those who perform the sonographic procedures and some of the challenges they face in the clinical setting. Before psychoanalysis of others takes place, however, it may be more beneficial to start with a look in the mirror.

Though it is an obvious statement to make, we are all different, and though your career paths have now aligned, your backgrounds vary drastically. Therefore, one cannot simply look at others, make blanket observations, and try to infer possible character traits without first asking some important questions about oneself. Thus, as you read this chapter, strive to learn more about yourself, and attempt to utilize this knowledge while you are in school and as you progress in the direction of and eventually past your established educational goals. And while this chapter will provide some common characteristics of successful healthcare workers, you must in the end apply your identified strengths to the goals that you set for yourself as you endeavor to become a registered sonographer.

KNOW YOURSELF BEFORE YOU KNOW OTHERS

Chinese philosopher Laozi once stated, "He who knows others is wise; he who knows himself is enlightened".[1] The following sections will provide information related to personality **typewatching**. You should strive to learn more about yourself as you progress through your education. There are two fundamental questions to ask yourself as you read the information in this section: (1) Do you know yourself? (2) If you know yourself, can you change the things you do not like? For patient care, identifying your personality type will assist you in understanding how you view others, how you can utilize your strengths in sonography, and how you can improve your interactions with everyone, especially patients.

Identifying Your Personality Type

Healthcare workers tend to have high satisfaction that results from career stability, the opportunity to serve, meaningful and interesting work, and prospects for advancement.[2] But have you ever been asked the question, "Why did you choose sonography?" Your truthful answers can differ from something noble like "to help patients," or something self-interested like "for the money" (neither of which is a wrong answer). Researchers have sought to find out why individuals choose to pursue careers in caring professions like nursing or sonography. One study of nurses with findings that may also be applicable to sonographers reported that nurses gave the following reasons for entering the nursing profession: opportunity for caring, rewarding career, stepping stone to another career, career security, previous work or socialization experience, job satisfaction, and the positive manner in which nurses are portrayed in the media.[3]

The Myers-Briggs Type Indicator is an approach to analyzing personality type that was created by Katharine Cook Briggs and Isabel Briggs Myers based on the previous work of Carl Jung.[4] This tool helps identify one's tendency toward a certain personality type, a process called typewatching. According to the theory, as a result of genetic and environmental factors, each of us has inclinations for definite personality types. These include varying components of the following: extroversion (E) or introversion (I); sensing (S) or intuition (N); thinking (T) or feeling (F); and judging (J) or perceiving (P) (Table 2-1). Consequently, there are 16 possible personality types according to Briggs and Briggs Myers that can include combinations of the above listed preferences. A free Myers-Briggs test can be accessed online at http://www.humanmetrics.com/cgi-win/jtypes2.asp.

Though most researchers agree that there is no single "type" of person who chooses a profession or work in a particular vocation, they do agree that there are particular combinations of personality traits that predispose people to certain professions and interests in life.[3] One large study of nurses

TABLE 2-1	The different components of Myers-Briggs personality typing
Preference	**Brief Explanation**
Extraversion	Extroverts: • Talk first, think later • Are approachable • Enjoy going to meetings and tend to voice their opinions freely • Need affirmation from everyone almost all of the time • Find listening more difficult than talking
Introversion	Introverts: • Enjoy being by themselves • May be perceived as shy • Like stating their thoughts without interruption • Like to share special occasions with just one person or a few friends • Are thought of as great listeners
Sensing	Individuals who prefer sensing: • Like to concentrate on one thing at a time • Prefer specific definite answers • Find jobs that yield some concrete results most satisfying • Agree with "if it ain't broke, don't fix it" • Would rather work with facts and figures than ideas and theories
Intuition	Individuals who prefer intuition: • Tend to think about several things at once • Believe time is relative • Like to figure out how things work • Would rather fantasize about spending their next paychecks than balancing their checkbooks • Are often more excited about where they are going instead of where they are
Thinking	Thinkers: • Would rather settle problems based on facts, fairness, and truth instead of making people happy • May be classified as cold and uncaring because they pride themselves on their impartiality • Feel that it is more important to be right than liked • Remember numbers and figures more than faces and names • Enjoy logic and science and are skeptical about things like typewatching
Feeling	Feelers: • Often consider others' feelings in decision making • Will overextend themselves meeting other people's needs • Enjoy helping others though they may feel that some people take advantage of them • Prefer harmony over clarity • May be accused of being vague in their decision making because they adjust their opinions often to not hurt others' feelings
Judging	Judgers: • Always wait on others because they are typically early • Prefer everything to be in their assigned places • Don't like surprises • Are sometimes accused of being angry when they are not • Keep lists and use them

(continues)

TABLE 2-1	The different components of Myers-Briggs personality typing (Continued)
Preference	**Brief Explanation**
Perceiving	Perceivers: • Are easily distracted • Have to depend on last-minute preparations to meet deadlines • Change the subject often in conversations • Turn most work into play • Love adventure and doing new things

Adapted from Kroeger O, et al. *Type Talk at Work: How the 16 Personality Types Determine Your Success on the Job*. New York, NY: Dell Publishing; 2002.

and nursing students sought to identify common personality traits using a psychobiologic model of personality devised by C. Robert Cloninger called the temperament and character inventory (TCI) (37). Much like the Myers-Briggs test, the TCI examines seven basic personality dimensions of temperament and character that theoretically interacts in ways to create the exclusive personality of an individual.[5] The study ultimately revealed that the nurses had an average ability to cope with uncertain situations; they perceived themselves as a valuable part of the community; they were modest risk takers and slightly impulsive; and they were high in sensitivity and sociability, hard-working, ambitious, realistic, resourceful, and team players.[5]

But why is it important to identify your personality type for a career in sonography? As many as 30% of all companies now use some form of personality testing as part of the interviewing processes.[2] For this reason alone, you should understand your personality type and be prepared for the interview process. Furthermore, once you are aware of your talents, you can look for situations in which you can best utilize your abilities to your advantage (Table 2-2). Hopefully, you have already recognized that sonography is the profession for you. Now, it is your obligation to find your strengths and use them to the best of your ability to provide patients with the best individualized care that *you* can afford.

Some critics of personality typing claim that a situation determines a certain behavior, and this is true, though they often explain this phenomenon through examples of extreme situations. None of us know how we would react to a bear chasing us until the bear starts to chase us. Thus, personality

TABLE 2-2	Advantages of different personality types
Personality Type	**Advantages**
ESTJ, ISTJ, ESFJ, ISFJ (~40% of American population)	Traditionalist, practical, very organized, solid, trustworthy, dependable
ESTP, ISTP, ESFP, ISFP (~30% of the American population)	Approach problems with flexibility, courage, and resourcefulness; risk takers and good negotiators
ENFJ, INFJ, ENFP, INFP (~15% of the American population)	Great motivators, conflict resolvers, great communicators, charismatic, accepting of others' opinions
ENTJ, INTJ, ENTP, INTP (~15% of the American population)	Have great vision and are innovators; big-picture people; good strategists, planners, and can understand and explain theories

From Tieger PD, Barron-Tieger B. *Do What You Are: Discover the Perfect Career for You Through the Secrets of Personality Type*. Boston, MA: Little, Brown and Company; 2001.[6]

trait recognition is valuable because life mostly consists of a wide-ranging list of perplexing but often routine situations.[7] Hopefully, personality testing will help you recognize your inclinations in routine situations as you deal with new people every day in school and in clinical settings.

Emotional Intelligence

The concept of **emotional intelligence** (EI) has been around for several years. EI has been thoroughly studied and consequently defined by many researchers; the fundamental thought is that those who have fully developed EI have an enhanced ability to recognize emotions in themselves and others, and they have the capacity to use those emotions to improve emotional and intellectual growth and decision making.[8] This view assumes that when done well, combining emotions and **cognition** facilitates decisions, manages emotions, improves relationships, and ultimately results in more intelligent decisions.[8]

One of the most widely accepted views of EI was described by Daniel Goleman. He claimed that EI is the strongest predictor of success in the workplace, even more important than academics, and he further asserted that we can improve our performance in the workplace by further developing our EI.[9] Goleman claimed that there are five components of EI: self-awareness, self-regulation, motivation, **empathy**, and social skills (Table 2-3).[9]

Sound Off

Some consider emotional intelligence to be the strongest predictor of success in the workplace.

Researchers have proven that high EI is essential for healthcare professionals. Many have claimed that EI represents a set of core competencies for identifying, processing, and managing emotions that enable nurses to cope with daily demands in a knowledgeable, approachable, and supportive manner.[8] EI has been proven to be important in decision making in the clinical environment and for professional relationship growth.[8] Furthermore, the ability for a healthcare worker to manage his or her interpersonal and intrapersonal skills increases both the capacity to cope with the stresses of work and job satisfaction.[10] There are two online tools that are useful for measuring EI: a measurement for judging how good someone is at reading other's expression and the emotions quotient test. These can be found in Table 2-4. The topic of EI as it relates to leadership will be returned to later in another chapter.

TABLE 2-3	The five components of emotional intelligence
Component	**Explanation**
Self-awareness	Having a thorough understanding of one's emotions, strengths, weaknesses, needs, and ambition
Self-regulation	An ongoing conversation we must have with ourselves that frees us from feelings
Motivation	To achieve beyond everyone's expectations, including one's own; to achieve for the sake of achieving
Empathy	Being aware of and considerate of other people's feelings
Social skills	Combining friendliness, cooperation, and effective communication to improve interactions

From Seema G. Emotional intelligence in classroom. *Adv Manage* 2012;5(10):16–23.

TABLE 2-4	Emotional Intelligence Online Resources
Emotional Intelligence Tests	**Online Resource**
How good are you at reading facial expressions?	http://greatergood.berkeley.edu/ei_quiz/
How high is your emotional intelligence?	http://www.edu-nova.com/apps/emotional_quotient.html

Now What?

Can you change at this point in your life? Our personalities are strongly influenced by both genetics and early events in our lives that we have absolutely no control over.[7] Consider the possibility that someone in your class also has your exact personality type (e.g., ISTP, ESTP, etc.). Are these people just like you? Certainly not; we are all, of course, different in many ways. At this point in your life, if you are classified as extroverted, you will most likely not resort to introversion, or vice versa.[7] However, we can control how our extroversion or other traits are expressed. For example, one of the possible interaction issues identified for an extrovert is to talk first and then listen. An extrovert who wanted to modify this supposed weakness in interaction could make a conscious attempt to listen first and sort thoughts carefully before talking. Essentially, this person would decide to listen, pause, reflect, and then talk. However, this person is still an extrovert, but he or she controls the trait with personal restraint and, as a result, most likely improves communication.

If a single part of your personality is causing you concern or difficulty with dealing with people during routine communications, you should find alternative ways in which to express those traits that are less destructive to your ultimate communication goal.[7] In essence, "you don't have to change yourself, you just have to change your self's outlet," and while no one can blame you for who you are, you are ultimately responsible for how you act.[7] Keep in mind that personality testing determines only a propensity toward certain behaviors in routine situations. Learning about your individual strengths and weaknesses is a lifelong challenge, and you should return to the task of acknowledging these traits, especially before applying for jobs.[11] People who have a well-defined identities know what they like, what they believe in and value, and how to utilize their strengths to enhance their lives and the people around them.[12] But ultimately the answer to whether or not you can change is up to you. If you recognize a perceived personality trait that you want to manage better, remember, you must first want to change to make a change.

ETHICS AT WORK

Though Chapter 6 will give further details about **ethics** in healthcare, a brief overview is needed at this point. Working in healthcare demands both physical and emotional **fortitude**. Though the physical demands are minimal in sonography relative to other occupations such as a lumber jack or plumber, the work ethic required to be successful in sonography is equivalent. Ethics at work is not only knowing the right thing to do, but doing it.[13] This means that most of us have the capability of knowing what is right or wrong, but our personal ethics require that we choose the right thing to do *always*. So what is the "right thing" to do?

Parents, teachers, and other adults all over the world teach children to smile and play nice, be prompt, look their best, do their best, obey the rules, tell the truth, and say "please" and "thank you."[13] Accordingly, it was no surprise when over 1,500 employers were asked what they expected from each and every employee; the survey findings revealed that:

Employers are searching for positive, enthusiastic people who are dressed and prepared properly, who go out of their way to add value and do more than what is required of them, who are honest, who will play by the rules, and who will give cheerful, friendly service regardless of the situation.[13]

In plain terms, employers want employees (in our case, sonographers) who demonstrate **honesty** and **integrity**, who have positive attitudes; who are reliable, professional, self-motivated, and respectful, and who demonstrate cheerfulness and friendliness.[13]

Patients expect the following from healthcare workers: competent care, someone who listens, clear communication, **courtesy**, **compassion**, empathy, understanding, **sincerity**, and **respect**.[2] If we compare the two lists of expectations between employers and patients, several common qualities manifest—respect, competence, honesty, and friendliness. The correlation makes sense however, if you understand that fundamentally, patients are customers, and hospitals are businesses trying to please those customers. Both employers (hospitals) and customers (patients) expect the same things, and as the employees, it is our obligation to simultaneously please both. To accomplish this, we must look closer at these expectations to recognize how **character** in healthcare is important.

Character

Character may be defined as the way a person thinks, feels, and acts.[14] It is something that is not always identifiable in a brief encounter, but rather it is a pattern of behavior that one demonstrates consistently.[15] **Personal values** are tenets that someone holds in high regard and that are highly desirable and worthy of esteem.[15] Combined, our character and personal values help form our **reputation**, or the ways in which others view us. It is important for individuals who pursue careers in healthcare to have certain character traits and personal values and to maintain a high-quality reputation, all of which contribute to one's ethics.

The demonstration of your personal values and the character traits that you exhibit to others help establish your personal reputation. It is exceedingly important to start off on the right foot in healthcare, because your reputation will follow you wherever you go. And though you may not recognize it now, the sonography profession is a small community in which sonographers know many other sonographers in the area. For this reason, your reputation as a student is important to your future success as a professional.

 Sound Off

It is exceedingly important to start off on the right foot in healthcare, because your reputation will follow you wherever you go.

For example, your social life is often put on display for everyone in the world to see. You must recognize that online activity and personal online social media, such as Facebook, Twitter, and Instagram, are often examined by prospective employers. Consequently, you need to be watchful concerning online posts of negative judgments and irresponsible behaviors that are perceived as unfavorable for someone pursuing a professional occupation such as sonography. For example, posts that display alcohol abuse, even if you do not chronically abuse alcohol, may be viewed by some as behavior that is counterproductive to professionalism. Be careful what you put on the Internet to protect your reputation.

 Sound Off

Be careful what you put on the Internet to protect your reputation.

The American Society of Echocardiography (ASE) further states that sonographers should have the following traits: flexibility, **enthusiasm**, and confidence.[16] Though the communication aspect of patient care will be discussed further in Chapter 9, it is important to examine these desires of our patients and a few other character traits that are invaluable to patient care.

Sound Off

Patients want the following from healthcare workers: competent care, someone who listens, clear communication, courtesy, compassion, empathy, understanding, sincerity, and respect.

Competent Care and Flexibility

Performing a sonographic procedure independently requires a certain level of **competence**. Competence is essentially the possession of necessary knowledge and skills to carry out a specific job appropriately and safely in a consistent manner.[15] For accredited sonography programs in association with the **Commission on Accreditation of Allied Health Education Programs** (CAAHEP) and the JRC-DMS, standards have been created to normalize competency and education in accredited sonography programs. Standards are the minimum requirement to which an accredited program is held accountable.[17] These standards include meeting competency requirements for sonography students in all specialty areas.[17]

To ensure proficient patient care, programs include clinical competencies, which are unassisted sonographic procedures that students perform on campus in a scan lab or in the clinical setting. Throughout the length of educational programs, students undergo competency testing in order to both meet standards of the accreditation and to ensure that a certain level of patient care can be provided upon graduation. With patient care, you should never "just wing it." It is your responsibility to be prepared and to keep up to date on current procedures, techniques, technology, and new equipment. It is also important to note that many employers require new hires to perform competencies as part of the orientation process. Employers may also require prospective employees to scan as part of the interview process to assess competency.

Sonography is a dynamic, constantly changing profession, and as a professional, it is your duty to remain competent. This requires that the sonographer has flexibility and be able to adjust to our continuously evolving healthcare system. New research studies and inventions regularly transform the role of the sonographer from altering protocols to technological advancement. Being flexible in your work schedule may also be needed, as oftentimes sonographers are required to stay late after hours and take call.

A competent person can accept **constructive criticism** and value the honest opinions of instructors, coworkers, and others.[18] While it does recognize weaknesses in judgment, this form of criticism mostly provides well-reasoned, valid opinions about the work of others. If you are insecure about your abilities, never hesitate to ask questions or ask for help. Sonographers are legally required to meet a certain standard of care, which includes being competent at the tasks they are performing.

Sound Off

Sonographers are legally required to meet a certain standard of care, which includes being competent at the tasks they are performing.

Courtesy and Respect

Healthcare needs to be delivered with **tact**. Tact means always being aware and considerate of the feelings of others.[18] Patients expect us to be courteous in the way that we interact with them. Courtesy can be defined as demonstrating polite behavior. Courtesy goes hand in hand with tact. Unfortunately, using good manners is not an inherent attribute for some people, but it is required in healthcare. An example of showing courtesy toward patients could be asking them if they need anything, like perhaps a warm blanket, before the exam begins.[19] Also, respecting those you encounter during the day demonstrates that you value others. You can demonstrate respect in patient care by being polite, shaking the patient's hand when you meet him or her, and paying attention when he or she is talking.

You should also verbally show respect by using the appropriate title, such as Dr., Mr., Ms., or Mrs., and by using the patient's last name.[19] Being courteous and respectful also includes using simple expressions like "please" and "thank you." Believe it or not, simple expressions like these can go a long way toward developing relationships with instructors, sonographers, physicians, and anyone else, especially during an initial encounter.

Compassion and Empathy

William Bennett once wrote, "Just as courage takes its stand *by* others in a challenging situation, so compassion takes its stand *with* others in their distress."[20] With compassion, we have a propensity to feel for our patients and their well-being. Compassion is an important part of patient care. **Compassion satisfaction** has been defined as the pleasure one gains from being able to help others and the feeling that one has the ability to make a positive difference in patients' lives.[21] We need to remind ourselves that our patients come to us with a certain need, and having compassion informs our obligation to help those who are ill. But with compassion, there is no attempt to feel or comprehend what the patient may be going through at the time.

Empathy is similar to compassion but on a higher level. Empathy demonstrates that you understand to the point of feeling how another person feels.[19] To develop empathy, one has to attempt to view the world through others' eyes.[2] Placing yourself in a patient's circumstances helps you appreciate what he or she is going through at the time. One author claims that empathy is perhaps the single most important restraint from immoral or antisocial behavior.[7] In sonography, you will encounter very ill patients, both young and old. An empathetic sonographer listens to patients without judging, demonstrates an honest attempt to understand the patient, and through identifiable actions, reveals a sincere willingness to help patients to the best of his or her abilities.

Sound Off

An empathetic sonographer listens to patients without judging, demonstrates an honest attempt to understand the patient, and through identifiable actions, reveals a sincere willingness to help patients to the best of his or her abilities.

Though having compassion for these individuals is warranted, it appears that multiple encounters that require extended amounts of compassion can actually lead to **burnout**. **Compassion fatigue** has been mentioned in the literature as a complication often discovered in people who work in helping professions, like sonography, for several years.[22] Compassion fatigue results from the combination of **traumatic stress** and burnout.[23] Traumatic stress is unique in that it is a consequence of "wanting to help a traumatized or suffering person."[22] Sonographers must often deal with patients undergoing traumatic events, such as heart attacks, miscarriages, strokes, or cancer, and they may certainly therefore suffer from compassion fatigue.

The short-term results of compassion fatigue may include nervousness, cynicism, pessimism, low self-esteem, anger at coworkers, and job dissatisfaction.[22] Long-term effects include weight issues, overall poor work performance, noticeable personality changes, and a desire to leave the profession.[22] There appears to be an innate self-preservation mechanism in which many people tend to build emotional barriers between themselves and their patients in order to fend off compassion fatigue, resulting in a decrease in empathetic feelings.[24] However, instead of reducing empathy, a sonographer can learn coping techniques that maintain the level of compassion while preventing the arduous effects of compassion fatigue (Table 2-5). One study indicates that those with high EI tend to have better coping abilities, are more in touch with their emotions, can regulate their emotions, and experience lower levels of distress and stress-related emotions.[24,25] Thus, the higher the EI you have, the less likely you are to suffer from compassion fatigue. You can test for compassion fatigue at http://www.healthy-place.com/psychological-tests/compassion-fatigue-self-assessment/.

TABLE 2-5	Coping with compassion fatigue

- Be informed and learn more about compassion fatigue at http://www.compassionfatigue.org/.
- Know that compassion fatigue is inevitable, and be prepared.
- Establish support groups.
- Encourage others to talk about traumatic events they experience at work in a weekly meeting.
- Consider seeking outside assistance, or visit employee health.

From Tellie M. Compassion fatigue—the cost of caring. *Nursing Update* [serial online] 2008;32(8):34–37. Available from: CINAHL with Full Text, Ipswich, MA. Accessed March 20, 2014.[25]

Accountability, Honesty, and Integrity

Healthcare workers must hold themselves accountable. **Accountability** means that one is responsible for one's actions. Sonographers are accountable to their patients, their employers, and their profession. The Society of Diagnostic Medical Sonography (SDMS), American Society of Echocardiography (ASE), and the Society of Vascular Ultrasound (SVU) have established a code of ethics for the sonographer. An analysis of codes of ethics is provided for you in greater detail in Chapter 6. The SDMS Code of Ethics consists of three primary principles promoting the well-being of patients: a high level of competence, **honesty** and **integrity** in communication, and maintaining the public trust.[26]

We have all heard the saying "honesty is the best policy." This idiom is particularly true in healthcare, where being dishonest can ultimately result in the loss of human life. For example, perhaps, a sonographer in a rush to leave on time haphazardly performs a liver sonogram, omits some protocol images, and unfortunately misses a small malignant tumor in the liver. The sonographer then reports to the radiologist that the liver appears within normal limits, even though the sonographer did not adequately image the liver. This is untruthful because the sonographer did not spend enough time analyzing the liver. As a result, instead of the cancer being imaged during a screening exam like sonography, it has a chance to spread further, possibly both extending the time of discovery and even reducing the lifespan of the patient. By taking the proper amount of time, the sonographer could have found the tumor, and immediate follow-up investigation and treatment could ensue.

Integrity and honesty go hand in hand. Integrity may be defined as thinking with honesty and choosing the best paths to follow based on high **standards**.[27] Standards are morals, ethics, or habits established by customs, authorities, or an individual that are deemed satisfactory.[14] One must recognize that second-rate standards never result in a first-rate person (Table 2-6).[27] Demonstrating

TABLE 2-6	First-rate standards in sonography

- Play by the rules of your college and your profession.
- Know your limitations and weaknesses in your character, and stay away from situations that challenge your integrity.
- Hold yourself to the same standards as you hold others.
- Set a good example for others.
- Practice in a way that you would be proud to have others see you.
- Look out for the interests of others, and make sure all patients are treated fairly and equally, regardless of who they are.

Adapted from Watson CE. *How Honesty Pays: Restoring Integrity to the Workplace.* Westport, CT: Praeger; 2005.[27]

integrity in every situation is a challenge for some, but choosing to have integrity is always the proper decision.

For example, a sonography student is assigned an online, at-home assignment and instructed to not use his or her textbook during the assignment. Realistically, there may be no manner in which the student would be caught for cheating if he or she used the textbook. The student could get away with cheating. However, does he or she really escape the repercussions of cheating? Who ultimately suffers in the end? Indeed, the student suffers eventually, as he or she may need to recall the material on a final examination or a registry. Cheating negates integrity, and it will inevitably catch up with you. What about the patients that the student encounters in the clinical setting? Couldn't this momentary lapse in integrity ultimately affect the life of a person?

These are candid questions about integrity and honesty that you need to consider. We are all faced with dilemmas in our lives that challenge our integrity. Making terrible decisions always affects someone. Some may argue that doing the right thing is not always easy. That is incorrect. Doing the right thing is always easy if you have integrity.

Sound Off

Some may say that doing the right thing is not always easy. This is incorrect. Doing the right thing is always easy if you have integrity.

Self-Motivation and Enthusiasm

Self-motivation could potentially be the characteristic that most influences a person's behavior.[18] Self-motivation is the ability to do what needs to be done without being influenced or initiated by someone else. It requires the perception to recognize a goal and the courage and strength to reach that same goal. Completing tasks without being told is vital in healthcare. Every day, sonographers complete work-related tasks that are not distinctly spelled out in their job descriptions—transporting patients, assisting patients with hygiene needs, calling physicians' offices, etc. Though not all job duties are clearly outlined sometimes, sonographers are often self-motivated independent workers who recognize tasks that must be done and complete them. Sonographers also demonstrate self-motivation by learning new equipment, procedures, and techniques, even if the job does not explicitly demand alterations in the routine. Self-motivators also take it upon themselves to constantly learn about their chosen profession.

Both sonographers in clinical and instructors in the classroom recognize your inclination toward self-motivation almost right away in your assignments and diligence in your work. In the classroom, you demonstrate self-motivation by being prepared for class, tests, and class discussions ahead of time. In clinical, consistently demonstrate your willingness to learn, and inquire often about assisting sonographers. Self-motivation is demonstrated by your initiative and **enthusiasm** to learn.

Enthusiasm is defined as an eagerness or excitement for what you are doing.[18] If we return to the list of employer/ASE-required traits for employees and sonographers, we can recognize that there is a common theme of enthusiasm, friendliness, and positive attitude. Demonstrating a positive attitude and enthusiasm about your career is important to professional work ethic, and you should make it evident in everything you attempt.[15] People are often classified as either optimists or pessimists. From the personality testing that you completed in this chapter, you can probably decipher how you would be classified. Do you think the glass is half empty (pessimist) or half full (optimist)? People who demonstrate consistent enthusiasm tend to be optimists. Which type of sonographer would you want to work with in clinical? Which type of sonographer would you want to perform a sonogram on you? Remember, you *chose* to enter sonography because you had an interest in the profession. You need to decide now that you are going to be enthusiastic about learning and fully dedicated to doing your best. If you have this enthusiasm for sonography now, the feeling can grow into a real love for our profession.

Sound Off

You need to decide now that you are going to be enthusiastic about learning and fully dedicated to doing your best. If you have this enthusiasm now for sonography, the feeling can grow into a real love for our profession.

Hunger for Knowledge

Sonographers should have a hunger for knowledge. Our profession demands that sonographers keep current with changes in healthcare through **continuing medical education** (CME) in order to maintain certification after one is registered. CME credits can be acquired through different means including articles, meetings, and lectures. Sonographers will also be required to accomplish **recertification** in the near future.[28] Even though sonographers must continue their education to maintain certification, successful sonographers continually learn outside of these demands. As you complete your didactic classes, an intrinsic enjoyment in learning about the human body should exist. As you scan more, you should develop an interest in learning more about pathology and how it affects normal function. There is always something new to learn in sonography, and the responsibility of the sonographer is to never stop learning.

Self-Confidence

Self-motivation plus a thirst for knowledge combined with enthusiasm results in **self-confidence**, another required trait mentioned by the ASE for sonographers. Self-confidence means that you believe in yourself and your abilities. It is typical for students to have dissimilar confidence levels. For example, you may have confidence in your ability to study for a hefty test and to do well. You gained this confidence through practice taking tests and doing well on tests. Like this, confidence in your abilities as a sonographer is something that comes with much practice, so you must be patient with the development of your skills, and gradually, you will gain more self-confidence. Essentially, self-confidence is something that cannot be taught, but rather gained with experience.

Competencies are used to gauge your level of training in certain sonographic procedures, and being successful with competencies is a good way to grow in self-confidence. But even if you are successful with a competency, only you can truly know if you are thoroughly competent, and thus, you are ultimately responsible for recognizing your weaknesses and correcting those weaknesses with more self-motivated practice while you are in school. There is a point, however, in which **assertiveness** can be perceived as aggression. Self-confidence to the point of arrogance can backfire, so be careful to not overstep your bounds as a student. Remember, throughout your career in sonography, you will never stop learning, so the task of building self-confidence is an ongoing task.

Final Thoughts on Character

From reading the information in this section, one can visualize the demands upon your character and moral fortitude that comes with working in a healthcare setting. A successful sonographer who consistently demonstrates the above mentioned traits or strengths provides such an example for you as a student to emulate. We have all worked with individuals who lack professionalism, and you will no doubt encounter sonographers and other healthcare workers who are lacking as well. What should you do? First, make sure that your character is obviously different from theirs—with patients, with coworkers, and all the time. One of the greatest things someone can do for other people is provide them with a good example.[29] Second, if the lack of professionalism negatively affects patient care, let your instructor or employer know. That is your responsibility. Remember, integrity counts.

Though the occupation of sonographer provides us with a respectable salary, you should visualize your future career in sonography as a dignified mission to help people. By doing this, your focus will not be on monetary gains alone, but rather the endless rewards gained from the knowledge that you have the daily opportunity to make immeasurable positive differences in patients' lives.

CLINICAL RESPONSIBILITIES AND WORKPLACE CHALLENGES FOR THE SONOGRAPHER

Everyone has their own individual strengths as discussed earlier. Some researchers suggest that while most people tend to focus on fixing weaknesses, we should rather focus on taking advantage of our strengths.[29] **Strength** is "an inner ability, something that can be displayed in a performance."[29] Let's return to the example of the extrovert mentioned earlier in this chapter. Though the extrovert may recognize that he or she lacks the ability to control his or her sociability, this individual could choose to hone it as a strength and use it to improve communication with others. An extrovert who is outspoken could certainly make a fine lead sonographer, department manager, spokesperson for the sonography profession, or sales representative for ultrasound equipment. But is the research applicable for a person who is required to perform a standard echocardiography examination when basically every cardiac sonographer must have this ability? There are required strengths as approved by CAAHEP and appraised by the **Joint Review Committee on Education in Diagnostic Medical Sonography** (JRC-DMS), which a sonographer must be capable of in order to perform an accurate sonographic examination (Table 2-7). From this list, it is evident that a sonographer must have the following: the ability to obtain a thorough clinical history; a thorough understanding of human anatomy, physiology, and pathology; an appreciation of normal and abnormal sonographic findings; and the skill to integrate data from sonographic findings and clinical findings.

Sonographic Reasoning and Clinical Correlation

One of the primary obligations of the sonographer is to "obtain, review, and integrate pertinent patient history and supporting clinical data to facilitate optimum diagnostic results."[30] In other words, obtaining a thorough clinical history is an imperative responsibility of a sonographer. Recall, from Chapter 1, that investigative imaging was defined as a technique used by sonographers whereby he or she obtains sonographic protocol images while simultaneously searching for and identifying abnormalities. Furthermore, while other technologists acquire clinical history and basically report the information to the interpreting physician, sonographers must be capable of integrating that data and applying the gained knowledge to the study at hand in order to "facilitate optimum diagnostic results,"

TABLE 2-7	Required strengths of the sonographer

The general sonographer, adult cardiac sonographer, pediatric cardiac sonographer, and vascular technologist are able to perform the following:

- Obtain, review, and integrate pertinent patient history and supporting clinical data to facilitate optimum diagnostic results.
- Perform appropriate procedures and record anatomic, pathologic, and/or physiologic data for interpretation by a physician.
- Record, analyze, and process diagnostic data and other pertinent observations made during the procedure for presentation to the interpreting physician.
- Exercise discretion and judgment in the performance of sonographic and/or other diagnostic services.
- Demonstrate appropriate communication skills with patients and colleagues.
- Act in a professional and ethical manner.
- Provide patient education related to medical ultrasound and/or other diagnostic vascular techniques, and promote principles of good health.

From Commission on Accreditation of Allied Health Education Programs. *Diagnostic Medical Sonography.* Accessed December 28, 2014 from http://www.caahep.org/Content.aspx?ID=23[30]

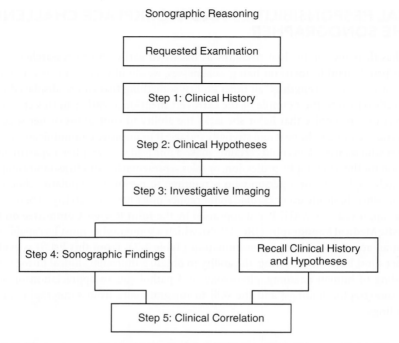

Figure 2-1. The sonographic reasoning method. Step 1: Clinical history—the information gathered by obtaining a clinical history; Step 2: Clinical hypotheses—educated guesses based on clinical history findings; Step 3: Investigative imaging—a technique used by sonographers whereby they obtain sonographic protocol images while searching for and identifying abnormalities; Step 4: Sonographic findings—information gathered by performing the sonographic examination; Step 5: Clinical correlation—the process of recalling clinical history and clinical hypothesis, contrasting that information with sonographic findings, and evaluating the information for connections.[31]

a method that may be referred to as **sonographic reasoning** (Figs. 2-1 and 2-2). Sonographic reasoning establishes a clear way of thinking that sonographers can use for every sonographic examination.

Whereas investigative imaging allows for a thorough examination of both normal and abnormal structures, it is **clinical correlation** that helps guide a sonographer toward a more targeted examination. Clinical correlation is the process of obtaining clinical history and contrasting that information with sonographic findings.[31] Essentially, this type of logical thinking is referred to as **inductive reasoning**. Inductive reasoning requires one to make an educated guess that is based on the facts of a clinical history. And though your educated guess may be correct, it is not always true, and therefore, your sonographic findings help establish or negate clinical hypotheses. For most clinical history findings, there are multiple diagnostic variables, but sonographic reasoning is a good place to start.

Sound Off
Steps in Sonographic Reasoning:
1. Clinical history
2. Clinical hypotheses
3. Investigative imaging
4. Sonographic findings
5. Clinical correlation

As explained in Chapter 1, clinical history includes a patient's signs and symptoms, pertinent illnesses, past surgeries, laboratory findings, the results of other diagnostic testing, and family history,

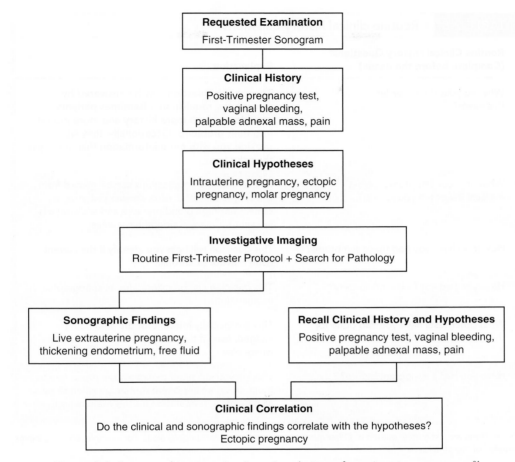

Requested Examination

First-Trimester Sonogram

Clinical History

Positive pregnancy test,
vaginal bleeding,
palpable adnexal mass, pain

Clinical Hypotheses

Intrauterine pregnancy, ectopic
pregnancy, molar pregnancy

Investigative Imaging

Routine First-Trimester Protocol + Search for Pathology

Sonographic Findings

Live extrauterine pregnancy,
thickening endometrium, free fluid

Recall Clinical History and Hypotheses

Positive pregnancy test, vaginal bleeding,
palpable adnexal mass, pain

Clinical Correlation

Do the clinical and sonographic findings correlate with the hypotheses?
Ectopic pregnancy

Figure 2-2. Sonographic reasoning in action during a first-trimester sonogram.[31]

if relevant. Though you will learn more about obtaining clinical history in themed classes (abdominal, adult echocardiography, vascular, etc.), there are some general questions that you can ask patients before every exam that are appropriate (Table 2-8). However, before you even enter the ultrasound room or question the patient, you can perform some clinical investigation by asking the patient relevant questions (Table 2-9). The importance of clinical correlation cannot be overstated in sonography. **Clinical correlation ambiguity** can manifest quickly if one is unaware of how to properly perform sonographic reasoning. Specifically, clinical correlation ambiguity is lacking the ability to obtain a thorough clinical history and relate the information with the sonographic findings of the examination.[31]

The purpose of collecting the clinical history before the examination is to develop clinical hypotheses. A clinical hypothesis is a conditional theory of pathology based on clinical history, and while a sonographer may be more apprehensive about the most common or severe pathology, other pathologies cannot be excluded without imaging. This preliminary framework helps the sonographer perform more targeted investigative imaging. Although the sonographer does not advance an official diagnosis, this exercise is similar to what the interpreting physician accomplishes as he or she analyzes the case (Figs. 2-3 and 2-4).

Figure 2-3 provides an example of how the physician correlates the information obtained by evaluating a sonographic study in which the clinical findings are as follows: elevated bilirubin and alkaline phosphatase (ALP); leukocytosis (elevated white blood cell count); sudden onset of right upper quadrant pain; nausea and vomiting; no past abdominal surgeries; and no previous imaging studies.

TABLE 2-8	Routine clinical history questions

Routine Clinical History Questions[a] (Complete before the exam.)	Explanation
Why did your doctor order this exam?	Though this question may be answered by viewing the requisition, oftentimes patients provide you with more history and more insight into their problems. Occasionally, they will provide you with more information than they give their doctors.
What are your symptoms? (What medical issues are you having?)	Relevant follow-up questions can be gained from this simple question. Also, knowing whether a patient has high blood pressure and is diabetic is relevant for many sonographic studies.
How long have you had these symptoms?	This question will help you identify if the current issue is **acute** or **chronic**.
Have you had any (relevant) surgery?	This question can be tailored for all sonographic examinations.
What other tests have you had done for this issue?	This is especially relevant for the area being imaged, even if the study was performed somewhere else.
Have you had a sonogram before?	Though you still need to explain the procedure to them, this is an important routine question to ask all patients in preparation for the examination.

[a]Note: These are just routine questions. Other questions can be applied for specialty areas. For example, obstetric exams require last menstrual cycle information.[31]

TABLE 2-9	Routine clinical investigation tasks

Routine Clinical Investigation Tasks (Complete before the exam.)	Explanation
Step 1: Examine the patient's chart and/or requisition.	The sonographer should look for information pertaining to the immediate study in the patient's chart, such as viewing the written order for indications, signs, and symptoms. The requisition for an outpatient procedure must contain an indication for the sonographic examination.
Step 2: Examine the patient's laboratory findings.	Laboratory findings, when available, should always be examined before the examination. For example, liver function test, renal function, and complete blood count (CBC) can be evaluated before the sonographic examination.
Step 3: Examine the reports from the patient's prior imaging studies.	The reports from the most relevant and recent imaging study examinations should be examined prior to the sonographic examination.

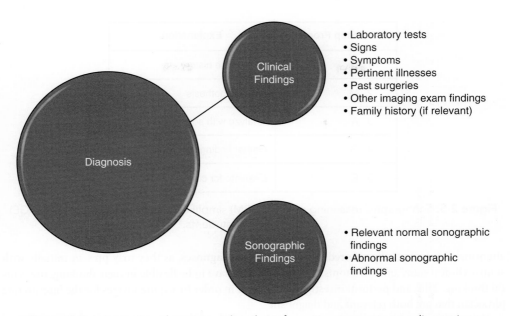

Figure 2-3. Interpreting physicians utilize this information to construct a diagnosis or a list of differential diagnoses.

Simply based on the clinical history, a physician would be capable of recognizing that the patient most likely has acute cholecystitis even before the sonogram is completed. During the sonogram, the sonographer identifies definite sonographic findings of cholecystitis, like a thickened gallbladder wall, fluid around the gallbladder, and tenderness over the gallbladder while scanning (Murphy sign). The diagnostic puzzle pieces fit, and the clinical findings correlate with the sonographic findings—a clinical correlation.

It does not always work this way however. For example, a different patient with the same symptoms could have gallstones and liver carcinoma instead of just acute cholecystitis. These two

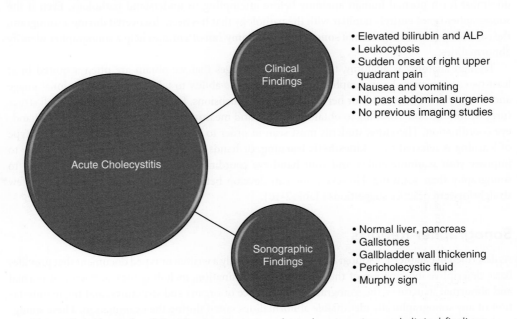

Figure 2-4. Example of the diagnostic process based on imaging and clinical findings.

Five-Step Process	Explanation
1. I	*Investigate history*
2. M	*Make hypothesis*
3. A	*Analyze with sonography*
4. G	*Gather findings*
5. E	*Evaluate for connections*

Figure 2-5. Sonographic reasoning method (SRM) simplified as a five-step process (IMAGE) for sonography students.[31]

abnormalities are actually referred to as **differential diagnoses**, as they may present initially with similar clinical signs and symptoms. So sonographers have to be flexible in their thinking, use critical thinking skills, and perform investigative imaging in order to acquire images for the interpreting physician that are both relevant and diagnostic.

Using sonographic reasoning may be overwhelming for new students, and therefore, a simplified version with a five-step, easy-to-remember mnemonic, *IMAGE*, is provided in Figure 2-5. IMAGE stands for (1) investigate history; (2) make hypotheses; (3) analyze with sonography; (4) gather all sonographic findings; and (5) evaluate for connections.[31]

Appreciating Anatomy, Physiology, and Pathology

Sonography education is typically divided between two chief training venues: didactic or classroom training and clinical or workplace training. As we can see in the list of requirements for a sonographer in this chapter, sonographers must have an appreciation of how the body works (**physiology**) and be able to apply that knowledge while they are performing sonographic exams. Consequently, one must learn normal human anatomy before attempting to understand pathology. Even if the sonographer is not entirely familiar with the pathology that has been discovered during a sonogram, the capability of knowing normal **sonographic anatomy** can oftentimes help a sonographer identify abnormalities.

Though anatomy is anatomy, the sonographic images that we obtain are often acquired in at least two scan planes. A sonographer must also have the ability to take the two-dimensional image and recreate that image in his or her mind in three dimensions. Furthermore, scanning small structures within the body, rotating to obtain an image, and measuring structures all require good hand-eye coordination. Therefore, students must scan in order to learn the art of sonography. This type of learning is referred to as **kinesthetic learning**, or hands-on learning. There is no better way to improve your scanning ability and your hand-eye coordination techniques that are applicable to sonography than scanning. However, one can develop better hand-eye coordination with a few straightforward practice suggestions (Table 2-10).

Sonographer Reports

As described in Chapter 1, a sonographer report is typically a written or typed document that provides basic descriptive information of the sonographic examination, including measurements of normal and abnormal structures, the sonographic appearance of organs and structures, and the manifestation of any sonographically identifiable abnormalities noted during the examination. These sonographer impressions of the examination, which include any alterations from the normal protocol in

TABLE 2-10	Tips to improve hand-eye coordination
Improving Hand-Eye Coordination	**Explanation**
Play video games (but study first).	Playing video games can help with hand-eye coordination. Both traditional gaming, in which a controller is involved and interactive games, in which hand gestures are used, like dancing or sports games, could improve coordination.
Start playing an instrument.	Learning a new instrument or one that you already know but have not played in a while may help improve hand-eye coordination.
Pick up a new sport, or play catch.	Playing a sport, especially one like ping pong, tennis, or racketball, can help with hand-eye coordination. Also, an occasional simple game of catch may help.
Pick up a new hand-eye hobby.	Find a new hobby that is both enjoyable, relaxing, and makes you use your hands like sewing, quilting, or painting.

patient position and the technical acquisition of images (i.e., special transducer frequency, technically difficult patient, etc.), are used to assist the interpreting physician in making an overall diagnosis. Sonographer reports do not include a diagnosis however, but rather provide comparisons between normally and abnormally appearing structures, in sonographic terms. For example, a report that notes a patient has a 3-cm gallstone is technically providing a diagnosis of cholelithiasis. In sonographic terms, one can describe a gallstone as a mobile, shadowing, echogenic structure within the lumen of the gallbladder. However, this does not reduce the requirement for the sonographer to be familiar with the distinctive sonographic appearance of cholelithiasis. Common sonographic terminology can be found in Table 2-11. You can become more familiar with sonographic jargon if you study and read what the sonographer writes on reports. For comparison, you can read the final dictated official report from the physician.

Occupational Stress for the Sonographer

The sonographer most certainly has physical demands placed upon him or her throughout the day. These physical demands and how they relate to proper scanning techniques will be closely analyzed in Chapter 5. However, sonographers encounter other forms of **occupational stress**, or stress related to job duties in the workplace, that result in negative psychologic and physiologic effects.[21] Though **role ambiguity**, or the frustration that arises when job expectations differ between employer and employee, is not as often an issue given the technical aspects of the occupation, there can be instances when additional job duties beyond performing sonograms can lead to stress.[32] For example, stressors in the sonography department include demanding work schedules and **taking call**.

For the student, gaining proficiency in sonographic examination is an ongoing process. For the sonographer, though he or she is proficient, he or she must also have the ability to work at a consistently high intellectual and physical level for eight or 12 hours at a time. The demanding work schedule often includes varying examinations that may include vascular, abdominal, and obstetric examinations all in the same day. Sonographers working in the hospital may have to complete inpatient, outpatient (with add-ons), and emergency patients throughout the day, requiring the sonographer to perform varying types of multiple exams per sonographer each day.[33] Taking call is the process by which a sonographer is paid a small amount of money to be on standby via telephone for emergency cases after regular department hours, including nights and weekends. Though taking call may not be profitable if one is not called in, the rewarding thing about **callback pay** is that it is

TABLE 2-11	Common sonographic descriptive terminology	
Common Descriptive Sonographic Terms	**Explanation**	**Examples**
Anechoic (Fig. 2-6)	• Without echoes • Dark on the image • Fluid-filled structures • Produces through transmission	• Gallbladder • Simple renal cyst • Urinary bladder
Hypoechoic (Fig. 2-7)	• Having few echoes • Dark but not black on the image • Comparative term	• Solid, dark tumors • Fresh blood clot in a vessel • Right kidney is more hypoechoic than the liver.
Hyperechoic (Fig. 2-8)	• Having many echoes • Bright or gray on the image • May produce posterior shadowing • Comparative term	• Solid, bright tumors • Hepatic hemangioma • Aged blood clot in a vessel • Gallstones
Echogenic (Fig. 2-9)	• Structure that produces echoes • Bright or gray on the image • Comparative term	• Diffusely bright (echogenic) liver • Pancreas is more echogenic than the liver. • May be used by some synonymously with hyperechoic
Isoechoic (Fig. 2-10)	• Having the same echogenicity • Comparative term	• Mass that is the same echogenicity as the surrounding tissue • Focal nodular hyperplasia
Complex (mass) (Fig. 2-11)	• Having mixed echogenicities • A structure that has both fluid and solid components	• Complex ovarian cysts • Hydatid cyst in the liver
Homogeneous (Fig. 2-12)	• Of uniform composition • Smooth structure with consistent echogenicity	• Normal liver • Normal spleen
Heterogeneous (Fig. 2-13)	• Of differing composition • Patchy structure with inconsistent echogenicity	• Liver with multiple masses • Thyroid gland affected by Graves disease
Shadowing (Fig. 2-14)	• Failure of the sound beam to pass through an object	• Seen posterior to a gallstone, rib, kidney stone
Through transmission (acoustic enhancement) (Fig. 2-15)	• The amount of the sound beam passing through a structure	• Seen posterior to fluid-filled structures • Cysts, urinary bladder, blood vessels

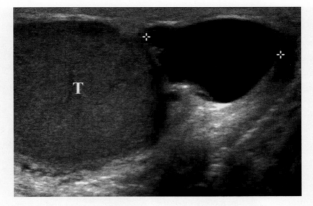

Figure 2-6. Anechoic. Cyst (between calipers) noted adjacent to the testicle (*T*).

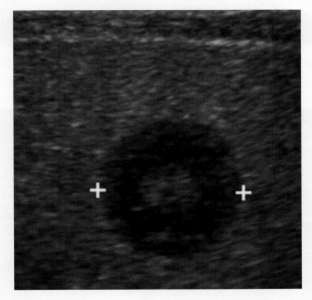

Figure 2-7. Hypoechoic. A hypoechoic, metastatic melanoma (between calipers).

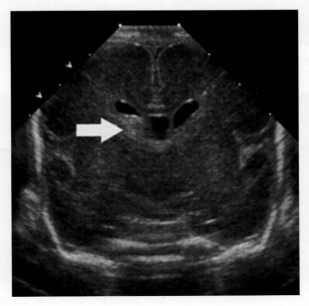

Figure 2-8. Hyperechoic. A hyperechoic Grade I germinal matrix bleed (*arrow*) in a neonatal brain.

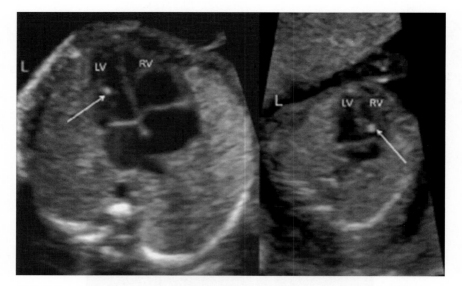

Figure 2-9. Echogenic. An echogenic intracardiac focus (*arrow*) within the fetal heart. *LV*, right ventricle; *RV*, right ventricle.

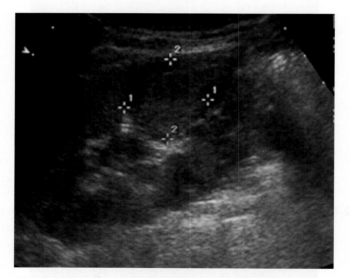

Figure 2-10. Isoechoic. An isoechoic tumor (between calipers) is noted on this pediatric kidney.

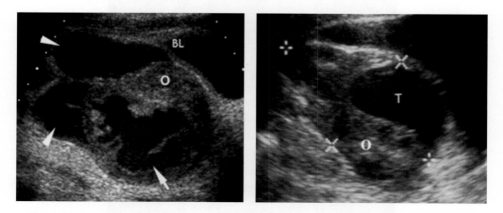

Figure 2-11. Complex (mass). This complex mass (*arrowheads* and *arrow*) within the female pelvis involved the ovary (*o*), fallopian tube (*T*), and bladder (*BL*).

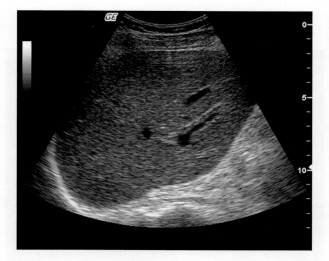

Figure 2-12. Homogeneous. The sonographic appearance of a normal, homogenous liver.

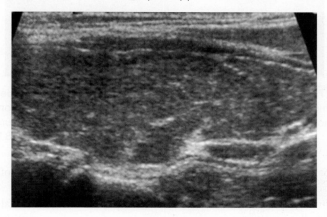

Figure 2-13. Heterogeneous. The sonographic appearance of a heterogeneous thyroid lobe due to Graves disease. (From Seigel JS. *Pediatric Sonography*. 4th ed. Philadelphia, PA: Lippincott William & Wilkins; 2010:157.)

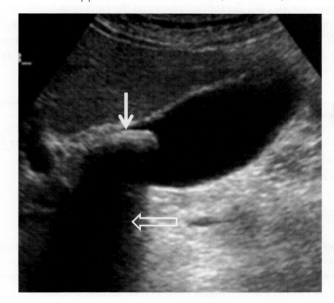

Figure 2-14. Acoustic shadowing. A gallstone (*solid arrow*) is noted within the gallbladder producing a posterior acoustic shadow (*open arrow*). (From Seigel JS. *Pediatric Sonography*. 4th ed. Philadelphia, PA: Lippincott William & Wilkins; 2010:281.)

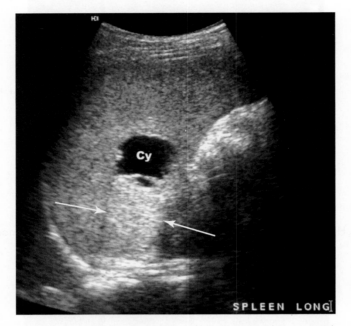

Figure 2-15. Through transmission (acoustic enhancement). This image demonstrates a simple splenic cyst (*Cy*) with through transmission (between *arrows*). (From Penny SM et al. Examination Review for Ultrasound: Sonographic Principles and Instrumentation (SPI). Philadelphia, PA; Lippincott Williams and Wilkins; 2011:88.)

typically substantially higher than regular shift work. Unfortunately, the abuse of callback and the demanding work schedule can ultimately lead to sonographer burnout.

Burnout is defined as the result of stress that leads to physical and emotional exhaustion, feelings of hopelessness, disconnectedness, and a reduction in professional accomplishment.[21] One study showed that sonographers and vascular technologist do experience moderate levels of burnout and that burnout can negatively affect the quality of both the sonographers' work and patient care.[34] Therefore, it is important for both the sonographers and the employers to recognize the symptoms of burnout and work together to make effective changes to the work environment. Like compassion fatigue, those with high EI tend to suffer less from burnout.[8] Also, to combat burnout, one study proposed that the development of empathy combats the effects of burnout and its harmful impact on the workplace.[35] Other preventive measures are provided in Table 2-12.

TABLE 2-12	Tips for reducing burnout on the job

- Take time for breaks between patients, even if only for a few minutes to rest your mind.
- Learn to manage your stress as discussed in Chapter 1.
- Get adequate sleep.
- Inquire often about job task clarification.
- Ask for others to help you if needed.
- Get a hobby.
- Reward yourself for accomplishments on the job, and even if your employer does not recognize you, share those accomplishments with friends and family.

From Haroun L. *Career Development for Health Professionals: Success in School and on the Job.* 3rd ed. Maryland Heights, MO: Saunders Elsevier; 2011.

STUDENT INTERACTION WITH SONOGRAPHERS

Now that we have closely examined the demands placed upon the sonographer, we can discuss how you as a sonography student can communicate with sonographers effectively. Establishing a good working relationship with a sonographer will afford you a great opportunity to learn. You should be persistent in your pursuit of knowledge. But although being persistent is important, being annoying is a distraction (Table 2-13). The following section will provide some communication tips to use as you interact with professional sonographers.

When and How to Communicate

The best place to talk to a sonographer is outside of the ultrasound room in an area where conversations cannot be overheard by patients. In fact, there can be serious legal repercussions that result from the violation of a patient's right to privacy under the **Health Insurance Portability and Accountability Act of 1996** (HIPAA). Though HIPAA will be explained in greater detail in Chapter 7, you should know that one should never discuss patient-related information in public.

Most sonography departments are centered around a work station at which images are viewed and sonographer reports are created. This area is presumably out of the patient care environment, and thus, it is a place where case-specific material may be discussed. Never discuss pathology or point at the ultrasound monitor while in the room in front of a patient, as this may cause unwarranted distress to the patient. It would behoove you to ask your sonographer where such information can be discussed.

TABLE 2-13	Ways to annoy sonographers
Six Ways to Annoy Sonographers	**Explanation**
1. Constantly complaining	Nobody wants to work with someone who is constantly complaining about school, scan time, other students, or practically anything.
2. Constantly talking	Learn when to be quiet, especially while a sonographer is performing an examination.
3. Being a know-it-all	Acting like you know everything as a student does not demonstrate humility. Even after school, you will continue to learn. If you know the answer to questions, answer them respectfully.
4. Being lazy	Work hard. Ask for tasks to complete. Stay busy. Do not sit around doing nothing.
5. Being the consummate rule-breaker	Breaking rules in school will get noticed and will most likely hurt your chances of getting a job later. Be there, be on time, and leave on time. People notice.
6. Getting personal	Try to stay out of personal conversations between sonographers, and keep a safe professional distance. Keep personal information to yourself. Don't get involved in departmental drama.

Adapted from Watson CE, Idinopulos TE. *Are You your Own Worst Enemy? The Nine Inner Strengths You Need to Overcome Self-defeating Tendencies at Work.* Westport, CT. Praeger; 2007.[36]

TABLE 2-14	Tips for getting more scan time
Acquiring More Scan Time	**Explanation**
Examine the schedule, and plan ahead.	Inform the sonographers of tasks or full exams that you would like to perform.
Make a list of daily tasks to accomplish.	Try to focus on specific anatomy to identify as you scan throughout the day to save time.
Scan before or after the exam for a few minutes.	Ask if you could begin the examination or scan after the sonographer finishes.
Know your protocols well.	Really understanding the protocol will increase your speed and help you acquire more scanning experience.

Many sonographers who you work with in the clinical setting are not compensated for helping teach you. Thus, you should view yourself as a guest in their workspace and approach interactions with respect, **humility**, and appreciation. Humility is a noticeable trait and one that can certainly position your relationship with a sonographer on the right path where both of you can learn together.

Acquiring Scan Time

As you have most likely surmised by now, there is a direct relationship between the time you spend scanning and enhancing your scanning skills. That is, the more you scan, the better the scanner you will become. But sometimes, it can be difficult to get your hands on the transducer in the clinical setting. Busy departments may not offer as much time to scan as you would like. And you certainly do not want to appear rude or aggressive to a sonographer. Table 2-14 provides some tips for acquiring more scan time.

STUDENT INTERACTION WITH INTERPRETING PHYSICIANS

Not all physicians are alike, some do not relate well with students and at times, even with sonographers and patients. However, interacting with a physician can be one of the most memorable learning experiences you will have in school and as a sonographer, especially if the physician is someone who likes to teach. If you are awarded the opportunity, watching the physician dictate reports or discuss cases is an outstanding way to learn, even if the study is not a sonogram.

Because physicians are highly dependent upon the sonographer's skills, sonographers must gain the trust of the physician. As a student, you will be in the unique position to observe and appreciate these professional interactions between the physician and the sonographer on a routine basis at some clinical facilities. Listen carefully to how sonographers present cases to the physician, especially questions that are unique to each examination. You will be able to witness the special relationship between the physician and sonographer and the mutual respect that is achieved with time.

When you speak with a physician, remain respectful and pay attention to him or her vigilantly. Be inquisitive and make mental notes of what he or she shares with you. Some physicians like to ask students questions. Answer them appropriately, and do not hesitate to tell them when you do not know the answer, but be sure to know the answer the next time. You may eventually be allowed to present cases to the physician while you are in school. Be prepared for questions, be confident, and do not be afraid to tell them what you do not know. You are still learning, and they know that. Remember, do not assume anything. Table 2-15 provides some information that should be known when presenting cases to a physician.

TABLE 2-15	Must-know information before presenting cases to a physician
Must-Know Information before Presenting Cases	**Essentials**
Demographic findings	Age Gender Race
Clinical history	Symptoms Signs Laboratory findings Related previous surgeries Related previous imaging findings Family history (if relevant)
Sonographic findings	Abnormal findings Measurements Related normal findings

SUMMARY

This chapter provides some insight into the ideal character, personality, and EI of a sonographer. Also, we examined the responsibilities of the sonographer in the clinical setting. While providing compassionate patient care is vital, there is a point at which compassion can be trying, leading to compassion fatigue. The sonographer's obligation in the clinical setting is to provide compassionate patient care while simultaneously performing complicated sonographic examinations. From the research, it is evident that although the occupation of sonographer is challenging, it is also highly respected, and it can be a rewarding job both professionally and personally.

REFERENCES

1. *Quotation #23998 from Classic Quotes.* Accessed on December 28, 2014 from http://www.quotationspage.com/quote/23998.html

2. Haroun L. *Career Development for Health Professionals: Success in School & on the Job.* 3rd ed. Maryland Heights, MO: Saunders Elsevier; 2011.

3. Eley D, et al. Why did I become a nurse? Personality traits and reasons for entering nursing. *J Adv Nurs* [serial online] 2012;68(7):1546–1555. Available from: CINAHL with Full Text, Ipswich, MA. Accessed March 19, 2014.

4. Kroeger O, et al. *Type Talk at Work: How the 16 Personality Types Determine Your Success on the Job.* New York, NY: Dell Publishing; 2002.

5. Eley D, et al. Exploring temperament and character traits in medical students; a new approach to increase the rural workforce. *Med Teach* [serial online] 2009;31(3):e79–e84. Available from: MEDLINE, Ipswich, MA. Accessed March 19, 2014.

6. Tieger PD, Barron-Tieger B. *Do What You Are: Discover the Perfect Career for You Through the Secrets of Personality Type.* Boston, MA: Little, Brown and Company; 2001.

7. Nettle D. *Personality: What Makes You the Way You Are.* Oxford: Oxford University Press; 2007.

8. Collins S. Emotional intelligence as a noncognitive factor in student registered nurse anesthetists. *AANA J* [serial online] 2013;81(6):465–472. Available from: CINAHL with Full Text, Ipswich, MA. Accessed March 19, 2014.

9. Seema G. Emotional intelligence in classroom. *Adv Manage* 2012;5(10):16–23.

10. Satija S, Khan W. Emotional intelligence as predictor of occupational stress among working professionals. *Aweshkar Res J* [serial online] 2013;15(1):79–97. Available from: Business Source Complete, Ipswich, MA. Accessed March 20, 2014.

11. Kaplan RS. *What to Ask the Person in the Mirror: Critical Questions for Becoming a More Effective Leader and Reaching Your Potential*. Boston, MA: Harvard Business Review Press; 2011.

12. Cloud H. *Integrity: the Courage to Meet the Demands of Reality*. New York, NY: Harper Collins; 2006.

13. Chester E. *Reviving Work Ethic: a Leader's Guide to Ending Entitlements and Restoring Pride in the Emerging Workplace*. Austin, TX: Greenleaf Book Group Press; 2012.

14. Merriam-Webster online. *Character*. Accessed December 23, 2014 from: http://www.merriam-webster.com/dictionary/character.

15. Makely S. *Professionalism in Health Care*. 3rd ed. Upper Saddle River, NJ: Pearson Prentice Hall; 2009.

16. American Society of Echocardiography online. *Sonographer FAQs*. Accessed December 28, 2014 from http://www.asecho.org/sonographer-faqs/

17. JRCDMS online. *Commission on Accreditation of Allied Health Education Programs: Standards and Guidelines for the Accreditation of Allied Health Programs in Diagnostic Medical Sonography*. Accessed December 28, 2014 from http://www.caahep.org/documents/file/For-Program-Directors/DMSStandards.pdf

18. Colbert BJ. *Workplace Readiness for Health Professions*. 2nd ed. Clifton Park, NY: Delmar Cengage Learning; 2006.

19. McCorry LK, Mason J. *Communication Skills for the Healthcare Professional*. Baltimore, MD: Lippincott Williams & Wilkins; 2011.

20. Bennett WJ. *The Book of Virtues*. New York, NY: Simon and Schuster; 1993.

21. Severn M, et al. Occupational stress amongst audiologists: Compassion satisfaction, compassion fatigue, and burnout. *Int J Audiol* [serial online] 2012;51(1):3–9. Available from: CINAHL with Full Text, Ipswich, MA. Accessed March 20, 2014.

22. Potter P, et al. Evaluation of a compassion fatigue resiliency program for oncology nurses. *Oncol Nurs Forum* [serial online] 2013;40(2):180–187. Available from: CINAHL with Full Text, Ipswich, MA. Accessed March 20, 2014.

23. Thieleman K, Cacciatore J. Witness to suffering: mindfulness and compassion fatigue among traumatic bereavement volunteers and professionals. *Social Work* [serial online] 2014;59(1):34–41. Available from: CINAHL with Full Text, Ipswich, MA. Accessed March 20, 2014.

24. Zeidner M, et al. Personal factors related to compassion fatigue in health professionals. *Anxiety, Stress, And Coping* [serial online] 2013;26(6):595–609. Available from: MEDLINE, Ipswich, MA. Accessed March 20, 2014.

25. Tellie M. Compassion fatigue—the cost of caring. *Nursing Update* [serial online] 2008;32(8):34–37. Available from: CINAHL with Full Text, Ipswich, MA. Accessed March 20, 2014.

26. Society of Diagnostic Medical Sonography online. *SDMS Position Statement: Code of Ethics for the Profession of Diagnostic Medical Sonography*. Accessed December 28, 2014 from http://www.sdms.org/about/codeofethics.asp

27. Watson CE. *How Honesty Pays: Restoring Integrity to the Workplace*. Westport, CT: Praeger; 2005.

28. American Registry of Diagnostic Medical Sonography online. *Recertification General Information*. Accessed December 28, 2014 from http://www.ardms.org/registrant_resources/recertification_general_information/

29. Clifton DO, Nelson P. *Soar with Your Strengths: a Simple Yet Revolutionary Philosophy of Business and Management*. New York, NY: Bantam Books; 2010.

30. Commission on Accreditation of Allied Health Education Programs. *Diagnostic Medical Sonography*. Accessed December 28, 2014 from http://www.caahep.org/Content.aspx?ID=23

31. Penny SM & Zachariason A. The Sonographic Reasoning Method, JDMS, 31(2), March/April 2015.

32. Blume G. Focusing on the issues. When caring hurts: the silent burnout of sonographers. *J Diagn Med Sonogr* [serial online] 2002;18(6):418–421. Available from: CINAHL with Full Text, Ipswich, MA. Accessed March 20, 2014.

33. SDMS News Wave, January 2013. Retrieved from http://www.sdms.org/members/news/NewsWave/NW-January-2013.pdf

34. Daugherty J. Burnout: how sonographers and vascular technologists react to chronic stress. *J Diagn Med Sonogr* [serial online] 2002;18(5):305–312. Available from: CINAHL with Full Text, Ipswich, MA. Accessed March 20, 2014.

35. Wilczek-Ru yczka E. Empathy vs. professional burnout in health care professionals. *J US-China Med Sci* 2011;8(9):529–532.

36. Watson CE, Idinopulos TE. *Are You your Own Worst Enemy? The Nine Inner Strengths You Need to Overcome Self-defeating Tendencies at Work*. Westport, CT: Praeger; 2007.

Thinking Critically

1. Discuss with your family members the results of your personality tests to see if they agree regarding your findings.
2. Based on your personality tests, are there certain strengths that can be applied to patient care and to your chosen profession?
3. Now that you are aware that burnout could be a problem for you in the future, how do you plan on preparing for it?
4. Which of the diagrams in Figure 2-16 would most likely represent you after you have failed an exam?
5. Obtain the necessary information (clinical and sonographic findings) of an interesting sonography case from your clinical site, and complete the sonographic reasoning diagram in Figure 2-17.

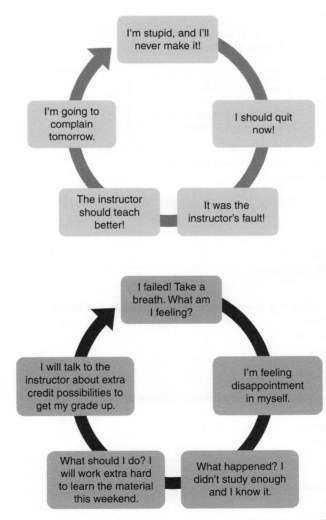

Figure 2-16. Varying responses to failing an anatomy exam. Which do you think demonstrates higher emotional intelligence?

Sonographic Reasoning Method Form

Requested Examination:
Age:
Gender:

Step in SRM	Explanation	Observations
*In*vestigate History	Investigate all pertinent clinical history (labs, imaging reports, patient complaints, etc.)	
*M*ake Hypotheses	Make educated guesses based on clinical history findings.	
*A*nalyze with Sonography	Perform the sonogram.	
*G*ather all Findings	Gather all sonographic findings for this case.	
*E*valuate for Connections	Compare clinical history with sonographic findings. Does a hypothesis correlate with imaging findings?	

1. Were you correct? (circle one) Yes   No
2. What did you learn?

Figure 2-17. Sonographic reasoning diagram.[31]

Chapter 2
Review Questions

1. **Which of the following is a valuable trait to have as a student?**
   a. Aggressiveness
   b. Overconfidence
   c. Assertiveness
   d. Arrogance

2. **Believing in yourself and your abilities defines the term**
   a. overconfidence.
   b. self-confidence.
   c. assertiveness.
   d. arrogance.

3. **What term is defined as to achieve for the sake of achieving?**
   a. Motivation
   b. Self-regulation
   c. Self-awareness
   d. Cognition

4. **Which of the following is the best definition for emotional intelligence?**
   a. The pleasure one gains from having the ability to help others and to make a difference in others' lives
   b. The courteous manner of offering well-reasoned positive and negative opinions about the work of others
   c. Demonstrating polite regard for others
   d. Having the ability to recognize the emotions of self and others and the capacity to use those emotions in the decision-making process

5. **Which of the following is not a reason why one should identify his or her personality type?**
   a. To make appropriate personality changes based on circumstances
   b. To be prepared for the interview process for a new job
   c. To recognize and utilize one's strengths better
   d. To recognize one's weaknesses

6. **Which of the following is defined as the pleasure one gains from being able to help others?**
   a. Compassion
   b. Compassion fatigue
   c. Compassion satisfaction
   d. Emotional intelligence

7. **The form of reasoning by which one makes an educated guess based on facts describes**
   a. cognitive reasoning.
   b. inductive reasoning.
   c. deductive reasoning.
   d. hypothetical reasoning.

8. **Which of the following is described as an educated guess based on clinical history findings?**
   a. Deductive reasoning
   b. Inductive reasoning
   c. Clinical hypothesis
   d. Clinical correlation ambiguity

9. **Fortitude is best described as**
   a. the strength of mind that allows someone to face difficult circumstances.
   b. a trait that demonstrates one's understanding of the feelings of others.
   c. something that one holds in high regards.
   d. demonstrating polite behavior and empathy.

10. **What sonographic term means without echoes?**
    a. Echogenic
    b. Hyperechoic
    c. Anechoic
    d. Hypoechoic

11. **What sonographic term means having few echoes?**
    a. Echogenic
    b. Hyperechoic
    c. Anechoic
    d. Hypoechoic

12. **What term describes a work-related condition in which one experiences physical and emotional exhaustion?**
    a. Chronic harshness syndrome
    b. Occupational stress
    c. Doubt syndrome
    d. Burnout

13. **Which of the following is the correct sequence of the sonographic reasoning process?**
    a. Sonographic findings, investigative imaging, clinical correlation, clinical history, clinical hypothesis
    b. Clinical history, clinical hypothesis, investigative imaging, sonographic findings, clinical correlation
    c. Clinical hypothesis, sonographic findings, clinical history, investigative imaging, clinical correlation
    d. Investigative imaging, sonographic findings, clinical history, clinical correlation, clinical hypothesis

14. **Which of the following is not provided on a sonographer's report?**
    a. Echogenicity of organs
    b. Appearance of abnormalities
    c. Measurement of normal and abnormal structures
    d. At least three differential diagnoses

15. **Which of the following would be least likely to disrupt your working relationship with a sonographer?**
    a. Constantly talking during an examination
    b. Getting personal
    c. Being chronically early
    d. Bringing a magazine to read during an extended vascular examination of a transplanted liver

16. **Which of the following would be the least helpful technique for acquiring extra scan time?**
    a. Being erratic with protocol images needed for an examination
    b. Making a list of daily tasks to accomplish
    c. Examining the schedule and making a list of tasks to accomplish
    d. Being assertive but not aggressive when asking to scan

17. **Which of the following questions would be a *routine* question that would not be asked before one started scanning a patient?**
    a. Do you have cancer?
    b. What are your symptoms?
    c. Have you had a sonogram before?
    d. What other tests have you had for this condition?

18. **Which of the following terms means having the same echogenicity?**
    a. Echogenic
    b. Isoechoic
    c. Hyperechoic
    d. Anechoic

19. **Which of the following is described as a set of values based on hard work and diligence?**
    a. Typewatching
    b. Cognition
    c. Thoroughness
    d. Work ethic

20. **Which of the following is not considered one of the first-rate standards in sonography?**
    a. Setting a good example for others
    b. Holding yourself to the same standards you expect of others
    c. Playing by your own rules
    d. Knowing your limitations

Historical and Current Applications of Ultrasound in Medicine

CHAPTER OBJECTIVES

- Explore the study of sound and the history of acoustics.
- Develop an appreciation for those individuals who made contributions to the study of sound.
- Provide an overview of the use of ultrasound in medicine.
- Analyze the specialties within the sonography profession.
- Offer some information regarding current and future applications of ultrasound in medicine.

KEY TERMS

Abdominal sonography – the medical use of ultrasound to analyze the abdomen, small parts, and other structures

Acoustic enhancement – useful ultrasound artifact that occurs when sound travels through a weakly attenuating structure like fluid resulting in an area of increased brightness distal to the weak attenuator

Acoustic radiation force impulse elastography – common form of elastography in which the ultrasound probe provides realtime B-mode imaging and focused pressure using shear waves to compress the tissue of concern

Acoustics – the study of sound

Adnexa – bilateral regions within the female pelvis adjacent to the uterus that contain the ovaries, fallopian tubes, and other structures

Amaurosis fugax – the temporary loss of vision in one eye due to a momentary lack of blood flow to the retina, which could indicate an impending stroke

Amenorrhea – lack of menstrual flow

American College of Radiology – the principal organization of radiologists, radiation oncologists, and clinical medical physicists in the United States that aims to serve patients and society by empowering members to advance the practice, science, and professions of radiologic care and also provides accreditation for many imaging modalities including ultrasound

American Institute of Ultrasound in Medicine – a medical association composed of physicians, sonographers, scientists, students, and other healthcare providers that is dedicated to advancing the safe and effective use of ultrasound in medicine through professional and public education, research, development of guidelines, and accreditation

A-mode – amplitude mode ultrasound display in which the depth of the returning echo is represented on the x-axis while the strength (amplitude) of the reflector is represented along the y-axis

Anechoic – echo-free or without echoes

Aneuploidy – having an abnormal number of whole chromosomes (e.g., trisomy 21, trisomy 18)

Arrhythmia – irregular heartbeat or rhythm

Arthritis – the inflammation of a joint

Ascites – abdominal fluid

Assisted reproductive therapy – artificial methods used to create a pregnancy

Ataxia – lack of muscle coordination that can result in the inability to perform routine voluntary movements like talking, walking, eye control, and swallowing

Atrial fibrillation – a quivering, irregular heartbeat that can lead to stroke and other heart-related complications

Automated biometry – software utilized by the ultrasound machine that automatically obtains biometric measurements of the fetus

Automated breast ultrasound – a computer system that mechanically steers the transducer and obtains sonographic images of the entire breast, ultimately reconstructing those images into 3D representations for interpretation

B-mode – brightness mode ultrasound display in which a dot with varying degrees of brightness is used on the screen; the stronger the returning echo, the brighter the dot; also referred to as grayscale sonography

Body habitus – body type

Breast Imaging Reporting and Data System – a scoring method of breast masses based on imaging characteristics including the size, shape, orientation, margin, echogenicity, lesion boundary, attenuation, special cases, vascularity, and surrounding tissue and can be applicable to sonography, mammography, and MRI of the breast

Breast sonography – sonographic specialty that includes female and male breast sonography

Cardiac sonographer – an echocardiographer who uses ultrasound to create images of the heart and surrounding structures

Cardiomyopathy – any disease of the musculature or the myocardium of the heart

Cardioversion – a procedure in which electricity is used to reorder the rhythm of the heart back to a normal pattern

Chromosomal anomaly – any alteration in the normal structure or number of chromosomes

Color Doppler imaging – doppler shift information presented as a color or hue superimposed over a grayscale image

Computer-aided diagnosis system – provides a computer analysis of diagnostic images often used in mammography

Congenital anomalies – an anomaly (defect) with which someone is born

Congestive heart failure – a condition caused by the inability of the heart to pump blood adequately throughout the body thus leading to a lack of blood supply and oxygen to vital tissues

Continuous-wave Doppler – a Doppler device that utilizes two elements—one element that continuously sends ultrasound waves into the body and another element to continuously listen for the returning signal

Contrast agents – substances ingested, injected, or in some way instilled into the body to improve visibility of specific organs, structures, or pathology

Contrast-enhanced ultrasound – the use of contrast agents in medical ultrasound

Coupling gel – a substance that is used to allow the transmission of sound into the body; also referred to as ultrasound gel

Crystal deposition disease – the accumulation of crystals of calcium pyrophosphate dihydrate in the connective tissues; also referred to as chondrocalcinosis

Cyanosis – the bluish discoloration of the skin because of decreased oxygen

Decubitus – lying down

Deep vein thrombosis – a blood clot (thrombus) in a deep vein, typically in the legs

Direct testing – a diagnostic test performed with direct visualization of the structures being examined

Doppler effect – theory that states that a frequency shift is created when sound impinges upon a moving object

Duplex imaging – the simultaneous viewing of a structure in B-mode while sampling assessment of the vessel occurs with pulsed-wave Doppler

Dysmenorrhea – painful menses

Echocardiogram – a sonogram of the heart

Echocardiographer – one who uses ultrasound to create images of the heart and surrounding structures; also referred to as a cardiac sonographer

Echocardiography – the medical use of ultrasound to examine the heart and surrounding structures

Ectopic pregnancy – a pregnancy located anywhere other than within the fundal portion of the endometrium of the uterus

Elastogram – the study that contains the images obtained with elastography

Elastography – a sonographic technique employed to evaluate a mass based on its stiffness, ultimately providing a prediction as to if the mass is more likely malignant or benign

Electrocardiogram – a non-invasive test that checks for abnormalities with the electrical activity of your heart

Endorectal transducer – an ultrasound transducer that is inserted into the rectum for the analysis of the prostate and other pelvic organs and structures

Endoscope – a camera device inserted into the body that is used to visually evaluate body cavities or organs

Endoscopic ultrasound – the use of an ultrasound transducer that is attached to an endoscope, which allows for the viewing of internal anatomy

Endovaginal sonography – technique used in gynecologic sonography in which an ultrasound transducer is inserted into the vagina for improved visualization of pelvic organs and structures; also referred to as transvaginal sonography

Ergonomics – the scientific study of creating tools and equipment that help the human adapt to the work environment

Exercise stress echocardiogram – a test that combines an exercise stress test, typically by using a treadmill, with an echocardiogram

Fetal echocardiography – the use of ultrasound to analyze the fetal heart for the diagnosis of fetal heart defects

Fetal hydrops – the excessive accumulation of fluid within at least two or more fetal body cavities

Fetal karyotyping – an analysis of fetal chromosomes

First trimester – gestational weeks 1 through 12

Focused assessment with sonography for trauma (FAST) – is a rapid ultrasound study performed in the emergency room, typically by an emergency room physician, which is used to determine if there is evidence of intra-abdominal trauma

Foley catheter – a urinary catheter placed into the bladder to assist in voiding

Four-dimensional ultrasound – the use of realtime imaging in three dimensions

Fremitus – a technique used in breast imaging in which the sonographer has the patient hum to evaluate the stiffness of a breast mass

Fusion imaging – a technique whereby the high-quality images and specific strengths of different imaging modalities can be overlain and exploited (e.g., the combination of images acquired with sonography and magnetic resonance imaging); also referred to as hybrid imaging

Graded compression – a technique used during realtime imaging of the bowel whereby the abdomen is gradually compressed by the transducer and then released with the hopes of differentiating normal, compressible bowel from abnormal bowel

Gravid – pregnant

Grayscale sonography – see B-mode

Gynecologic sonography – the medical use of ultrasound to analyze the non-gravid female patient

Hemi-paralysis – paralysis occurring in only one side of the body

High-intensity focused ultrasound – a non-invasive surgical method that uses ultrasound to perform tissue ablation (destruction)

Hybrid imaging – see fusion imaging

Hydrophone – an instrument based on the piezoelectric transducer that was designed to be used underwater for recording or listening to underwater sound

Hyperechoic – displayed echoes that are relatively brighter than surrounding tissue and may also be referred to as echogenic

Hypoechoic – displayed echoes that are relatively darker than surrounding tissue

Hypoxic – a decrease in oxygen

Incontinence – lacking the ability to control urination

Indirect testing – a diagnostic test in which an analysis of one part of the body is performed in order to obtain information about another area of suspected disease in the body

Intercostal – between the ribs

Intraoperative sonography – the medical use of ultrasound within the operating room

Intrauterine pregnancy – a pregnancy located within the fundal portion of the endometrium, the optimal location of a pregnancy

Intravascular ultrasound – the medical use of ultrasound that employs a miniature ultrasound probe placed on a catheter and inserted into the circulatory system

Invasive procedures – procedures that include an imaging modality to treat disease and typically involve the use of catheters, needles, and surgical asepsis techniques (sterile techniques)

Ipsilateral – the same side of the body

Ischemic – a decrease in blood supply to part of the body

Joint effusion – the pathologic buildup of fluid within a joint

Keepsake imaging – non-diagnostic sonography performed to provide the obstetric patient with keepsake photos and videos of the fetus

Lead zirconate titanate – the element or crystal found within the face of the transducer that is used to create ultrasound waves

Maternal – mother

Medium – a solid, liquid, or gas

Menometrorrhagia – excessive irregular bleeding

Menorrhagia – abnormal heavy and prolonged menstruation

Metrorrhagia – irregular menstrual bleeding between periods

Miniaturization – the process of making technology smaller and more lightweight

M-mode – motion mode that captures the movement of structures along a single scan line represented over time, with depth along the y-axis and time along the x-axis

Murmur – an abnormal sound heard during a heartbeat

Musculoskeletal sonography – the medical use of ultrasound to analyze the musculoskeletal system

Myocardial infarction – death of the muscle tissue of the heart secondary to a lack of blood supply; also referred to as a heart attack

Neurosonography – the medical use of ultrasound to analyze the nervous system, including the neonatal brain and spine

Non-gravid – not pregnant

Nothing by mouth – NPO or nothing to eat or drink

Nuchal translucency – an anechoic space along the posterior aspect of the fetal neck that can be measured with sonography; increased thickness has been linked with multiple fetal anomalies

Obstetric sonography – the medical use of ultrasound to analyze the fetus and its environment

Ophthalmic ultrasound – the medical use of ultrasound in ophthalmology

Pebble theory – theory recognized by Boethius in which he hypothesized that sound waves travel in a manner equivalent to what is observed when waves are created by dropping a pebble into water

Pediatric echocardiography – the medical use of ultrasound to analyze the pediatric heart and surrounding structures

Pedoff probe – a continuous-wave non-imaging transducer

Pericardial (pericardium) – small space located between the visceral and parietal coverings around the heart

Pericardial tamponade – a serious medical condition resulting in heart dysfunction caused by an increase in pressure as a result of the excessive accumulation of blood or fluids around the heart

Pericarditis – inflammation of the pericardium

Pharmacologic stress echocardiogram – a test that combines an echocardigram and the use of a drug to artificially stress the heart; replaces the exercise stress echocardiogram when a patient is unable to perform physical exercise

Photoplethysmography – a non-invasive test that uses infrared sensors to detect skin color changes that occur with each heartbeat

Piezoelectric effect – the process whereby a material, such as a crystal or element within an ultrasound transducer, generates electricity and changes shape when pressure is applied to it

Piezoelectric materials – a material, such as lead zirconate titanate, that has piezoelectric properties

Plethysmography – a lung test that is performed to see how much air the lungs can hold; also known as a pulmonary function test

Polyps – abnormal growths of tissue that project from the mucous membrane and can be benign or malignant or have variable malignant potential

Power Doppler – amplitude mode of Doppler where it is not the shift itself that provides the signal but rather the strength (amplitude) of the shift

Probe cover – a device used to cover the ultrasound transducer and may be latex or non-latex and sterile or non-sterile

Propagate – to transmit

Pulmonary hypertension – an increase in blood pressure in the blood vessels of the lungs

Pulsed-wave Doppler – doppler technique that uses pulses of sound to obtain Doppler signals from a user-specified depth

Radiofrequency ablation – a procedure that utilizes radio waves or electric current to generate sufficient heat to interrupt nerve conduction on a semi-permanent basis

Radioiodine ablation – a treatment used for hyperthyroidism or thyroid cancer in which a radioactive isotope is administered orally in order to gradually shrink the thyroid gland

Realtime scanners – ultrasound imaging technique that allows continual imaging of the body as if one were watching a movie

Reflectoscope – an instrument that uses ultrasound to detect flaws in metals

Saline infusion sonohysterography – an invasive procedure that utilizes the installation of saline into the uterine cavity and/or the fallopian tubes to assess these areas for pathology; may also be referred to simply as sonohysterography

Second trimester – gestational weeks 13 through 26

Sequela – a pathologic condition resulting from a disease, injury, therapy, or other trauma

Small parts – aspect of abdominal sonographic imaging that includes the breast, thyroid gland, male pelvis, and genitalia, and other superficial structures

Sonohysterography – see saline infusion sonohysterography

Sound – a traveling variation in pressure and a form of energy that is produced when a vibrating source causes molecules within a medium to move back and forth

Spectral analysis – the quantitative analysis method used to display the distribution of frequencies whereby Doppler shift frequencies are presented in frequency order

Spectral waveform – the visual display or graph of the way the pressure changes between the wave fronts during spectral analysis; may be referred to as the spectral display

Spinal dysraphism – a spectrum of congenital spinal defects including various forms of spina bifida

Stand-off device – a manufactured aqueous gel pad, a large amount of gel, or a bag of saline that is used to provide some distance between the transducer and the skin surface, thereby typically allowing superficial structures to be imaged more clearly

Stress echocardiogram – a sonogram that employs either exercise or a pharmacologic agent to increase heart rate in order to assess how the heart functions with exertion

Stroke – the loss of brain function as a result of the lack of blood supply to that region; may also be referred to as a cerebrovascular accident

Subluxation – the incomplete dislocation of a joint

Synechiae – an adhesion resulting in an abnormal bond between two structures

Synovitis – inflammation of the synovial membrane

Teratogen – any substance or mechanism that causes a fetal malformation

Third trimester – gestational weeks 27 through 42

Therapeutic ultrasound – medical treatment used to increase the blood supply to certain areas in the body by heating the tissue, which in turn reduces healing time and provides for a quicker recovery following soft tissue damage

Three-dimensional ultrasound – ultrasound imaging mode that allows the viewer to see width, height, and depth; also referred to as volume scanning

Thromboembolism – the formation of a blood clot within a blood vessel that dislodges and is carried by the bloodstream to obstruct another blood vessel

Tissue harmonic imaging – ultrasound technique that utilizes additional frequencies (harmonics) other than the transmitted frequency sent into the body in order to create a crisper, higher-resolution image

Transabdominal approach – sonographic scanning approach utilizing the surface of the abdomen

Transesophageal echocardiogram – sonogram that requires the insertion of an ultrasound transducer on the end of an endoscope into the esophagus in order to acquire image of the heart

Transthoracic echocardiogram – an echocardiogram acquired through the chest

Transvaginal sonography – see endovaginal sonography

Triplex imaging – the combination of B-mode, spectral, and color Doppler information on the screen at the same time

Ultrasound elastography – see elastography

Ultrasound-guided brachytherapy – an invasive procedure that utilizes sonographic guidance to administer radioactive material close to or within a cancerous tumor for treatment

Uterine myomas – benign solid tumors of the uterus; also referred to as fibroids and uterine leiomyomas

Vacuum-assisted breast biopsy – a tissue sampling technique that uses specialized equipment and imaging guidance to remove samples of breast tissue with a vacuum through a single, small skin incision

Vascular sonographer – one who uses ultrasound to create images of vascular structures within the body

Vascular sonography – the medical use of ultrasound to analyze the circulatory system

Vasoconstriction – the narrowing of the blood vessels by the contraction of the muscles within their walls

Volumetric imaging – the use of an offline work station to do post-processing of acquired volumes

Wireless transducer – an ultrasound transducer that is not directly connected to the ultrasound machine by a wire but rather utilizes wireless technology to relay sonographic data to the machine

INTRODUCTION

As we discovered in Chapter 1, sonography is a profession that includes sonographers, physicians, and, now, you. But in order to gain a fundamental understanding of sonography, we must both look to the past at our profession's modest beginnings and look forward into the possibilities provided by an evolving healthcare system, which will illustrate how this outstanding screening modality has become a permanent diagnostic instrument used by providers all over the world. This chapter will offer a brief history of acoustics and list those individuals who advanced the theories of sound, ultimately guiding our profession toward marvelous diagnostic capabilities and vast medical applications. Concurrently, this chapter will also provide the sonography student with an overview of the various specialties within the sonography profession.

THE STUDY OF SOUND

Technically, **sound** has been defined as a form of energy that is produced when a vibrating source causes molecules within a **medium** to move back and forth. The back and forth motion of the molecules create waves of sound energy that are allowed to travel, or **propagate**, through the medium. Sound must have a medium—solid, liquid, or gas—through which to travel. It cannot travel in a vacuum. Since sound always requires a medium through which to travel, and the human body is certainly an ensemble of different mediums, it is allowed to propagate through the human body. In fact, the average speed through which sound travels in the soft tissue of the body is 1,540 meters per second (m/s) or 1.54 millimeters per microsecond (mm/μs).

The scientific study of sound is referred to as **acoustics**. The Franciscan friar Marin Mersenne was the first to measure the velocity of sound and has since been referred to as the "father of acoustics."[1] However, long before the time of Mersenne, the recognized study of sound perhaps began around the time of Pythagoras in the 6th century, as he has often been referred to as the "father of music" and the "father of harmony."[2] Pythagoras once noted, "there is geometry in the humming of the strings, there is music in the spacing of the spheres."[3]

Sound Off

Acoustics is the scientific study of sound.

There were several other well-known individuals, many of them better acknowledged for other ventures, who provided supporting concepts and theories concerning sound, such as Aristotle, Boethius, Leonardo da Vinci, and Galileo. Among this list, the most notable are Boethius and da Vinci. Boethius identified the **pebble theory**, which he recognized by dropping a pebble into water. He imagined that sound waves traveled in a similar manner to the waves that were produced by the pebble dropping into the water.[4] Da Vinci also assumed that sound traveled in waves and is credited as the person who identified that the angle of reflection equaled the angle of incidence.[4]

Robert Boyle was a physicist who, in the 1600s, recognized that in order for sound to propagate, there must be a medium through which the sound could travel.[1] His research indeed laid the groundwork for the use of **coupling gel** during all diagnostic sonographic procedures today. Coupling gel, often simply referred to as ultrasound gel, provides a means whereby the sound emitted by the transducer can be sent through the body.

Though acoustics includes medical applications, like the use of ultrasound to create an image, it also includes the study of how animals utilize sound, architectural acoustics, musical acoustics, and more.[5] In fact, as many of us learned in elementary school, animals like the bat and dolphin utilize sound to both communicate with each other and search for prey. In the 1700s, Abbe Lazzaro Spallanzani, often credited as the "father of ultrasound," studied how bats utilized sound waves to detect their victims and to guide their flight.[1] By recalling this fundamental information, we can actually recognize how the ultrasound transducer utilizes the pulse-echo technique (discussed in Chapter 1), the fundamental basis whereby an image within the human body is created with sound and displayed on the monitor.

Sound Off

A bat uses the pulse-echo technique to identify its prey and guide its flight.

Christian Johann Doppler discovered that the pitch of a sound wave varies if the source of the sound was moving, a principle referred to as the **Doppler effect**.[1] Doppler recognized that a frequency shift or change is created when sound impinges upon a moving object, like the moving blood cells within an artery or vein (Fig. 3-1).[1] Radar detectors, meteorologists who predict the weather, and even burglar alarms use the Doppler effect.[6]

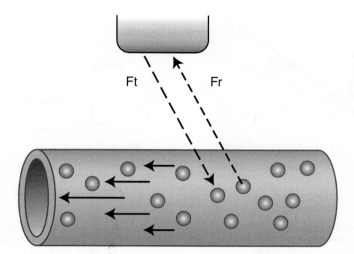

Figure 3-1. Doppler frequency shift. The transmitted Doppler sound beam (*Ft*) encounters red blood cells (RBCs) moving toward the transducer within the blood vessel. The RBC motion causes an increase in frequency of the returning echo (*Fr*) due to the Doppler effect. The ultrasound instruments detect and measure the frequency of the returning Doppler signal, confirming the presence of blood flow and the direction in which the blood is traveling.

Sound Off

The Doppler effect states that a frequency shift is created when sound impinges upon a moving object.

But to initially appreciate just how an image is created on our monitors, one must appreciate the principle of piezoelectricity. The Currie brothers, Pierre and Jacques, are credited with recognizing the **piezoelectric effect**, or the principle of piezoelectricity.[1] This is the process whereby a material, such as a crystal or element within an ultrasound transducer, generates electricity and changes shape when pressure is applied to it (Fig. 3-2). These crystals within the ultrasound transducer are referred to as **piezoelectric materials** and are most likely some derivative of **lead zirconate titanate**. It is these crystals that ultimately produce ultrasound waves that are utilized for diagnostic purposes. The piezoelectric effect formed the foundation from which the ultrasound uses in medicine originated.

Sound Off

The principle of piezoelectricity states that a material, such as a crystal or element within an ultrasound transducer, generates electricity and changes shape when pressure is applied to it.

ULTRASOUND IN MEDICINE

During World War I, with research developed by L.F. Richardson, Paul Langevin used ultrasound to detect submarines with the **hydrophone**, ultimately leading to the development of SONAR—sound navigation and ranging.[1] The sonar technology utilized sound that was sent through the water, bounced off of an object, and then returned to the source. The object's location was then displayed on a monitor. Between 1929 and 1942, with research developed by Sergei Sokolov, Floyd Firestone worked to utilize the **reflectoscope**, an instrument that used ultrasound to detect flaws in metals.[1,4] It was Firestone's flawed technique that ultimately was used first in medicine.[1,4]

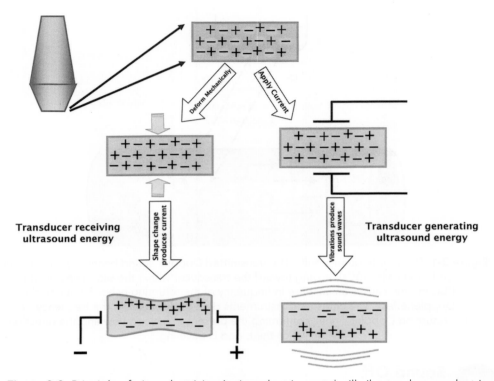

Figure 3-2. Principle of piezoelectricity. A piezoelectric crystal will vibrate when an electric current is applied to it, resulting in the generation and transmission of ultrasound energy. On the other hand, when reflected energy encounters a piezoelectric crystal, the crystal will change shape and produce an electrical impulse.

When researchers first began to apply ultrasound for medical purposes, they understood that ultrasound could be transmitted through the human body. In fact, the first application of ultrasound for medical diagnosis was in 1941, when Karl Dussik used the technology to image the lateral ventricles in the brain.[1] Furthermore, in 1950, W.D. Keidel, a German physiologist, used transmitted ultrasound to examine the heart on the other side of the body, using an additional transducer as a receiver.[1] As the research progressed, the pioneers began to recognize that not only ultrasound waves could be transmitted through the body but that these ultrasound waves returned to the transducer, and therefore, they postulated that an image could be acquired from those returning waves. Consequently, the beginnings of pulse-echo technique were established.

The pulse-echo technique sought to exploit the reflected sound back from within the body to create an image. Essentially, with the pulse-echo technique, the sound must be pulsed or allowed to be alternated rapidly on and then off so the transducer has time to listen for the returning echo. First, the ceramic crystal within the transducer is electronically stimulated, creating a pulse of sound, which is sent into the body. Secondly, the sound wave travels into the body, interacts with a structure, and then returns to the transducer. Lastly, the machine listens for the returning echo. When the transducer hears the echo, the machine calculates the distance from the reflector based on the time it took to return to the transducer and promptly presents the reflector's location on the monitor.[7]

The first effort to utilize pulse-echo ultrasound was in the late 1940s and early 1950s. Douglass Howry, John Wild, and George Ludwig, who was the first to demonstrate reflections from a gallstone, worked to utilize the piezoelectric effect and the pulse-echo technique.[4] Taking advantage of the earlier work and the postulations of Firestone and his associates, Carl Helmut Hertz, a Swedish physicist, and Inge Edler, a Swedish cardiologist, managed to borrow a sonar device from a local shipyard,

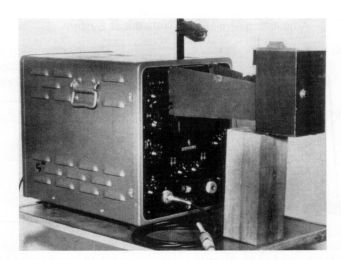

Figure 3-3. Edler and Hertz used an ultrasonoscope, seen here, to record their early echocardiograms.

tailored it, and recorded the first echoes from Hertz's own heart (Fig. 3-3).[8] Though the two worked collaboratively to develop clinical echocardiography, Edler is considered the "father of echocardiography."[8] In the 1960s, Dr. Harvey Feigenbaum and others worked diligently to advance echocardiography, publishing articles and proving the usefulness of this developing imaging instrument. One author noted that the discovery of echocardiography is among the 10 greatest discoveries of the 20th century.[8]

In order to further advance the medical use of ultrasound, research led the pioneers to develop varying working models of ultrasound systems, including the B-52 gun turret tank, which used a transducer that rotated around the patient who was partially submerged in water, the water bath scanner, and the articulated arm scanner (Figs. 3-4 and 3-5).

Sound Off

Echocardiography has been noted among the 10 greatest discoveries of the 20th century.

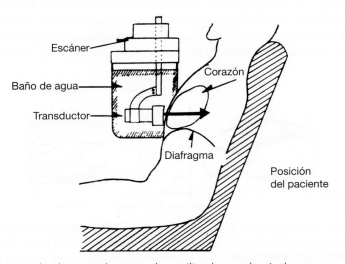

Figure 3-4. An early ultrasound system that utilized a mechanical sector scanner, with a transducer submerged in a water bath, to obtain images of the heart.

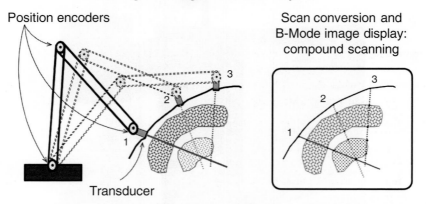

Figure 3-5. Articulating arm B-mode scanning produced an acoustic tomographic image slice of the body. This type of early ultrasound scanning, termed compounding, was performed manually, which required the building of an image over several seconds to ensure that the ultrasound beam was perpendicular to the boundary at some point during the scan.

Imaging Modes and Doppler

There have been many advances for the medical use of ultrasound since its inception, most of which ultimately lie beyond the necessary scope of understanding required for the novice student. However, it is important to have an appreciation of where our modality originated and also the sacrifices and insight of those who managed to develop our profession into what it is today. Consequently, the following section will provide some brief insight into imaging modes, their origins, the uses of Doppler, and several noteworthy pioneers.

Display Options

There are several display options used in sonography (Fig. 3-6). Beginning in the 1950s and 1960s, **A-mode**, or amplitude mode, was one of the earliest methods of displaying the returning echo for medical uses. With A-mode, the depth of the returning echo was represented on the x-axis while the strength (amplitude) of the reflector was represented along the y-axis. A pulse of sound was sent out to create one scan line of information. Thus, this line was interpreted to represent both the depth and amplitude of the reflector.[7] Essentially, A-mode examines the range, location, and amplitude of ultrasound signals.[8] A-mode is utilized in echocardiography and **ophthalmic ultrasound**. For example, in ophthalmology, A-mode is often used prior to cataract surgery for biometric assessment.[9]

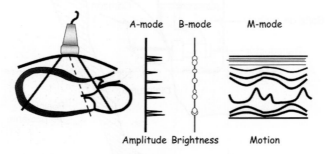

Figure 3-6. Several sonographic display options. **From left to right:** A transducer is placed on the chest, and the ultrasound beam is directed through the heart. The returning ultrasound echoes can be displayed in amplitude mode (A-mode) in which the amplitude of the spikes corresponds to the strength of the returning echo. Brightness mode (B-mode) demonstrates the strength of the echoes at various depths by depicting them as dots of varying brightnesses. Motion mode (M-mode) plots the B-mode display against time.

B-mode, or brightness mode, displays the returning ultrasound signal as a dot on the monitor. In 1951, Douglas Howry, William Roderic Bliss, and Gerald J. Posakony developed the first two-dimensional (2D) B-mode compound scanner called the immersion tank ultrasound system.[4] With B-mode, the dot displayed on the screen has varying degrees of brightness, based on the strength of the returning echo. Thus, the stronger the returning echo, the brighter the dot displays on the monitor. The brightest dots will appear almost white—**hyperechoic**. The mid-shade echoes appear more gray—**hypoechoic**—while those without any echoes, **anechoic**, appear black. This is why B-mode may also be referred to as **grayscale sonography**; and currently, several display options are available and may be chosen by the sonographer (Fig. 3-7).[7]

Joan Baker was one of the first non-physicians allowed to use the early B-scans in 1969.[8] Furthermore, Baker went on to help found the American Society of Ultrasound Technical Specialist, which would later be known as the Society of Diagnostic Medical Sonography (SDMS).[8] In the hopes of reducing repetitive strain injuries in the sonography profession, she is currently a strong advocate for the use of proper ergonomics.[10]

M-mode, or motion mode, documents the movement of structures within the body. Recall it was Dr. Helmut Hertz and Inge Edler, in 1954, who described the first M-mode technology (Fig. 3-8).[4] With motion mode, the movement of structures along a single scan line is documented.[7] Thus, the single scan line is represented over time, with depth along the y-axis and time along the x-axis.[7]

B-Mode (Grayscale) Image Display Options

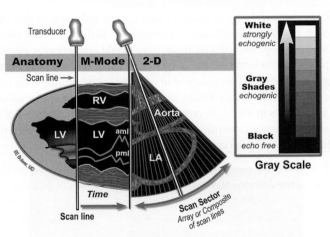

Parasternal Long-Axis Views

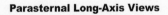

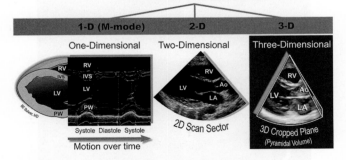

Figure 3-7. B-mode or grayscale display options. **Upper panel, from left to right:** Imaging of cardiac anatomy can be optionally displayed as M-mode or as a 2D image. Both M-mode and 2D are image display options that are based on grayscale or brightness modulation (B-mode). **Lower panel, from left to right:** The amplitudes of the received echoes can be processed into B-mode data that can be displayed using M-mode, 2D (cross-sectional anatomy), or 3D formats.

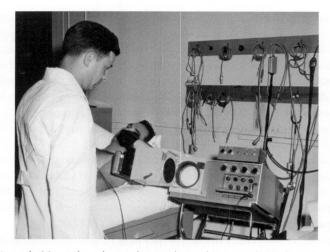

Figure 3-8. This early M-mode echocardiograph machine used a Polaroid camera to record images of the heart.

M-mode is utilized in obstetrics to demonstrate fetal heart rate (Fig. 3-9). It is also utilized in echocardiography as a critical part of standard protocols. For example, M-mode is used to demonstrate the myocardial wall thickness during both systole and diastole.[7]

The original ultrasound machines or scanners were considered static, in that they provided still-frame images. Though the systems' resolution was improving in the 1950s and 1960s, the researchers decided to push the technology toward a technique that would revolutionize medical imaging. They sought to allow an operator to visualize the human body using **realtime scanners**, much like fluoroscopy in radiography. Essentially, they wanted to use ultrasound to image the body as if one were watching a movie. Developed by Walter Krause and Richard Soldner, realtime sonography started to be manufactured by Siemens in 1965.[4] To create realtime sonography, an array of detectors is used. Realtime equipment is what we currently use in diagnostic sonography. From that point on, the ultrasound machine and the transducer technology have expanded immensely.

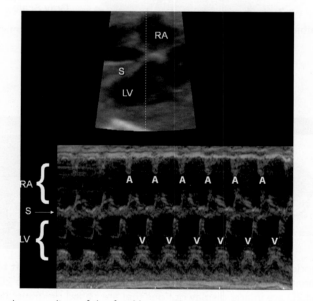

Figure 3-9. M-mode recording of the fetal heart. The M-mode cursor line intersects the right atrium (*RA*), the interventricular septum (*S*), and the left ventricle (*LV*). The M-mode recording shows the atrial contractions (*A*) and the corresponding ventricular contractions (*V*).

Sound Off

Realtime equipment is what we currently use in diagnostic sonography.

Doppler Technology

As mentioned earlier, Doppler recognized the frequency shift resulting from moving objects. Researchers such as Shigeo Satomura and Yasuhara Nimura from Japan studied Doppler principle application for vascular assessment.[4] Other researchers from Japan described Doppler instrumentation relative to direction of flow within vessels.[4] It was Robert Rushmer and his colleagues that established the varying uses of both **continuous-wave** (CW) **Doppler** and **spectral analysis** in 1963.[4]

CW transducers, which may also be referred to as **Pedoff probes**, utilize two elements—one element that continuously sends ultrasound waves into the body and another element to continuously listen for the returning signal (Fig. 3-10). A CW transducer does not pause and listen to the returning echo as does a pulsed-wave (PW) transducer, and they are not capable of depth discrimination or producing a 2D image (Figs. 3-11 and 3-12).[7] For this reason, sampling of a specific blood vessel among many blood vessels can be challenging, simply because there is no image provided and one cannot select the depth. However, CW transducers do provide a **spectral waveform** and are capable of measuring high velocities accurately. A spectral waveform provides the time, velocity, frequency shift, flow direction, and amplitude of the returning signal from within the blood vessel. CW technology is still used today in both vascular and echocardiography. In fact, both PW technology and CW technology can be housed in a single transducer.

Pulsed-wave Doppler was initially introduced in 1970 by Donald Baker.[4] Baker and his colleagues worked to further develop the use of a handheld duplex pulsed Doppler system, or **duplex imaging**, which allowed for the simultaneous viewing of a structure in B-mode while sampling assessment of the vessel occurred (Fig. 3-13).[4,7] In the 1970s, great advancements of **color Doppler imaging** and instrumentation propelled the use of ultrasound technology into numerous medical specialties that needed an effective tool that could successfully analyze the vascular and tissue characterization of disease processes.[4] Color Doppler imaging is a colorization of the Doppler shift information superimposed on the grayscale image, providing both direction and mean velocity information about the flow (Fig. 3-14).[7] While duplex imaging utilizes both B-mode and pulsed-wave Doppler, **triplex imaging** is the combination of B-mode, spectral, and color Doppler information on the screen

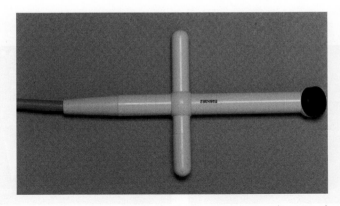

Figure 3-10. A Pedoff continuous-wave Doppler transducer. The transducer contains two elements: one for transmitting and one for receiving. These transducers are not used for imaging.

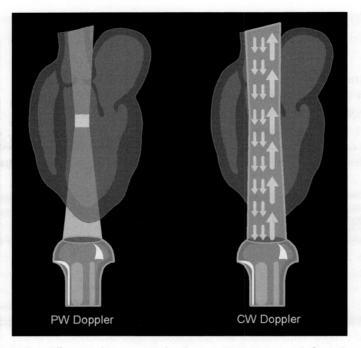

Figure 3-11. The difference between pulsed-wave (PW) Doppler (*left*) and continuous-wave (CW) Doppler (*right*). CW Doppler uses a constant ultrasound beam (*large arrows*) and continuously senses the reflected ultrasound energy (*small arrows*). PW Doppler intermittently transmits the ultrasound beam in pulses and detects the reflected energy between those pulses. With PW Doppler, the ultrasound system can focus on the reflections occurring within a single area of interest at a specified distance from the transducer.

at the same time (Fig. 3-15).[7] Lastly, **power Doppler**, also referred to as color Doppler energy or power angio, provides information about the amplitude of the returning signals only (Fig. 3-16).[7] However, power Doppler is highly sensitive and ideal for identifying slow flow within organs or structures.

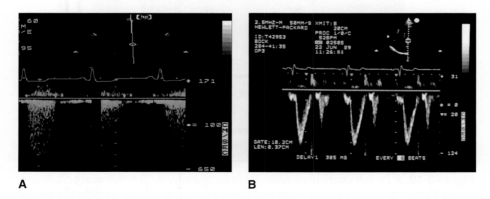

Figure 3-12. A. Continuous-wave Doppler image. B. Pulsed-wave Doppler image.

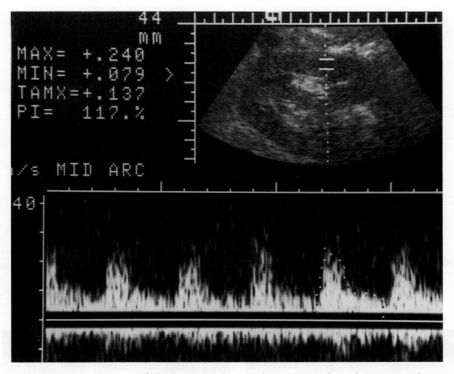

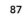

Figure 3-13. The use of duplex Doppler combines B-mode with PW Doppler.

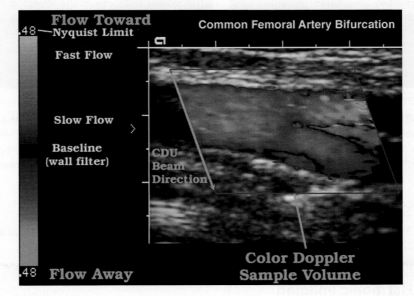

Figure 3-14. Color Doppler (CD) image.* This CD image shows the bifurcation of the common femoral artery. The color map on the left side of the image demonstrates that red is the dominant color above the baseline indicating flow relatively toward the transducer. Blue is the dominant color below the color map baseline indicating flow away from the transducer. Higher-flow velocities are displayed in brighter colors transitioning to yellow in the "toward" direction and to green in the "away" direction. The CD sample volume is indicated in the image by an angled box (parallelogram). The orientation of the CD ultrasound beam is shown by the angled sides of the box. *Images in color are provided for the student online in student resources.

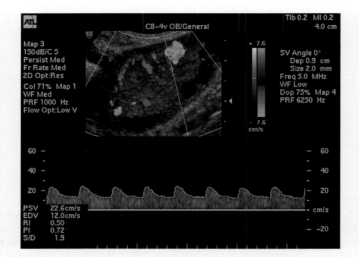

Figure 3-15. Triplex imaging of the ovary.* Triplex includes grayscale, color Doppler, and pulsed-wave Doppler. *Images in color are provided for the student online in student resources.

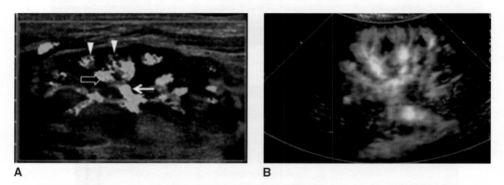

A   B

Figure 3-16. Color Doppler sonography.* A. Color Doppler image demonstrates the various sections of the renal vasculature (*open and closed arrows*). B. Power Doppler, which is much more sensitive than color Doppler, enhances visualization of the vascularity within the kidney. *True color images are provided for the student online in student resources.

Sound Off

Triplex imaging is the combination of B-mode, spectral, and color Doppler information on the screen at the same time.

Tissue Harmonic Imaging

Though the physics behind **tissue harmonic imaging** (THI) is really beyond the scope of this book, it is important to note that harmonics is a valuable component of sonographic imaging. Essentially, additional frequencies, other than the transmitted frequency sent into the body, are generated by the differing human body tissues. These frequencies are referred to as harmonics. Harmonic frequencies are collected by the transducer and used to create a crisper, higher-resolution image (Figs. 3-17 and 3-18). Harmonics also allow for artifacts—which are classically produced—to be reduced and in some cases removed completely from the image.[7]

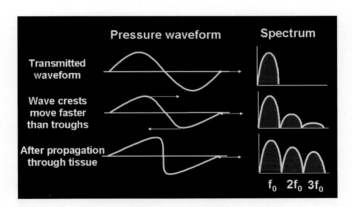

Figure 3-17. Tissue harmonics. The propagation of sound through tissue causes gradual changes in the shape of the ultrasound wave as it travels through the body. Harmonics are multiples of the fundamental frequency that is sent into the body. These harmonics can be collected and used to create a better image.

3D and 4D Technology

Three-dimensional ultrasound (3D), also referred to as volume scanning, was developed in the early 1990s at Duke University, when researchers created a matrix array transducer.[4] 3D allows one to see the width, height, and depth of images and has many applications in sonography, with the most commonly recognized use of the technology in obstetrics for clear visualization of the form of the fetal face. However, 3D can be used in other specialties, including breast, vascular, gynecologic, and abdominal sonographic imaging (Fig. 3-19).

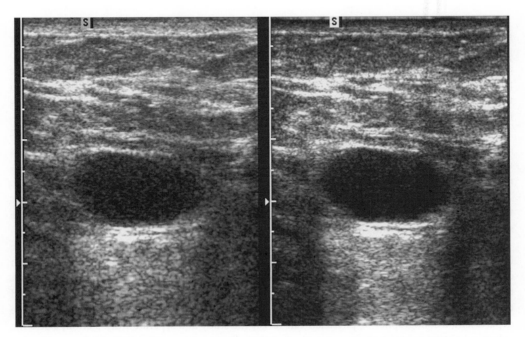

Figure 3-18. Tissue harmonic imaging (THI) of a simple cyst. **Left.** The initial image without harmonics demonstrates artifactual or false low-level echoes within the cyst. **Right.** THI removes most of the false echoes.

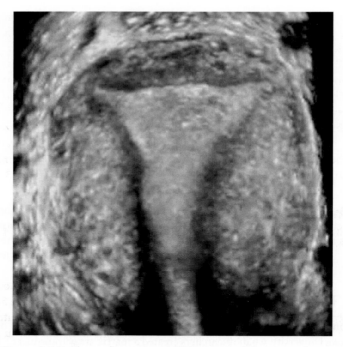

Figure 3-19. Three-dimensional (3D) image of the normal uterus.

Sound Off

3D allows one to see the width, height, and depth of images.

3D ultrasound images are made up of two 2D images placed next to each other, and the computer system within the ultrasound machine reconstructs the 2D information provided by the transducer into a 3D format.[7] There are several ways in which a 3D image can be created with ultrasound. To acquire a 3D image manually, the sonographer must select and move the transducer across a specific path while image frames are acquired by the transducer to create a final 3D image. The problem with the free-hand method is that the size of the volume is determined by the speed at which the sonographer moves the transducer.

Another method to acquire a 3D image is with a mechanical 3D transducer. These transducers consist of a linear or sequenced array transducer contained within housing. The transducer is mounted on a motor that moves back and forth. In this way, the 3D acquisition is automated, permitting accurate measurement of 3D volumes. The final type of 3D method is with a 2D transducer. This transducer looks like a phased array probe but acquires data in two planes simultaneously. It has the ability to not only produce realtime multiplanar and volume scans but can show anatomy in two scan planes at the same time.

One of the concerns of sonography is the dependence upon the skill of the sonographer to acquire diagnostic imaging. A newer application of volume scanning or **volumetric imaging** is the use of an offline work station to do post-processing of acquired volumes after the patient is discharged from the department. This type of scanning is much like CT imaging in that the 2D transducer is used to acquire multiple volumes instead of individual slices. After the patient is discharged from the department, a sonographer or physician can revisit the study at a separate work station, assess the volumetric information, and process the images digitally. For volumetric imaging, the sonographer finds a good window, completes one sweep from lateral to medial, and that is it. The computer can recreate 3D images from 2D images.[11]

There are some limitations to 3D technology, however. For example, in obstetrics, to acquire the most optimal 3D image of the fetal face, oftentimes, a substantial amount of amniotic fluid must be located adjacent to the fetal face, and the fetus must be in a favorable position. Also, for some applications of 3D, a 2D image can provide enough information for diagnostic purposes while 3D simply offers confirmation. However, the uses of 3D, especially in obstetrics and gynecology, are expanding. For example, in obstetrics, it is thought that a 3D image of the fetal skull can provide a more accurate measurement than can 2D.[11]

While 3D technology is limited to motionless images, **four-dimensional ultrasound** (4D) offers realtime imaging in 3D. In other words, the difference between 3D and 4D sonography is the ability of the sonographer to scan realtime in 3D, where, fundamentally, the fourth dimension is time.[6] Realtime multiplanar imaging and surface rendering are options with mechanical 3D probes.

Sound Off

The difference between 3D and 4D is the ability of the sonographer to scan realtime in 3D, where, fundamentally, the fourth dimension is time.

Though there are some benefits for the application of 4D technology in diagnostic sonography, the use of the technology is still evolving. There has been some exploitation of both 3D and 4D ultrasound technology by some non-diagnostic obstetric centers for economic and entertainment purposes. These may be referred to as **keepsake imaging** centers. The American Institute of Ultrasound in Medicine's official statement calls for certified professionals to perform ultrasound examinations and licensed physicians to interpret those examinations to ensure that appropriate patient care standards are upheld. The statement emphasizes "that all imaging requires proper documentation and a final report for the patient medical record signed by a physician."[12] This topic will be revisited in the ethics section of this book, Chapter 6.

SPECIALTIES IN SONOGRAPHY

It is common for individuals unfamiliar with the sonography profession to assume that students in sonography school just learn about scanning pregnant women. No doubt, sonography has made an enormous impact in the obstetric profession. However, as you know, sonography is utilized by many medical fields, and as a result, sonography reverberates throughout the medical profession. The following sections will provide an overview of the various sonography specialties, including discussions of individuals who have helped establish the use of ultrasound in that specialty. Furthermore, Chapter 14 provides the essential components to include in protocols with relevant anatomy and structures recommended by the **American Institute of Ultrasound in Medicine** (AIUM) in conjunction with the **American College of Radiology** (ACR) and other professional organizations.

Abdominal Sonography

As mentioned earlier, the first use of diagnostic ultrasound in the United States can be traced back to George Ludwig in the 1940s.[4] Ludwig used pulse-echo ultrasound waves to detect gallstones in animal tissue.[13] He used A-mode to detect the gallstones with a device he made called the ultrasonic locator.[13] He was also vital in the establishment of clinical applications of ultrasound, and we still utilize his reported velocity of sound transmission in soft tissue—recall this figure was 1,540 m/s.[13] **Abdominal sonography** has evolved greatly over the years, and abdominal sonographers have adapted and honed their skills, making sonography of the abdomen a mainstay in diagnostic imaging.

Abdominal sonographers must appreciate the relevant normal abdominal anatomy and pathology of each organ and system within the abdomen and **small parts**. Though equipment varies

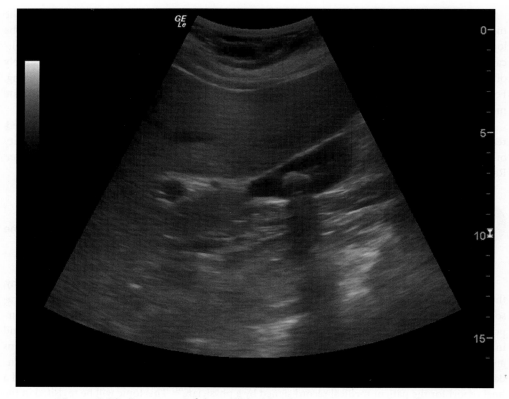

Figure 3-20. Sonogram of the gallbladder that contains a single gallstone.

between procedures, transducer frequency ranges between 2 and 5 MHz for general adult abdominal imaging with higher frequencies preferred for better resolution and for pediatric abdominal imaging and superficial structures. CW and PW Doppler are often utilized to assess vascular structures and provide evidence of blood flow within abdominal masses and organs.

Abdominal sonographic imaging includes a wide variety of abdominal structures, such as the liver, spleen, gallbladder, biliary tree, pancreas, abdominal vasculature, and the kidneys and bladder (Fig. 3-20). Thus, abdominal sonograms can be ordered for numerous reasons (Table 3-1). Common sonographic procedures for the abdominal sonographer consist of the complete abdomen sonogram; right upper quadrant sonogram; abdominal aorta and inferior vena cava sonogram; sonography of the urinary tract, often referred to as a renal sonogram; and targeted organ studies, like a sonogram of the appendix (Table 3-2). Abdominal sonographers may assist the physician in **invasive procedures** as well, including thoracentesis, paracentesis, mass biopsies, and core biopsies of organs.

Patient preparation for abdominal sonographic imaging is typically **nothing by mouth** (NPO) for at least six hours prior to the scheduled exam. However, some institutions encourage patients to be NPO after midnight the night before or for a minimum of eight hours while others only require four hours, especially for emergency indications. For renal sonograms, there may be no preparation needed, though patients may be asked to be well hydrated for the exam. Other studies, like the pyloric sonogram, require the infant patient to drink a clear liquid while realtime scanning is performed of the distal stomach.

Sonographers practicing abdominal sonography should have a thorough understanding of Doppler principles and hemodynamics, because occasionally, they must perform studies that include Doppler interrogation of various organs. Common vascular structures of the abdomen that are often evaluated with sonography include the portal veins, hepatic artery, hepatic veins, abdominal aorta

TABLE 3-1	AIUM indications for an abdominal and/or retroperitoneal sonogram

- Abdominal, flank, and/or back pain
- Signs or symptoms that may be referred from the abdominal and/or retroperitoneal regions such as jaundice or hematuria
- Palpable abnormalities such as an abdominal mass or organomegaly
- Abnormal laboratory values or abnormal findings on other imaging examinations suggestive of abdominal and/or retroperitoneal pathology
- Follow-up of known or suspected abnormalities in the abdomen and/or retroperitoneum
- Search for metastatic disease or an occult primary neoplasm
- Evaluation of suspected congenital abnormalities
- Abdominal trauma
- Pretransplantation and posttransplantation evaluation
- Planning for and guiding an invasive procedure
- Searching for the presence of free or loculated peritoneal and/or retroperitoneal fluid
- Suspicion of hypertrophic pyloric stenosis or intussusceptions
- Evaluation of a urinary tract infection

From AIUM Practice Guideline for the Performance of an Ultrasound Examination of the Abdomen and/or Retroperitoneum. Retrieved January 25, 2015 from http://www.aium.org/resources/guidelines/abdominal.pdf.[14]

TABLE 3-2	Components of an abdominal sonographic imaging exam

Abdominal Sonographic Imaging[14]	Organs or Structures Included
Abdominal aorta	Abdominal aorta, IVC, and possibly both kidneys
Abdominal wall	Specific area of a palpable mass or the evaluation for hernias and/or hematomas
Appendix or bowel	Appendix (right lower quadrant), affected bowel, and additional quadrant evaluation
Complete abdomen	Pancreas, liver, gallbladder, biliary tree, kidneys, adrenal glands,[a] abdominal aorta, inferior vena cava, spleen, urinary bladder (if needed)
Thyroid or neck	Thyroid lobes, parathyroid glands (if seen), lateral neck (for lymphadenopathy), salivary glands
Peritoneal fluid search	**Ascites** search in the peritoneal spaces
Renal	Kidneys, adrenal glands,[a] urinary bladder, abdominal aorta (possibly)
Right upper quadrant	Pancreas, liver, gallbladder, biliary tree, right kidney, right adrenal gland,[a] inferior vena cava, abdominal aorta (possibly)
Scrotum	Testicles, epididymis, scrotum, spermatic cord, inguinal canal (if needed)

[a]Though the adrenal glands are often not visualized in adult patients, they are readily seen in pediatric patients. Therefore, sonographers should analyze the region of the adrenal glands in all patients.

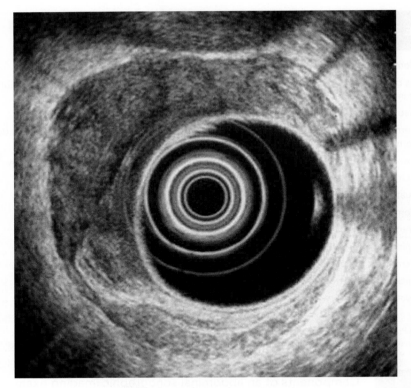

Figure 3-21. An endorectal sonogram image.

and its tributaries, and the inferior vena cava. Also, liver, kidney, pancreas, and other organ transplants can be assessed with sonography for signs of transplant rejection and other posttransplant complications. Some abdominal sonographers may be asked to evaluate for renal artery stenosis, perform **intraoperative sonography**, or assist a physician during **endoscopic ultrasound** (EUS). With EUS, the transducer is attached to an **endoscope**, which allows for the viewing of internal anatomy; this is used in many settings, including the analysis of the gastrointestinal tract and lungs (Fig. 3-21). Additional EUS applications will be discussed later in this chapter. Current trends for abdominal sonography can be found in Table 3-3.

Small Parts Sonography

Structures referred to as small parts, such as the thyroid, scrotum, and prostate gland, are often additional required studies that must be performed by sonographers practicing abdominal sonography (Tables 3-4, 3-5, and 3-6). They may also be required to perform breast sonography in many radiology

TABLE 3-3	Current trends in abdominal sonography

- **Fusion imaging**
- Elastography
- Musculoskeletal sonographic imaging
- Use of contrast
- Volumetric imaging

From Orenstein BW. Current trends in abdominal sonography. SDMS News Wave, March 2010:1–4.

TABLE 3-4	AIUM indications for a scrotal sonogram

- Evaluation of scrotal pain, including but not limited to testicular trauma, ischemia/torsion, and infectious or inflammatory scrotal disease
- Evaluation of palpable inguinal or scrotal masses
- Evaluation of scrotal asymmetry, swelling, or enlargement
- Evaluation of potential scrotal hernias
- Detection/evaluation of varicoceles
- Evaluation of male infertility
- Follow-up of prior indeterminate scrotal ultrasound findings
- Localization of undescended testes
- Detection of occult primary tumors in patients with metastatic germ cell tumors
- Follow-up of patients with prior primary testicular neoplasms, leukemia, or lymphoma
- Evaluation of abnormalities noted on other imaging studies (including but not limited to computed tomography, magnetic resonance imaging (MRI), and positron emission tomography)
- Evaluation of intersex conditions

From AIUM Practice Guideline for the Performance of Scrotal Ultrasound Examinations. Retrieved January 25, 2015 from http://www.aium.org/resources/guidelines/scrotal.pdf.[15]

TABLE 3-5	AIUM indications for a thyroid and parathyroid sonogram (neck)

- Evaluation of the location and characteristics of palpable neck masses, including an enlarged thyroid
- Evaluation of abnormalities detected by other imaging examinations, (e.g., a thyroid nodule detected on computed tomography, positron emission tomography-computed tomography, or magnetic resonance imaging) or seen on another ultrasound examination of the neck (e.g., carotid ultrasound)
- Evaluation of laboratory abnormalities
- Evaluation of the presence, size, and location of the thyroid gland
- Evaluation of patients at high risk for occult thyroid malignancy
- Follow-up imaging of previously detected thyroid nodules when indicated
- Evaluation for regional nodal metastases in patients with proven or suspected thyroid carcinoma before thyroidectomy
- Evaluation for recurrent disease or regional nodal metastases after total or partial thyroidectomy for thyroid carcinoma
- Evaluation of the thyroid gland for suspicious nodules before neck surgery for non-thyroid disease
- Evaluation of the thyroid gland for suspicious nodules before **radioiodine ablation** of the gland
- Identification and localization of parathyroid abnormalities in patients with known or suspected hyperparathyroidism
- Assessment of the number and size of enlarged parathyroid glands in patients who have undergone previous parathyroid surgery or ablative therapy with recurrent symptoms of hyperparathyroidism
- Localization of thyroid/parathyroid abnormalities or adjacent cervical lymph nodes for biopsy, ablation, or other interventional procedures
- Localization of autologous parathyroid gland implants

From AIUM Practice Guideline for the Performance of a Thyroid and Parathyroid Ultrasound Examination. Retrieved January 25, 2015 from http://www.aium.org/resources/guidelines/thyroid.pdf.[16]

TABLE 3-6	AIUM indications for a prostate sonogram

- Guidance for biopsy in the presence of an abnormal digital rectal examination or elevated prostate-specific antigen (PSA)
- Assessment of gland and prostate volume before medical, surgical, or radiation therapy
- Symptoms of prostatitis with a suspected abscess
- Assessment of **congenital anomalies**
- Infertility
- Hematospermia

From AIUM Practice Guideline for the Performance of Ultrasound Evaluation of the Prostate (and Surrounding Structures). Retrieved January 25, 2015 from http://www.aium.org/resources/guidelines/prostate.pdf.[17]

departments and in the outpatient setting (see the "Breast Sonography" section for more information). Moreover, abdominal sonographers may be asked to evaluate the penis, chest, specific painful joints or tendons, bowel, the abdominal wall for hernias, and palpable masses or to confirm evidence of shrapnel, splinters, and other foreign bodies. Essentially, abdominal sonographers may be required to scan any external body part to which both acoustic gel and the transducer can be applied.

Sound Off

Essentially, abdominal sonographers may be required to scan any external body part to which both acoustic gel and the transducer can be applied.

The majority of small parts, because of their more superficial locations, require the use of a linear transducer and, in some cases, the use of an acoustic **stand-off device.** A stand-off device may be a manufactured aqueous gel pad, a large amount of gel, or a bag of saline, or even submerging the anatomic structure in water (Figs. 3-22 and 3-23). The stand-off device places some distance between the transducer and the skin surface, thereby typically allowing superficial structures to be imaged more clearly. Conversely, if small parts, such as the testicles or thyroid glands, are enlarged, a curved

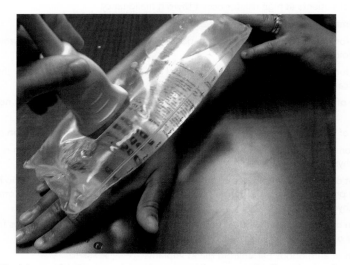

Figure 3-22. A bag of saline can be substituted for a stand-off pad in order to visualize superficial structures anywhere in the body. Sonographers may also use excess gel as a stand-off method.

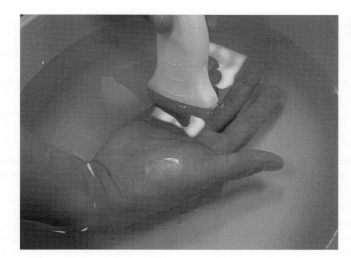

Figure 3-23. Because fluid acts as a sound beam enhancer, submerging the area of interest in a pan of water, as seen here, can be used as a stand-off mechanism as well.

linear transducer may be required to image the entire structure. The prostate may be visualized with the transducer placed on the abdomen—the **transabdominal approach**—but for detailed prostate imaging, an **endorectal transducer** is frequently employed (Fig. 3-24).

Challenges arise for abdominal sonographers resulting from large patient **body habitus**, bowel gas, surgical bandages, and patient preparation, lack of compliance, or intolerance. With many bowel studies, excluding pyloric stenosis examinations for the infant, the sonographer employs a technique called **graded compression**, whereby the sonographer pushes down on the patient's abdomen

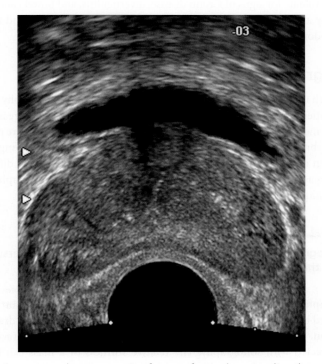

Figure 3-24. A transrectal sonogram is often performed to visualize the prostate gland (*arrowheads*).

TABLE 3-7	AIUM indications for a breast sonogram

- Evaluation and characterization of palpable masses and other breast-related signs and/or symptoms
- Evaluation of suspected or apparent abnormalities detected on other imaging studies, such as mammography or MRI
- Initial imaging evaluation of palpable masses in women under 30 years of age who are not at high risk for development of breast cancer and in lactating and pregnant women
- Evaluation of problems associated with breast implants
- Evaluation of breasts with microcalcifications and/or architectural distortion suspicious for malignancy or highly suggestive of malignancy in a setting of dense fibroglandular tissue, for detecting an underlying mass that may be obscured on the mammogram
- Guidance of breast biopsy and other interventional procedures
- Treatment planning for radiation therapy
- As a supplement to mammography, screening for occult cancers in certain populations of women (such as those with dense fibroglandular breasts who are also at elevated risk of breast cancer or with newly suspected breast cancer) who are not candidates for MRI or have no easy access to MRI
- Identification and biopsy guidance of abnormal axillary lymph node(s), for example, in patients with newly diagnosed or recurrent breast cancer or with findings highly suggestive of malignancy or other significant etiology

From ACR practice parameter for the performance of a breast ultrasound examination. Retrieved January 25, 2015 from http://www.acr.org/~/media/ACR/Documents/PGTS/guidelines/US_Breast.pdf

with the transducer during the examination to discern normal from abnormal bowel. In adults, the sonographer can evaluate for signs of Crohn disease, diverticulitis, and bowel cancer. See the section "Neurosonography and Pediatric Sonography" for changes to certifications and more information about pediatric abdominal imaging.

Breast Sonography

In conjunction with mammography and physical examination, breast sonography currently plays an essential role in patient care. Though mammography is the gold standard for breast imaging, sonography is the initial modality of choice for patients under 30 and for those who are pregnant or lactating.[18] Also, dense breast tissue on a mammogram can camouflage underlying pathology while sonography is often minimally hindered. Mammography is often incapable of differentiating cystic versus solid masses as well, while this task is readily accomplished with sonography.[18] Consequently, there are several unique indications for a breast sonogram (Table 3-7).

 Sound Off

Mammography is often incapable of differentiating cystic versus solid masses, though this task is readily accomplished with sonography.

Breast sonography is also utilized for possible breast implant rupture, during needle placement for a standard breast biopsy, **vacuum-assisted breast biopsy**, breast cyst drainage, and **radiofrequency ablation**.[18] **Elastography** has proven effective in the additional characterization of solid breast masses detected with sonography. The relative stiffness of a mass can be provided with elastography, with stiffer masses more likely to be malignant. Elastography is discussed further in this chapter.

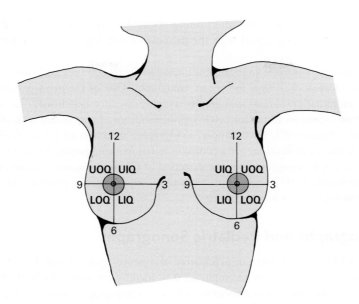

Figure 3-25. For breast sonography, each breast is imaged based on the face of a clock. The breast may also be divided into an upper inner quadrant (UIQ), upper outer quadrant (UOQ), lower inner quadrant (LIQ), and lower outer quadrant (LOQ).

Sonography of the breast should be performed with a high-resolution, realtime linear array transducer with a frequency of at least 10 MHz, though a higher frequency is preferred for improved resolution. Harmonic imaging and spatial compounding increase resolution as well. Occasionally, for shallow masses, a stand-off device may be utilized. Sonographers can perform breast sonography in various positions, but a supine-oblique position, which requires the patient to be rolled up 30 to 45 degrees toward the breast being examined with the **ipsilateral** arm raised, is often used to minimize the thickness of the portion of the breast that is to be examined.[18]

For sonography of the breast, the breast is visualized like the face of a clock, with each breast having its own clock face (Fig. 3-25). Imaging of the breast can be performed in transverse and longitudinal planes or radial and antiradial planes. Also, breast sonographers may incorporate special labeling for the location of masses such as *fingers from the nipple*. Furthermore, special techniques may be employed, such as **fremitus**, a task that requires the patient to hum while the breast is imaged with color Doppler to further assess the stiffness of a breast mass. Some facilities may also utilize zonal and depth labeling for breast masses as well. Therefore, as a student, you should recognize the variability of labeling between institutions, adjust your protocol, and be prepared.

Sound Off

For sonography of the breast, the breast is visualized like the face of a clock, with each breast having its own clock face.

To better appreciate the method in which sonography of the breast is performed, breast sonographers should have a thorough appreciation of mammographic techniques and breast pathology noted on a mammogram, as the ability to correlate the location of abnormalities seen on mammography is vital for adequate patient care. Correlation of abnormalities noted among imaging modalities, including MRI of the breast, is ultimately performed by the interpreting physician who often integrates a scoring method of breast masses referred to as the **Breast Imaging Reporting and Data System** (BI-RADS). The BI-RADS sonography characteristics include the size, shape, orientation, margin, echogenicity, lesion boundary, attenuation, special cases, vascularity, and surrounding tissue.[19] Ultimately, the interpreting physician assigns a score, based on BI-RADS, as part of the breast imaging report with the purpose of relaying pertinent information to the ordering physician.

Though sonography has made an invaluable impact in the recognition and management of breast disease, there are several challenges for breast sonography. One of the main concerns is that, like all sonography examinations, breast sonography is highly operator-dependent. The advent of automated whole breast scanners allows for better reproducibility and correlation with other modalities (see "Automated Ultrasound"). Furthermore, sonographic detection of microcalcifications in the breast is limited. Microcalcifications are a common initial mammographic finding of breast cancer. Improving resolution in sonography for the detection of microcalcifications is currently underway. The future is optimistic, as 3D imaging and computer-assisted detection programs are furthering the applications of sonography in breast imaging.[18]

Neurosonography and Pediatric Sonography

Recall it was Karl Dussik, an Austrian psychiatrist and neurologist, who first used ultrasound for medical diagnostic purposes when he employed it to identify the ventricles in the brain in 1941.[1] **Neurosonography**, also referred to as neurosonology, is a sonographic specialty that includes neonatal brain imaging, newborn infant spine imaging, and intraoperative sonography (Fig. 3-26). Premature infants often require sonographic imaging because they can suffer from intracranial hemorrhage at the time of birth, though there are multiple indications (Table 3-8).

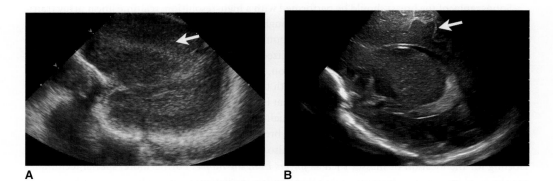

A   B

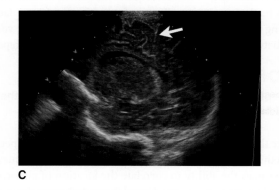

C

Figure 3-26. Head sonography is the most frequent means of neonatal brain imaging, especially in premature infants. Normal neonatal neurosonography. Postnatal sonographic parasagittal images of normal 26-week (**A**), normal 35-week (**B**), and normal-term (**C**) infants. The *arrows* are demonstrating the normal progressive development of the cerebral sulci.

TABLE 3-8	AIUM indications for neurosonography in neonates and infants

- To evaluate for hemorrhage
- To evaluate for hydrocephalus
- To evaluate for the presence of vascular abnormalities
- To evaluate for possible or suspected **hypoxic-ischemic** encephalopathy
- To evaluate for the presence of congenital malformations
- To evaluate patients with signs and/or symptoms of central nervous system disorders (e.g., seizures) and facial malformations
- For follow-up or surveillance of previously documented abnormalities, including prenatal abnormalities
- For screening before surgical procedures

From AIUM Practice Guideline for the Performance of Neurosonography in Neonates and Infants. Retrieved January 25, 2015 from http://www.aium.org/resources/guidelines/neurosonography.pdf.[20]

Sonography provides a portable, high-resolution, economic alternative to other imaging studies that are more expensive and require the patient to be transported from the neonatal intensive care unit. In the unit, sonographers must be mindful of surgical asepsis techniques to prevent the spread of infections between neonates. The sonogram is typically performed with a small footprint, high-frequency, sector or curved linear array transducer, and images are obtained routinely through the anterior fontanelle. However, other fontanelles may be utilized and Doppler interrogation can be conducted of the neonatal and infant brain. Neonatal brain sonographic imaging may also be performed in an outpatient setting as a follow-up for previously discovered pathology or upon the suggestion of the child's pediatrician.

The infant spine can be easily imaged with sonography, most often with a high-frequency linear array transducer with frequency ranges between 7 and 10 MHz, though higher frequencies afford better resolution. For this examination, the patient is placed prone, and the spinal contents are imaged. Infants often present with signs or symptoms of some form of **spinal dysraphism**— specifically findings suggestive of closed spina bifida. These signs include a sacral dimple, sacral tuft of hair, or a sacral hemangioma, among other clinical findings (Table 3-9). Infants may be scanned also as the result of suspicious intrauterine findings during an obstetric sonogram. In the recent past, neurosonology existed as a distinct certification offered by the ARDMS. However, in 2015, the

TABLE 3-9	AIUM indications for an infant spine sonogram

- Lumbosacral stigmata known to be associated with spinal dysraphism, including but not limited to skin tags, hair tufts, midline hemangiomas, and sacral dimples
- The spectrum of caudal regression syndrome
- Evaluation of suspected defects such as cord tethering
- Detection of **sequelae** of injury
- Hematoma after spinal tap or birth injury; sequelae of prior instrumentation, infection, or hemorrhage
- Posttraumatic leakage of cerebrospinal fluid
- Visualization of fluid with characteristics of blood products within the spinal canal in patients with intracranial hemorrhage
- Guidance for lumbar puncture
- Postoperative assessment for cord re-tethering

From AIUM Practice Guideline for the Performance of Neurosonography in Neonates and Infants. Retrieved January 25, 2015 from http://www.aium.org/resources/guidelines/neurosonography.pdf.[20]

ARDMS began to replace the NE certification (neurosonology) with pediatric sonography (PS), which includes all pediatric imaging—neurosonology, abdomen, small parts, pelvic, and various other procedures explicitly distinct to PS.[22]

Sound Off

In 2015, the ARDMS began to provide a pediatric sonography certification.

Though some distinctive images may be required for pediatric imaging of the abdomen, the abdomen and small parts are often imaged in the pediatric patient using protocols similar to that of the adult patient. Because radiation exposure should be minimized for pediatric patients, sonography provides an outstanding non-invasive, non-ionizing imaging tool to evaluate the abdomen in infants and children.

Renal sonography is an example of how our modality can provide such a valuable service. Pediatric renal sonography is critical for the appropriate care of the pediatric patient presenting with urinary tract symptoms and is often used as an initial screening tool in pediatrics because of its straightforwardness, accuracy, and non-invasive nature. Often, renal sonography is ordered before more invasive radiographic procedures, such as the voiding cystourethrogram (VCUG), to assess the overall architecture of the urinary tract in the symptomatic child. Sonographers may be asked to scan parts of the bowel as well. Furthermore, in the pediatric patient, sonographers can evaluate for pyloric stenosis, intussusception, and appendicitis.

Musculoskeletal Sonography

One of the most rapidly advancing applications of ultrasound in medicine is the use of sonography to evaluate the musculoskeletal (MSK) system—**musculoskeletal sonography** (Fig. 3-27). This ever-expanding specialty includes the evaluation of the shoulder, wrist, knee, and essentially any other joints, tendons, and muscles of the extremities (Table 3-10). The search for foreign bodies may also be a requirement while practicing MSK sonography. MSK sonographers may be employed in hospitals, orthopedic clinics, chiropractic offices, and in other outpatient settings. They may also assist the physician in interventional procedures, like joint aspirations. The ARDMS offers certification in MSK sonography, though both specific didactic and hands-on training may be required.

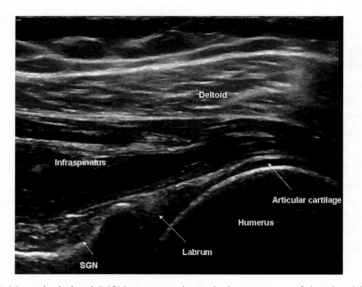

Figure 3-27. Musculoskeletal (MSK) sonography includes imaging of the shoulder, which is the most popular joint examined with sonography. SGN = spinoglenoid notch.

TABLE 3-10	AIUM indications for a musculoskeletal sonogram

- Pain or dysfunction
- Soft tissue or bone injury
- Tendon or ligament pathology
- **Arthritis, synovitis**, or **crystal deposition disease**
- Intra-articular bodies
- **Joint effusion**
- Nerve entrapment, injury, neuropathy, masses, or **subluxation**
- Evaluation of soft tissue masses, swelling, or fluid collections
- Detection of foreign bodies in the superficial soft tissues
- Planning and guiding an invasive procedure
- Congenital or developmental anomalies
- Postoperative or post-procedural evaluation

From AIUM Practice Guidelines for the Performance of a Musculoskeletal Ultrasound Examination. Retrieved January 25, 2015 from http://www.aium.org/resources/guidelines/musculoskeletal.pdf.[21]

Gynecologic Sonography

Gynecologic sonography has greatly impacted patient care of the female **non-gravid** uterus and pelvis. In association with the American College of Obstetrics and Gynecology (ACOG) and other groups, the AIUM has established indication for a pelvic sonogram (Table 3-11). Current trends in gynecologic sonography can be found in Table 3-12.

TABLE 3-11	AIUM indications for gynecologic sonography

- Pelvic pain
- **Dysmenorrhea** (painful menses)
- **Amenorrhea** (lack of menses)
- **Menorrhagia** (excessive menstrual bleeding)
- **Metrorrhagia** (irregular uterine bleeding)
- **Menometrorrhagia** (excessive irregular bleeding)
- Follow-up of a previously detected abnormality
- Evaluation, monitoring, and/or treatment of infertility
- Delayed menses, precocious puberty, or vaginal bleeding in a prepubertal child
- Postmenopausal bleeding
- Abnormal or technically limited pelvic examination
- Signs or symptoms of pelvic infection
- Further characterization of a pelvic abnormality noted on another imaging study
- Evaluation of congenital anomalies
- Excessive bleeding, pain, or signs of infection after pelvic surgery, delivery, or abortion
- Localization of an intrauterine contraceptive device
- Screening for malignancy in patients at increased risk
- Urinary **incontinence** or pelvic organ prolapse
- Guidance for interventional or surgical procedures

From AIUM Practice Guidelines for the Performance of Ultrasound of the Female Pelvis. Retrieved January 25, 2015 from http://www.aium.org/resources/guidelines/femalePelvis.pdf.

TABLE 3-12	Current trends in gynecologic sonography

- **Sonohysterography**
- 3D imaging for uterine malformations and ovarian masses
- Ovarian cyst management
- Stand-alone women's health/imaging centers
- Reproductive medicine

From Orenstein BW. Current trends in OB/GYN sonography. *SDMS News Wave*, April 2010:1–4.

Patient preparation for a transabdominal pelvic sonogram includes filling of the urinary bladder, often accomplished by drinking 32 oz of water an hour before the examination is scheduled. The reason for this preparation is to allow the patient's bladder to be distended (full), ultimately providing the sonographer with an acoustic window for visualizing the uterus, ovaries, and other structures in the **adnexa**. In essence, a urine-filled bladder provides an acoustic window and **acoustic enhancement**, thereby offering better imaging of pelvic organs. Patients who present with emergency indications may require that their bladders be retro-filled with saline using a **Foley catheter**. A preliminary task for students may be to check patients who are presenting for pelvic sonograms for appropriate bladder filling. Keep in mind, for an adequate study to be performed, the uterine fundus should be clearly identified. Typically, transabdominal sonography employs a transducer that is 3.5 MHz or higher.[23]

Though other techniques, such as transrectal, transperineal, and translabial scanning, may be performed, one of the most popular scanning techniques for gynecologic indications is **transvaginal sonography**, also referred to as **endovaginal sonography** (Fig. 3-28). For transvaginal sonography, a high-resolution transducer that has been draped with a protective wrap—**probe cover**—is placed in the patient's vagina after receiving her consent. The transducer should have a frequency of 5 MHz or higher.[23] After the examination is completed, the transducer is rinsed and sterilized. More about how to sterilize transducers can be found in the patient care section of this book.

Transvaginal sonography has several advantages over transabdominal pelvic sonography. One of the primary limitations of the transabdominal approach is patient body habitus, as obese patients present unique challenges. However, transvaginal sonography offers better resolution of organs and structures in large patients. Furthermore, transvaginal sonography does not typically require that the patient has a distended bladder, so the examination can be performed faster as well.

One of the early limitations of traditional transabdominal and endovaginal sonography was that they both lacked clear visualization of the endometrium in some cases, as well as the internal components of the uterine cavity. For example, some women may have complaints of irregular vaginal bleeding, which results from endometrial polyps or intracavitary fibroids. These abnormalities could possibly be missed with routine sonographic imaging. However, sonohysterography, also referred to as **saline infusion sonohysterography** (SIS), offers superb distinction of these types of masses and allows for clear visualization of the endometrial lining and uterine cavity (Table 3-13). For a SIS, using a catheter, sterile saline is injected through the cervix and into the uterine cavity (Fig. 3-29). The fluid is maintained in the uterine cavity with the help of a small catheter balloon. The sonogram is performed during the procedure. Sonohysterography may also be used to assess for fallopian tube patency and pathology.

Sound Off

Saline infusion sonography offers clear visualization of the endometrial lining and uterine cavity.

Gynecologic sonography has moreover made a significant impact on **assisted reproductive therapy** (ART) and fertility treatment. Sonography can be employed to assess the endometrium for cyclical changes and the ovaries for the evaluation of follicle size and cyst aspiration and to monitor for possible side effects of fertility drugs. Also, other ART methods, including embryo transfer, may use sonographic guidance.

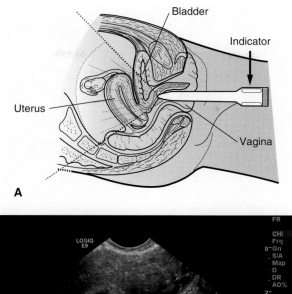

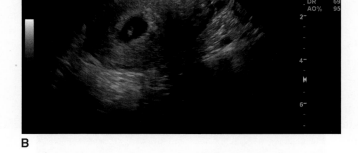

Figure 3-28. A. The transvaginal or endovaginal sonographic technique requires that the ultrasound transducer be inserted into the vagina for improved resolution. **B.** Sonography of the early pregnancy using the transvaginal or endovaginal technique is a valuable component of perinatal care.

Conversely, gynecologic sonography is an excellent imaging tool that is used to evaluate the postmenopausal female, especially when a patient presents with postmenopausal bleeding, as there is an established connection between postmenopausal bleeding and endometrial carcinoma. Current trends in gynecologic sonography include the use of 3D imaging for endometrial assessment, the identification of uterine congenital malformations, ExAblate therapy for fibroids (which combines MRI

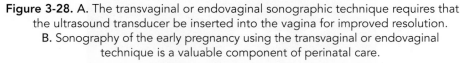

TABLE 3-13	AIUM indications for sonohysterography

- Abnormal uterine bleeding
- Uterine cavity, especially with regard to **uterine myomas, polyps, and synechiae**
- Abnormalities detected on endovaginal sonography, including focal or diffuse endometrial or intracavitary abnormalities
- Congenital abnormalities of the uterus
- Infertility
- Recurrent pregnancy loss

From AIUM Practice Guidelines for the Performance of Sonohysterography. Retrieved January 25, 2015 from http://www.aium.org/resources/guidelines/sonohysterography.pdf.[24]

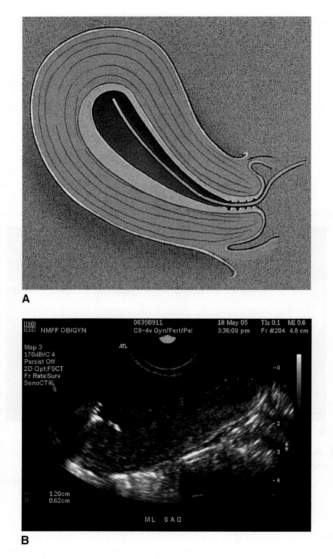

Figure 3-29. Saline infusion sonography utilizes saline that is instilled into the endometrial cavity by a catheter (**A**) to better visualize masses that are located within or adjacent to the uterine cavity (**B**).

and ultrasound), the assistance of guided invasive procedures, and for follow-up of intrauterine device implants such as the Essure device, which is an intrafallopian tube permanent birth control solution.[25]

Obstetric Sonography

Undoubtedly, **obstetric sonography** is one of the most established and recognizable applications of ultrasound in medicine. In 1957, Dr. Ian Donald (1910–1987) and Tom Brown worked to build the first known obstetric scanner, which was referred to as a contact compound scanner.[4] Since then, the technology has blossomed, and sonography has become a crucial component of care for the **gravid** patient, especially those patients who are considered to have a high risk for premature delivery, multiple gestations, and fetal anomalies. Consequently, sonographers practicing obstetrics must be familiar with both fetal abnormalities and maternal complications. Current trends in obstetric sonography can be found in Table 3-14.

TABLE 3-14	Current trends in obstetric sonography

- First-trimester screening examinations (nuchal translucency screening)
- Fetal biometry measurements utilizing 3D
- 3D and 4D technology

From Orenstein BW. Current trends in OB/GYN sonography. *SDMS News Wave*, April 2010:1–4.

There are several stages in pregnancy during which a sonogram may be required. In the first trimester, a sonogram may be performed for numerous reasons, including to confirm the presence of an **intrauterine pregnancy**, for vaginal bleeding, if an **ectopic pregnancy** is suspected, or for screening secondary to high-risk clinical history findings (Table 3-15). A routine **first-trimester** sonogram may be performed transabdominally or transvaginally, and it typically just includes a general assessment of both **maternal** and fetal anatomy. The first-trimester measurement of the fetal crown-rump length (CRL) is the most accurate measurement used for dating a pregnancy (Fig. 3-30).

Sound Off

Sonographers practicing obstetrics must be familiar with both fetal abnormalities and maternal complications.

The first trimester is also a time in which the fetus and mother can be screened for genetic complications, both clinically and sonographically. First-trimester maternal blood sampling can assist in the initial identification of possible fetal anomalies, which can then be quickly evaluated and followed with sonography. Also, in the first trimester, typically between 11 and 14 gestational weeks, a **nuchal translucency** measurement can be obtained. The nuchal translucency is a measurement taken of the posterior neck of the fetus. This measurement, if thickened or determined abnormal, is a valuable indicator for the presence of an **aneuploidy**, such as Down syndrome, or other fetal anomalies.

Perhaps one of the most likely times when a sonogram may be ordered for a routine anatomic survey is between 18 and 20 weeks, as most fetal anatomy can be thoroughly visualized adequately with sonography in the **second trimester**. Also, in the second and **third trimesters** of pregnancy, sonograms may be indicated when a detailed anatomic survey is warranted, as in the case where there is suspicion of maternal or fetal complications (Table 3-16, Fig. 3-31).

TABLE 3-15	AIUM indications for a first-trimester sonogram

- Confirmation of the presence of an intrauterine pregnancy
- Evaluation of a suspected ectopic pregnancy
- Defining the cause of vaginal bleeding
- Evaluation of pelvic pain
- Estimation of gestational (menstrual) age
- Diagnosis or evaluation of multiple gestations
- Confirmation of cardiac activity
- Imaging as an adjunct to chorionic villus sampling, embryo transfer, and localization and removal of an intrauterine device
- Assessing for certain fetal anomalies, such as anencephaly, in high-risk patients
- Evaluation of maternal pelvic masses and/or uterine abnormalities
- Measuring the nuchal translucency (NT) when part of a screening program for fetal aneuploidy
- Evaluation of a suspected hydatidiform mole

From AIUM Practice Guidelines for the Performance of Obstetric Ultrasound Examinations. Retrieved January 25, 2015 from http://www.aium.org/resources/guidelines/obstetric.pdf.[26]

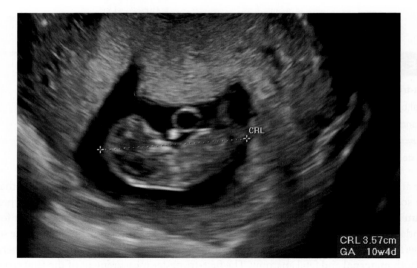

Figure 3-30. Early first-trimester sonogram of a 10-week, four-day gestation demonstrating the crown-rump length (CRL) measurement, which is the most accurate measurement used for aging a pregnancy.

TABLE 3-16	AIUM indications for second- and third-trimester sonograms

- Screening for fetal anomalies
- Evaluation of fetal anatomy
- Estimation of gestational (menstrual) age
- Evaluation of fetal growth
- Evaluation of vaginal bleeding
- Evaluation of abdominal or pelvic pain
- Evaluation of cervical insufficiency
- Determination of fetal presentation
- Evaluation of suspected multiple gestation
- Adjunct to amniocentesis or other procedure
- Evaluation of a significant discrepancy between uterine size and clinical dates
- Evaluation of a pelvic mass
- Evaluation of a suspected hydatidiform mole
- Adjunct to cervical cerclage placement
- Suspected ectopic pregnancy
- Suspected fetal death
- Suspected uterine abnormalities
- Evaluation of fetal well-being
- Suspected amniotic fluid abnormalities
- Suspected placental abruption
- Adjunct to external cephalic version
- Evaluation of premature rupture of membranes and/or premature labor
- Evaluation of abnormal biochemical markers
- Follow-up evaluation of a fetal anomaly
- Follow-up evaluation of placental location for suspected placenta previa
- History of previous congenital anomaly
- Evaluation of the fetal condition in late registrants for prenatal care
- Assessment for findings that may increase the risk for aneuploidy

From AIUM Practice Guidelines for the Performance of Obstetric Ultrasound Examinations. Retrieved January 25, 2015 from http://www.aium.org/resources/guidelines/obstetric.pdf.[26]

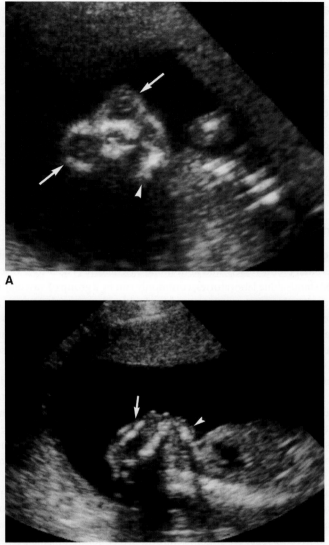

Figure 3-31. Anencephaly, demonstrated in these two images, is one of the most common fetal neural tube defects. **A.** It is characterized by "frog-like" orbits (*arrows*), though the lower face and mandible (*arrowhead*) is normally formed. **B.** A sagittal image of the same fetus reveals absence of the forehead and cranium (*arrow*). The mandible (*arrowhead*) and lower face appear normal.

Obstetric sonographers may be required to assist physicians with interventional perinatal procedures, including amniocentesis, chorionic villus sampling, and cordocentesis. These tests are often used in conjunction with sonography for **fetal karyotyping**, which is a manner of definitively distinguishing fetal chromosomal abnormalities by obtaining fetal blood, maternal blood, or amniotic fluid. Amniocentesis and all interventional or invasive obstetric procedures carry risks and benefits for both mother and fetus; thus, the physician and the patient must discuss these prior to the procedure taking place.

Fetal Echocardiography

An advanced branch of obstetric sonography in which sonographers can specialize is the field of **fetal echocardiography**. Though obstetric sonographers investigate the heart of the fetus, typically visualizing the heart in at least one plane for a four-chamber view, a fetal echocardiographer examines the heart in much more detail. Some fetal heart defects can be missed on the routine four-chamber heart view, however, like transposition of the great vessels, a potentially fatal defect if left undiscovered in utero (Fig. 3-32). Frequently, if the mother or father has a family history of congenital heart defects, or if an initial obstetric sonogram yielded suspicions for heart defects, a fetal echocardiogram will be performed (Table 3-17). Fetal echocardiographers must have an appreciation for the finer details of congenital heart defects, including the application of PW Doppler, M-mode, and color Doppler. They may also be involved with assisting a physician during interventional fetal procedures.

Vascular Sonography (Contributed by Traci B. Fox)

The **vascular sonographer** examines the arterial and venous systems of the arms and legs, the intracranial and extracranial blood vessels, and abdominal vasculature (Fig. 3-33). Vascular departments in hospitals may be stand-alone laboratories, commonly run by a group of vascular surgeons, or parts of radiology or imaging departments, thus combined with other specialties, such as in conjunction with general abdominal sonography. However, other arrangements of departments are possible, such as a cardiovascular laboratory, which performs both echocardiography and vascular exams. These studies are all considered to be non-invasive vascular exams, and in fact, vascular sonographers may work within a department referred to as a "non-invasive vascular lab."

The most common indications for different vascular sonograms are provided in Table 3-18 while Table 3-19 provides current trends in vascular sonography. In addition to the ultrasound machines found in most other sonography departments, the vascular sonographer also uses dedicated equipment to inspect the blood vessels. Many studies performed in the vascular lab are performed with standard ultrasound equipment and a 5- to 7-MHz linear transducer. However, some non-imaging arterial and venous studies are performed with blood pressure cuffs and a CW transducer.

Imaging vascular studies are often performed with a combination of PW spectral and color Doppler. When performing PW Doppler studies, it is crucial that angle correction be used whenever velocity measurements are needed. As stated earlier, vascular sonography is non-invasive and may be direct or indirect. **Direct testing**, like carotid artery sonograms, is performed with direct visualization of the structures being examined, like a carotid sonogram, whereby a sonographer places a transducer over the part of the body from which information is desired. With **indirect testing**, the transducer is placed over one body part in order to obtain information about another area of suspected disease. For example, with arterial **plethysmography**, the CW probe is placed at the ankle while blood pressure cuffs are inflated over the areas of interest higher in the leg. You may notice that some sonography departments that perform vascular examinations, especially peripheral arterial exams, are kept relatively warm. This is to avoid **vasoconstriction** that can occur in cold climates.

There is typically no patient preparation required for peripheral vascular sonographic exams or for intracranial or extracranial studies. Abdominal Doppler studies require the same patient preparation as for sonography of the upper abdomen, which is most likely six to eight hours NPO prior to the exam. For ultrasound involving the neck, it is recommended that the patient remove any necklaces and clothing that might obscure the examination area.

For lower extremity arterial and venous studies, the patient should remove his or her pants, shoes, and socks. If the patient is wearing underwear that is tight-fitting or limits access to the inguinal crease, these should be removed as well. Upper extremity vascular studies necessitate the removal

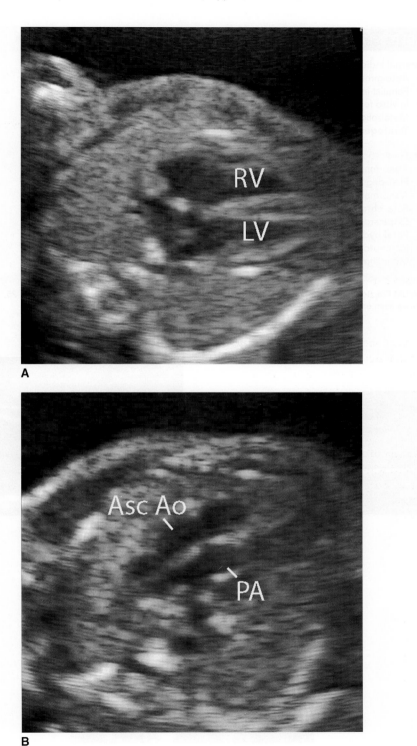

Figure 3-32. Fetal echocardiogram of transposition of the great arteries, a potentially fatal heart defect. **A.** A normal four-chamber view is present (*LV*, left ventricle; *RV*, right ventricle). **B.** The outflow tracts and proximal great arteries—pulmonary artery (*PA*) and ascending aorta (*Asc Ao*)—appear to be parallel instead of demonstrating the normal crossing pattern.

TABLE 3-17	AIUM indications for fetal echocardiography

Maternal indications
- Autoimmune antibodies
- Familial inherited disorders
- In vitro fertilization
- Metabolic disease
- **Teratogen** exposure

Fetal indications
- Abnormal cardiac screening examination
- First-degree relative of a fetus with congenital heart disease
- Abnormal heart rate or rhythm
- Fetal **chromosomal anomaly**
- Extracardiac anomaly
- **Fetal hydrops**
- Increased nuchal translucency
- Monochorionic twins

From AIUM Practice Guidelines for the Performance of Fetal Echocardiography. Retrieved January 25, 2015 from http://www.aium.org/resources/guidelines/fetalEcho.pdf.[27]

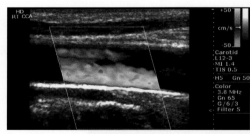

A

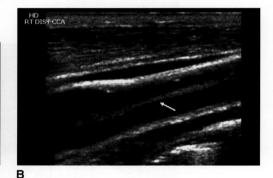

B

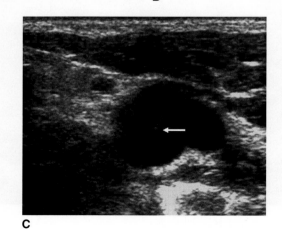

C

Figure 3-33. A. A common carotid artery dissection. **B.** Sagittal image of the distal common carotid artery demonstrates an intraluminal defect (*arrow*). **C.** Transverse at the level of the carotid bifurcation demonstrates the dissected lumen (*arrow*) visible within the internal carotid artery.

TABLE 3-18	Indications for vascular sonography
Sonographic Examination	**Indications**
Lower extremity venous	Clinical indications: Swelling, redness, warmth History of: Trauma, stasis, recent surgery, pregnancy, previous **deep vein thrombosis**, oral contraceptive use, cancer
Lower extremity arterial	Clinical indications: Claudication, cold or pale leg, lack of hair on leg History of: Arterial disease or previous arterial bypass or dialysis graft
Upper extremity arterial	Clinical indications: Cold hands, dialysis graft evaluation, mapping for coronary bypass graft surgery
Upper extremity venous	Clinical indications: Swelling, pain History of: Peripheral line or dialysis graft placement
Intracranial (TCD)	Clinical indications: Stroke, suspected vasospasm
Extracranial (carotid and vertebral arteries)	Clinical indications: **Stroke, amaurosis fugax, hemi-paralysis** or numbness, **ataxia**
Abdominal Doppler	Clinical indications depend on exam ordered. May include pain with eating (mesenteric studies), abnormal renal function (renal artery Doppler), and abnormal liver function tests (portal venous Doppler)

of the patient's shirt. In all exams, when the patient should be provided proper gowning to protect modesty and provide warmth.

Types of exams typically performed in a vascular lab include the following:

- Peripheral lower arterial exams can include pulse volume recording, usually performed in conjunction with segmental plethysmography, also referred to as a pressure test, **photoplethysmography** (PPG), and duplex Doppler exams. An exercise test is a segmental plethysmography exam that utilizes a treadmill or "toe lifts" as part of the exam.
- Peripheral lower venous exams include venous plethysmography and PPG (not as common anymore) and duplex Doppler.
- Peripheral upper extremity venous examinations can include segmental plethysmography, PPG, and duplex Doppler.

TABLE 3-19	Current trends in vascular sonography

- **Intravascular ultrasound**
- Elastography in vascular
- Sonography's role in aortic aneurysm repair
- Ultrasound-guided interventional procedures
- Vascular imaging in the hybrid room
- Transcranial Doppler techniques
- Carotid intimal-medial thickness scans
- Potential use of contrast media (currently not FDA approved)

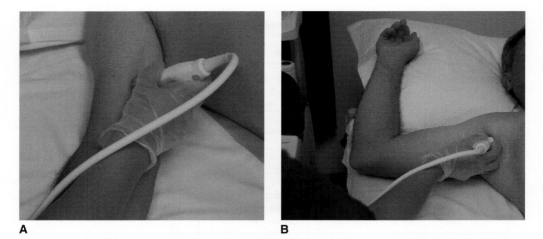

A   **B**

Figure 3-34. An example of a scanning technique (A) and positioning (B) for an upper extremity vascular sonographic examination.

- Peripheral upper extremity venous examinations are typically limited to duplex Doppler (Fig. 3-34).
- Extracranial and intracranial cerebrovascular Doppler are performed with duplex Doppler, although transcranial Doppler (TCD) may be performed with dedicated, non-imaging PW Doppler devices.
- Abdominal Doppler is performed with duplex Doppler.

Echocardiography (Contributed by Maureen McDonald)

The **cardiac sonographer**, also known as an **echocardiographer**, examines and assesses the anatomical structures of the heart as well as its hemodynamics, utilizing many different windows (Fig. 3-35). To perform a complete **echocardiogram**, the sonographer utilizes realtime 2D imaging, M-mode,

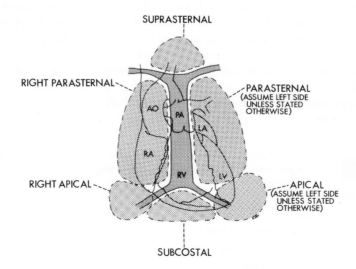

NOMENCLATURE FOR TRANSDUCER LOCATION

Figure 3-35. Common transducer nomenclature used in echocardiography to demonstrate various structures including the aorta (*Ao*), pulmonary artery (*PA*), right atrium (*RA*), left atrium (*LA*), right ventricle (*RV*), and left ventricle (*LV*).

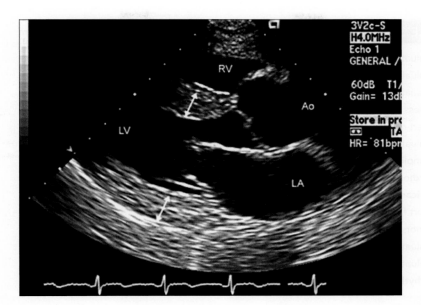

Figure 3-36. Transthoracic 2D echocardiogram recorded in a parasternal long-axis view demonstrating the right ventricle (*RV*), left ventricle (*LV*), left atrium (*LA*), and proximal aorta (*Ao*), as well as septal and posterior wall thickness (*double-headed arrows*).

and Doppler echocardiography. The most common test performed by the echocardiographer is a **transthoracic echocardiogram** (TTE), commonly referred to as an echo (Fig. 3-36). But echocardiographers may also assist other healthcare professionals in performing the **stress echocardiogram** (SE) and **transesophageal echocardiogram** (TEE). The following sections will discuss each of these. Current trends in echocardiography are provided in Table 3-20.

Sound Off

The most common test performed by the echocardiographer is a transthoracic echocardiogram, commonly referred to as an echo.

TABLE 3-20	Current trends in echocardiography
Echocardiography Specialty	**Current Trends**
Fetal echo	• Extended basic examination (includes outflow tracts) • 3D and 4D sonography • ARDMS fetal echocardiography certification examination now offered (since 2010)
Pediatric echo	• Digital storage • Pediatric TEE probes
Adult echo	• 2D and 3D speckle tracking for assessment of heart function and strain imaging • 3D and 4D technology • Cardiac resynchronization therapy • Contrast studies

From Orenstein BW. Current trends in echocardiography. *SDMS News Wave.* February 2010: 1–4.[28]

TABLE 3-21	Common indications for a transthoracic echocardiogram

- Evaluate chest pain
- Evaluate and monitor progression of valvular disease
- Evaluate and assess congenital heart disease
- Assess overall function of the heart
- Heart murmur
- Evaluate for the presence of wall motion abnormalities
- Complications from a **myocardial infarction**
- **Cardiomyopathy**
- **Pericardial** disease, **pericarditis**
- Heart failure
- Tumors
- Evaluate the effectiveness of therapy and surgical interventions
- Evaluate progression of heart disease
- **Arrhythmia**

Transthoracic Echocardiograms

A TTE can be performed on both outpatients and inpatients. For this reason, echocardiograms can be completed in a physician's office, a dedicated echo lab, or in a patient's hospital room. Common indications for a TTE can be found in Table 3-21. Given the limitations of ultrasound sonography and the fact that the heart sits behind the ribs and lungs, the cardiac transducer requires a small footprint as most images are obtained between the narrow windows provided between the ribs—the **intercostal** spaces. Typically, low-frequency phased array transducers are utilized for adult TTE, with frequencies ranging between 2 and 3.5 MHz. A dedicated 2-MHz CW probe is also often utilized during the examination as well.

Generally, there are no specific patient preparation needs for the TTE exam. Patients are asked to remove clothing from the waist up. The patient is provided a gown, which can be worn open in the front or back, dependent upon the preference of the sonographer. Usually, if the gown is open in the back, the left arm is taken out, allowing the sonographer access to the patient's chest. Additional towels, sheets, or blankets may also be used to cover the patient and provide additional warmth. The ultimate goal of draping the patient should be to provide the most accurate examination while maintaining patient modesty.

Cardiac ultrasound machines are equipped with basic **electrocardiogram** (ECG or EKG) capabilities. The ECG assists with timing of events to the cardiac cycle. More about ECGs can be found in Chapter 10 and Appendix 4. Three electrodes are placed on the patient's chest—typically the regions of the left shoulder, right shoulder, and left abdomen (Fig. 3-37). Care must be taken not to place the leads in regions where the images will be acquired. Since male patients are not typically shaved prior to the placement of the electrodes, it is also important to avoid as much chest hair as possible when placing the leads on the chest, because the leads may not stick well. Your patient will thank you in the end, because this will prevent some of the discomfort when the leads must be removed after the examination. If the patient has a pacemaker, the ECG electrode should not be placed on or adjacent to the implant and should instead be relocated to another area, possibly the right abdominal region. When attaching the ECG electrodes, it is valuable to visually survey the patient's chest, noting midline scars (clue to previous cardiac surgery) or any open wounds you may wish to avoid.

For a TTE, the patient is typically in the left lateral **decubitus** position—lying on his or her left side. In addition, the left arm is raised above the patient's head or placed under his or her head for comfort, and the right arm should be placed on his or her right side. This position spreads the chest tissue and

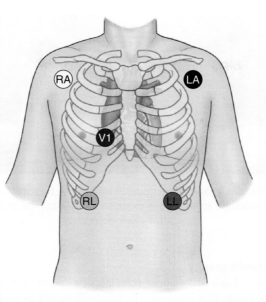

Figure 3-37. Electrode placement used in continuous electrocardiographic monitoring for the three-lead system, placement on RA, LA, and LL; four-lead system, placement on RA, LA, RL, and LL; and five-lead system, placement on RA, LA, RL, LL, and V1. *RA*, right arm; *LA*, left arm; *RL*, right leg; *LL*, left leg; *V1*, chest or precordium.

expands the rib cage, ultimately creating a better acoustic window for obtaining images. The patient will typically maintain this position for the entire exam, which may last up to 35 to 40 minutes. It may be necessary to place a wedge, towels, or several pillows behind the patient's back for support. This is especially true for patients who are sedated and unable to stay on their sides on their own.

The quality of the images is determined by the location of the heart in relation to the ribs and lungs. Several breathing techniques are employed during the examination to enhance visualization of the heart and reduce lung movement. It is important to note that patients with respiratory or heart complications may have difficulty controlling respirations.

Stress Echocardiography

SEs employ either exercise or a pharmacologic agent to increase heart rate in order to assess how the heart functions with exertion. Indications for a stress echo can be found in Table 3-22. Essentially, an **exercise stress echocardiogram** combines an exercise stress test with an echocardiogram. Exercise is completed on either a treadmill or stationary bike. If the patient is unable to perform physical stressing of the heart, then this test is not for them, and a **pharmacologic stress echocardiogram** should be considered.

TABLE 3-22	Indications for stress echocardiograms

- Assess myocardial viability
- Detect myocardial ischemia and possibility of coronary artery disease
- Evaluate valvular disease
- Assess response to therapy and procedures
- Assess response and effectiveness of medical treatment plan
- Identify abnormal arrhythmias
- Preop evaluation (more so pharmacologic)

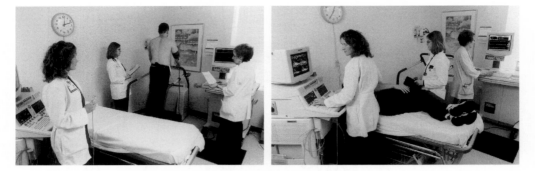

Figure 3-38. For a treadmill exercise echocardiogram, the treadmill must be located near the ultrasound machine so that post-exercise images can be acquired immediately after exercise ends.

Exercise Stress Echocardiography

The exercise SE is performed in a stress lab, an echo lab, or a doctor's office. Room layout is important especially when the treadmill is involved. The treadmill should be positioned so as to limit the number of steps to the bed (Fig. 3-38). Cables for the ECG and a blood pressure cuff should be long enough to reach from the treadmill to examining bed. When a stationary bike is utilized, there should be enough room for the ultrasound machine to be placed adjacent to the bike. Emergency equipment and a crash cart should always be located nearby.

In preparation for the procedure, the patient is typically asked to be NPO for at least four hours, though the patient may be allowed to have some water prior to the test to help avoid nausea during the exercise. All caffeinated products should be avoided for at least 12 hours prior to the test. In addition, medications such as beta blockers (unless evaluating their effects on the heart), nitrates (nitroglycerin, Isordil, etc.), carvedilol (Coreg), metoprolol (Lopressor, Toprol), propranolol (Inderal), or any other heart medications are not to be taken the day of the test. However, the ordering physician is ultimately responsible for altering any drug administration that could impact the study.

Two healthcare professionals are required to perform the stress test—the echocardiographer and another medical professional who is responsible for monitoring the patient and evaluating the symptoms. This individual can be a stress technician, a properly trained nurse, or a cardiology fellow. A physician, who is required to be present either in the room or in the immediate area, supervises the stress test.

A signed consent must be obtained prior to the start of the test. The physician explains the procedure and risks to the patient and answers any questions he or she may have. Once consent is obtained, the patient is supplied a gown and asked to remove everything from the waist up, as the heart is constantly monitored throughout the test with an ECG. In order to assure good adherence, the areas where the electrodes are attached are lightly scrubbed with a mild abrasive soap in order to clear the skin of any oils. In addition, men may also require their chest hair to be shaved. The echocardiographer must ensure that the placements of the leads do not obstruct the imaging windows. A resting ECG, heart rate, and blood pressure are taken, as well as a baseline echocardiogram. The same patient positioning as the TTE is followed.

It is best to assess the patient's ability to walk on a treadmill prior to the start of the procedure. Some patients, especially the elderly, have never walked on a treadmill and thus may find it both awkward and alarming. Therefore, demonstration of how to use a treadmill may be necessary to ease anxiety. The patient walks on the treadmill while the ECG monitors his or her heart rate. Prior to the examination, a patient-specific target heart rate is established by the physician.

As with any sonographic examination, a thorough explanation is warranted, as these procedures require the patient to move from the treadmill to the bed as quickly as possible so that the heart can be accurately assessed following exercise. Post-exercise images should be obtained within the first minute after exercise. If the stationary bike is used, the second set of images may be obtained once the patient has reached the target heart rate and is still peddling. Besides reaching target heart rate, exercise may be terminated for other reasons, including angina, dizziness, concerning ECG changes, and arrhythmias. It is important to ask the patient throughout the test how he or she is feeling.

Pharmacologic Stress Echocardiogram

The pharmacologic stress echocardiogram is performed by those patients who cannot exercise due to physical or medical limitations. A pharmacologic SE utilizes drugs such as adenosine, dipyridamole (Persantine), or dobutamine to increase blood flow to the heart, mimicking exercise. Dobutamine is probably the most widely used exercise-mimicking drug agent. An additional drug atropine is often used in conjunction with dobutamine. Atropine may be administered to augment heart rate response when the maximum dobutamine dosage has been given, though the target heart rate has not yet been achieved. Prior to the test, it is important to know if the patient has glaucoma or a symptomatic urinary obstruction as atropine cannot then be used. Patient prep is basically the same as it is for an exercise stress with the following exceptions:

- An IV is required for drug administration.
- Nothing to eat or drink at least eight to 12 hours prior.
- No caffeinated products 12 to 24 hours prior (dependent upon the drug used).
- The patient is not allowed to take beta blockers or calcium channel blockers (verapamil, diltiazem) 24 hours prior to a dobutamine stress test.
- Persantine and adenosine stress tests require some cardiac medications to be held for 72 hours; these may also include drugs for peripheral vascular disease such as Trental and Pletal.

Patient positioning for the imaging component of the test is also the same as with the exercise stress. Heart rate, blood pressure, and the ECG are monitored throughout the test. The medication is administered through an intravenous drip, and dosage is increased at regular intervals until the target heart rate is achieved or the maximum dosage of medication is met. Reaching target heart rate is considered peak stress. Once this level is achieved, the pharmacologic drip is turned off. The patient will continue to be monitored for approximately 10 to 15 minutes until heart rate returns to baseline. If the patient's heart rate does not return to a reasonable rate (less than 100 beats per minute) after a few minutes following peak stress, a reversal agent (propranolol or diltiazem) may be given.

The sensation of a high heart rate is uncomfortable for most patients. Some patients may experience side effects of the medication used. Some of these include chest pain, dizziness, headache, and nausea. If the symptoms become intolerable, significant ECG changes occur, or significant tachycardia occurs, the test may be terminated prior to peak stress. Four sets of images are acquired with the pharmacologic stress echo. The video clips are synced by the ECG and reviewed in a quad screen format for easy comparison and evaluation by the physician. The echo images are then evaluated along with the ECG and patient symptoms.

Transesophageal Echocardiography

The TEE is considered an invasive procedure. The technique dates back to the 1970s, when an M-mode tracing was obtained by inserting a transducer into a patient's esophagus.[1] Though the technique did not become popular, it did persuade the pioneers to search for a means whereby 2D images of the heart could be obtained from within the esophagus.

The patient who requires a TEE will most likely have a TTE before the examination, because many times, based on the TTE examination, a TEE will be ordered.

The patient should have nothing to eat or drink at least six hours prior to the exam. Since the TEE is considered invasive, a consent form must be signed by the patient prior to the examination and a clear explanation of possible complications provided.

Patient positioning requires that the patient be placed in left lateral decubitus with the chin tilted down toward the chest (see Fig. 1-1). If the patient has dentures, the dentures should be removed and a bite block inserted into the mouth. The patient's throat is sprayed with a numbing medicine. The patient will also be asked to wear a nasal cannula for oxygen administration. Blood pressure, heart rate, and ECG monitoring are performed throughout the test. Suction should be available during the test, and an emergency crash cart should be located nearby.

A TEE examination requires intravenous access for medication administration because sedation must be utilized. Some patients may require full anesthesia but most are put under conscious sedation with Versed, which is used to relax the patient, making him or her drowsy. Versed also allows the patient to follow instructions during the examination, though afterward, he or she typically has little recollection. Typically, there are three professionals in the examination room at the time of the test: the physician who performs the test, a properly trained nurse who monitors the patient and assists with patient care, and the echocardiographer.

For a TEE, the patient swallows a long tube similar to an endoscope. The scope, in this case, is about the width of the average index finger and lubricated to ease swallowing. The TEE transducers used today are located on the tip of the endoscope and can rotate from 0 to 180 degrees. Images acquired during a TEE have excellent resolution since the probe is located within the esophagus, thus allowing the transducer to be directed behind the heart, removing all interference from the ribs and lungs. Many TEE transducers utilize 5 MHz of frequency, but some have a range of frequencies—from 7 to 2 MHz—thereby allowing more penetration and resolution variability.

The TEE exam can be performed in any area with the appropriate equipment, including the echocardiography laboratory, heart catheterization laboratory, electrophysiology laboratory, and the operating room. During the TEE, the role of the sonographer is to assist the physician with machine operations, image optimization, and image acquisition. A TEE can be ordered on inpatients or outpatients, including patients who are considered to be critically ill. Typical indications for a TEE are found in Table 3-23.

Pediatric Echocardiography

Pediatric echocardiography can be performed on newborns, neonates, infants, and children, including adolescents up to the age of 17. Like the adult patient, pediatric patients may require a TTE or TEE. Common indications for pediatric echocardiograms can be found in Table 3-24. Pediatric imaging on newborns and infants requires higher-frequency transducers ranging from 5 to 12 MHz. Dependent upon the size of the patient, lower frequencies may be needed, ranging from 2 to 5 MHz. A dedicated 2-MHz CW transducer should also be available.

Pediatric TTEs can be performed in a physician's office, a hospital department, or an intensive care unit. Most infants can be scanned in the supine position, as many of the images in pediatric echocardiography are obtained from the abdomen and neck regions. Children and adolescents are scanned supine or in the left lateral decubitus position.

TABLE 3-23	Indications for a transesophageal echocardiogram

- Source of embolus (endocarditis, thrombus, mass)
- **Atrial fibrillation/cardioversion**
- Valvular disease/prosthetic valves
- Congenital heart disease
- Issues involving the aorta (aneurysm, dissection)
- Ablations
- Surgical monitoring/assess outcome prior to closure of the chest

TABLE 3-24	Indications for a pediatric transthoracic echocardiogram

- Congenital heart disease
- **Cyanosis**
- Acquired heart disease (cardiomyopathy, pericarditis)
- **Murmur**
- Cardiomegaly
- Arrhythmias
- Respiratory distress
- **Pulmonary hypertension**
- **Thromboembolism** (endocarditis)
- **Congestive heart failure**
- Follow-up to surgery/interventions
- Disease progression/structural growth

One challenge for pediatric imaging, as with all modalities, is patient movement. Younger children may become agitated easily, thus resulting in poor image acquisition and increased procedure time. Therefore, sedation may be required. Similar to the adult TTE, an NPO requirement is necessary, though for the infant, this could be a minimum of four hours.

Setup and administration of the pediatric TEE follow the same fundamental procedure as the adult description of the test. The shaft of the pediatric TEE probe is typically thinner than the adult probe, and the frequency range is from 3 to 7 MHz. Like the adult patient, many patients who require a TEE have already undergone a TTE. Many of the indications for a pediatric transthoracic echo apply to the pediatric TEE.

ADDITIONAL TECHNOLOGIES AND FUTURE APPLICATIONS

Sonography and the medical uses of ultrasound are constantly growing. One of the professional obligations of a sonographer is to be informed about changes that impact patient care and the uses of ultrasound in medicine. Therefore, the following section will provide an overview of other technologies, several relatively new diagnostic ultrasound uses, and potential future functions of ultrasound in medicine.

Therapeutic Ultrasound

Therapeutic ultrasound is the use of ultrasound in the healing process. In the early 1900s, Wood and Loomis reported the biologic effects of high-intensity ultrasound, leading to the evolution of therapeutic ultrasound techniques.[29] Therapeutic ultrasound is not used for imaging purposes but rather to increase the blood supply to certain areas in the body by heating the tissue, which in turn reduces healing time and provides for a quicker recovery following soft tissue damage.[29] Traditionally, qualified physicians and physical therapists utilize therapeutic ultrasound for joint injuries and muscle therapy. However, current studies have suggested that ultrasound therapy may be effective in bone fracture repair as well, though lower intensities are utilized compared to normal ultrasound therapy secondary to the potential for overheating bone tissue.[30]

High-Intensity Focused Ultrasound

High-intensity focused ultrasound (HIFU) is a technique that also heats the tissue, though the point of heating results in focal areas of tissue destruction (necrosis).[29] Basically, HIFU is a non-invasive surgical method that uses high-intensity—though focused—ultrasound to destroy tissue, called tissue ablation. Furthermore, the technique allows the physician to target a specific structure to be destroyed within the body without damaging adjacent tissue.[29] HIFU and normal sonographic techniques can be combined in one device, allowing both the realtime imaging and treatment.[29]

ExAblate therapy, mentioned earlier in this chapter, is another example of HIFU that combines MRI and HIFU to destroy the tissue of symptomatic though benign uterine leiomyomas or fibroids.[31] ExAblate is an FDA-approved procedure and offers an additional option for women who would prefer a less invasive means of fibroid treatment. HIFU is also used in the treatment of malignant tumors in the liver, prostate, and other organs, and it is currently being investigated for uses in glaucoma, thrombolysis, arterial occlusion, and drug and gene delivery.[9,29]

Contrast-Enhanced Ultrasound and Ultrasound-Guided Brachytherapy

The use of contrast in echocardiography was initially introduced in 1969 by Gramiak and Shah when they utilized an indocyanine green dye within the heart to visualize the chambers.[8] Most **contrast agents** today consist of small stabilized microbubbles of gas-liquid emulsions surrounded by either a soft or hard shell.[32] The microbubbles are typically smaller than red blood cells (RBCs), measuring between 1 and 4 μm, and are thus allowed to move through the vascular channels freely when injected into the venous system.[32] The contrast circulates throughout the body, and it enhances the echogenicity of vessels, improves tumor border recognition, and fills cardiac chambers (Figs. 3-39 and 3-40).[6]

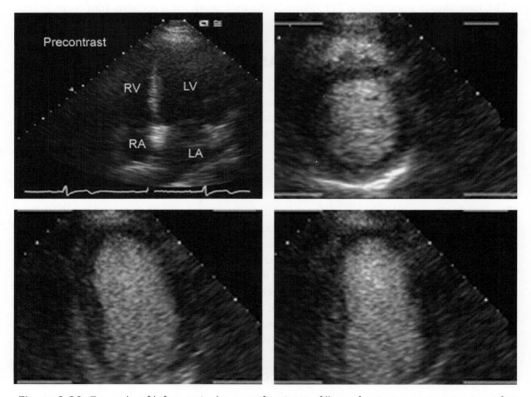

Figure 3-39. Example of left ventricular opacification or filling after intravenous injection of a contrast agent. *RV*, right ventricle; *RA*, right atrium; *LV*, left ventricle; *LA*, left atrium.

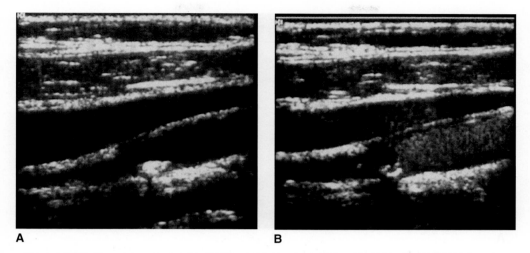

A **B**

Figure 3-40. Carotid artery occlusion. An initial image of the carotid bulb (A) demonstrates an echogenic plaque. After injection of contrast (B), contrast enhancement of flow is identified in the functional lumen of the common carotid artery, but no enhanced flow is seen distal to the plaque.

Contrast-enhanced ultrasound is employed in echocardiography, and other clinical application studies are currently underway in the US and other countries. Several unique contrast imaging techniques, referred to as ultrasound molecular imaging, have shown some promise in trials for early cancer detection, tumor characterization, guided cancer treatment therapies or guided chemotherapy, and gene therapies.[32] One working theory suggests that microbubbles can be utilized to administer cancer treatment by permeating the cancer with microbubbles containing chemotherapy and then bursting them by increasing the ultrasound power, resulting in targeted treatment.[32]

Ultrasound-guided brachytherapy is another technique used to treat cancers under ultrasound guidance. However, brachytherapy is an invasive procedure that utilizes sonography to administer radioactive material close to or within a cancerous tumor for treatment. One of the more common applications of brachytherapy is for the treatment of prostate cancer in which radioactive seeds are placed into the prostate gland. Researchers are finding other applications for brachytherapy, including 3D ultrasound technology integration treatment for other types of tumors as well, including rectal and anal cancers.[33]

Ultrasound Elastography

Ultrasound elastography (UE) has been used in sonography for several years now as an add-on to routine protocols. Though the physics and instrumentation behind UE are multifaceted, the theory is straightforward. Essentially, the tissue that comprises a malignant tumor tends to be stiffer compared to the tissue that comprises a benign tumor. UE evaluates a mass based on its stiffness and ultimately provides a prediction as to if the mass is more likely malignant or benign. The image obtained is referred to as an **elastogram** (Fig. 3-41).

Nonetheless, there are two fundamental ways in which UE can be performed. First, the manual technique, which is the older method, is performed by the sonographer. The sonographer applies manual pressure with the transducer to the suspicious area. The image provides a color spectrum, with certain colors indicating the stiffness properties of the mass. Based on the color indicator, an interpreting physician can predict with some accuracy whether or not a mass is more likely malignant or benign.

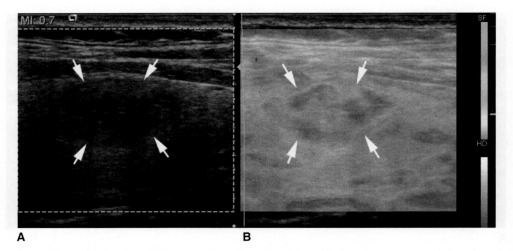

Figure 3-41. Elastography scan of a thyroid nodule *(arrows)*.* A. Representative grayscale image of a hypoechoic indeterminate nodule. B. Color depiction of the strain results. Correlation with the color scale on the right reveals that this nodule is stiffer than the rest of the thyroid gland, which theoretically increases the risk of malignancy. *Images in color are provided for the student online in student resources.

The second and most current method of UE is referred to as **acoustic radiation force impulse elastography** (ARFI). With ARFI, the ultrasound probe provides realtime B-mode imaging and focused pressure using shear-waves to compress the tissue of concern.[34] ARFI removes the variability of applied pressure of the manual technique between sonographers. Elastography has proven to be highly effective for differentiating breast, thyroid, prostate, lymph nodes, MSK, and pancreas tumors, with the most current research scrutinizing the accuracy of the technique in other organs, such as for the diagnosis of fibrosis and cirrhosis of the liver.[35] The software and instrumentation are not inherent in all ultrasound machines, nor is the technique utilized at all institutions.

Fusion Imaging

For correlation between imaging modalities, the high-quality images and specific strengths of the different modalities can be overlain and exploited, a technique referred to as fusion imaging or **hybrid imaging** (Fig. 3-42). Fusion imaging allows the ultrasound machine to communicate with the PACS system of the institution to call up MRI or CT scans performed previously. The MRI images can be "fused" or superimposed over the sonographic images in order to take advantage of the unique information provided by both modalities. A tracking system allows the MRI or CT image to move on the screen as the operator moves the transducer. The images stay in sync, permitting the studies to either overlap or be placed side by side. For example, if a liver lesion is visualized better with MRI, but the lesion is adjacent to the diaphragm in close proximity to the lung, the physician may prefer the realtime nature of ultrasound over the static image of MRI. With fusion, the physician may superimpose the MRI and the sonographic image, allowing for more accurate sampling of the tissue and also reducing the risk of complications.

Intravascular Ultrasound

Intravascular ultrasound (IVUS) is performed with a miniature ultrasound probe placed on a catheter and inserted into the circulatory system (Fig. 3-43). IVUS is used at the time of vascular intervention to identify vascular abnormalities, including plaque development (Fig. 3-44).[36] Though the

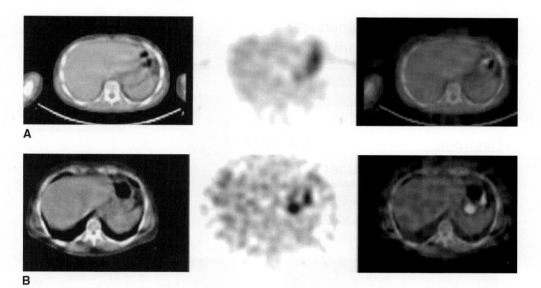

Figure 3-42. An example of hybrid or fusion imaging.* This study combined SPECT (nuclear medicine) and CT. *Images in color are provided for the student online in student resources.

technique is typically performed using 2D imaging, current research is geared toward improving 3D imaging during IVUS.[36] 3D IVUS techniques are suggested to improve diagnosis and treatment for vascular disease.[36]

Automated Ultrasound

As mentioned previously in the breast section of this chapter, mammography has limited accuracy at detecting abnormalities in dense breast tissue, making sonography an efficient supplement to screening mammography. Taking ultrasound breast imaging toward a more mechanized approach is a technique referred to as **automated breast ultrasound** (ABUS). Though a sonographer is still required to perform the pre-procedural setup of the examination, a computer system mechanically steers the transducer and obtains sonographic images of the entire breast, ultimately reconstructing those images into 3D representations for interpretation.[37] Diagnosis can then further be improved when the images are evaluated with a **computer-aided diagnosis** (CAD) **system**. A CAD system provides a computer analysis of diagnostic images. Though a CAD system is often used by some mammography units, a CAD has been proposed to read the ABUS images as well.[37]

Though other automated measurement software currently exists in vascular and echocardiography, there are other proposed and working automated techniques in sonography, such as **automated biometry**, in which the machine automatically obtains biometric measurements of the fetus. The research has proven thus far that automated biometry in obstetrics increases accuracy while reducing scan time.[38]

Focused Assessment with Sonography for Trauma

Although CT may be the preferred method of imaging for diagnosing abdominal trauma, **focused assessment with sonography for trauma** (FAST) scanning offers the emergency room physician a relatively quick and sensitive method of determining if there is evidence of intra-abdominal trauma

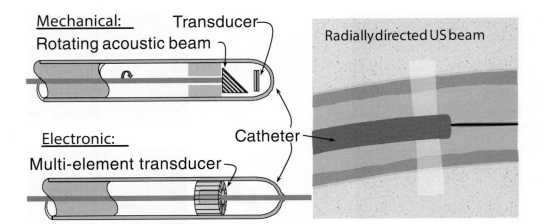

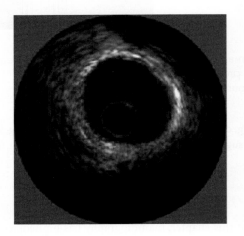

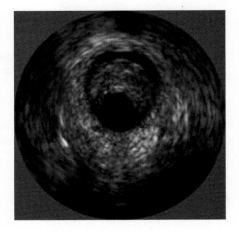

Normal vasculature   Elliptical stenosis

Figure 3-43. Intravascular ultrasound. Catheter-mounted transducer arrays provide an acoustic analysis of the vessel lumen and wall from the inside out. Images show a normal vessel lumen (**lower left**) and reduced luminal stenosis and plaque buildup (**lower right**).

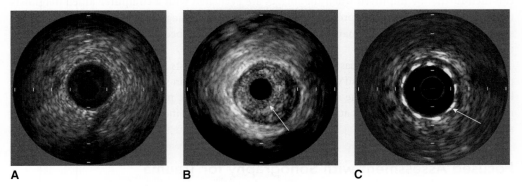

A   B   C

Figure 3-44. Intravascular ultrasound. A. Normal coronary artery. B. Atherosclerotic plaque inside coronary artery with notable plaque (*arrow*). C. Coronary artery after stent placement (*arrow*).

without the patient leaving the trauma unit. Prior to FAST scanning, the only other alternatives for diagnosing blunt abdominal trauma were open surgery, deep peritoneal lavage, or CT, all of which are either extremely invasive or, in the case of CT, not always optimal for the critically injured patient. FAST scanning is the scanning of the liver and spleen for laceration as well as the midline and the four quadrants of the abdomen in search of free peritoneal fluid, ascites. In addition, the heart may be scanned for a quick evaluation of **pericardial tamponade**. Though sonographers may be involved, the FAST examination is often performed by a physician in the emergency room, utilizing a small lightweight ultrasound machine.

Miniaturization

Most ultrasound machines that you will encounter in clinical are rather bulky. Through the years, ultrasound machines have become much smaller and lighter, examples of **miniaturization** (Fig. 3-45). Ultrasound technology has certainly come a long way since the B-52 gun turret. With a growing trend toward the use of proper **ergonomics** in sonography, the progression was both imminent and necessary. Most machines now have higher-definition monitors, an intuitive keyboard, and smaller computer system housing, all geared toward both advancing the technology and simultaneously minimizing chronic workplace injuries caused by awkward ultrasound machinery with cumbersome transducers. Currently, ultrasound machines can be the size of a laptop computer, and there is now technology that is even compatible with smartphones.

Wireless Technology: It's Here!

Since ultrasound was invented, the cord connecting the transducer to the machine has been a nuisance for many sonographers. Besides being heavy and disruptive to proper ergonomics, it is prone to contamination by body fluids, floor dirt, and other substances, which is good for neither the operator nor the patient. Cords also have the propensity to get crushed by careless sonographers, causing degradation of the image and costly repairs. Transducer cords also serve as a tether, forcing the sonographer to always be in close proximity to the ultrasound machine.

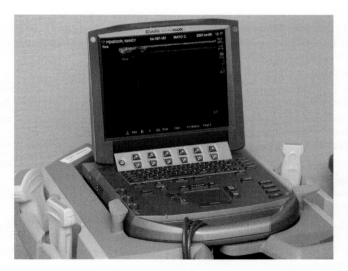

Figure 3-45. SonoSite is one company that produces smaller, more portable ultrasound machines.

Years ago, a wireless, voice-based system was developed for taking images from the side of the bed opposite the machine in an attempt to eliminate reaching across the patient. Although the ergonomic considerations behind the thought process were excellent, the technology ultimately floundered because it still required the transducer cord. In 2012, Siemens Healthcare introduced the ACUSON Freestyle ultrasound system that featured a **wireless transducer**, eliminating the impediment of cables in ultrasound imaging.[39]

Although commercially available, it is too early in development to know if the technology will provide the optimal image quality of a corded machine. Nevertheless, the future of wireless transducer technology is both exciting and promising for medicine and for the next generation of sonographers.

SUMMARY

This chapter provided you with plenty of information regarding your chosen specialty in sonography, including some historical foundations of our profession and the future possibilities. However, it is just a starting point for you to begin your studies. It should be apparent from the reading that our profession is constantly growing. One vital role of the sonographer is to maintain a thorough knowledge base regarding the sonography profession. Knowing that the medical uses of ultrasound are constantly evolving should provide you with both enthusiasm about your opportunities going forward and reassurance that you have chosen a wise career path.

REFERENCES

1. Armstrong WF, Ryan T. *Feigenbaum's Echocardiography*. 7th ed. Philadelphia, PA: Lippincott Williams & Wilkins; 2010.
2. Gong sound healing. Pythagoras. Accessed January 21, 2015 from http://gongsoundhealing.com/sound-therapy/pythagoras/
3. Brainy quote. Pythagoras quotes. Accessed January 21, 2015 from http://www.brainyquote.com/quotes/authors/p/pythagoras.html#OuRoCag6gVtiCFeT.99
4. Hagen-Ansert SL. *Textbook of Diagnostic Sonography*. 7th ed. St. Louis, MO: Elsevier; 2012.
5. Explore sound. What is acoustics? Accessed January 21, 2015 from http://www.exploresound.org/home/what-is-acoustics/
6. Kremkau FW. *Diagnostic Ultrasound: Principles and Instruments*. 7th ed. St. Louis, MO: Saunders Elsevier; 2006.
7. Penny SM, et al. *Examination Review for Ultrasound: Sonographic Principles & Instrumentation (SPI)*. Philadelphia, PA: Lippincott Williams & Wilkins; 2011.
8. Myer, RA (2004). History of ultrasound in cardiology. *J Ultrasound Med* 23:1–11.
9. Aptel F, Lafon C. Therapeutic applications of ultrasound in ophthalmology. *Int J Hyperther* [serial online]. 2012;28(4):405–418. Available from: Academic Search Complete, Ipswich, MA. Accessed May 20, 2014.
10. Sound ergonomics: about us. Joan P. Baker. Accessed January 22, 2015 from http://www.soundergonomics.com/information/about-us.html
11. Orenstein BW. Current trends in abdominal sonography. *SDMS News Wave*, March 2010:1–4.
12. AIUM Keepsake Fetal Imaging statement. Retrieved January 22, 2015 from http://www.aium.org/resources/viewStatement.aspx?id=31
13. Woo J. *A short history of the development of ultrasound in obstetrics and gynecology*. 2002. Retrieved January 25, 2015 from http://www.ob-ultrasound.net/history1.html
14. AIUM Practice Guideline for the Performance of an Ultrasound Examination of the Abdomen and/or Retroperitoneum. Retrieved January 25, 2015 from http://www.aium.org/resources/guidelines/abdominal.pdf
15. AIUM Practice Guideline for the Performance of Scrotal Ultrasound Examinations. Retrieved January 25, 2015 from http://www.aium.org/resources/guidelines/scrotal.pdf

16. AIUM Practice Guideline for the Performance of a Thyroid and Parathyroid Ultrasound Examination. Retrieved January 25, 2015 from http://www.aium.org/resources/guidelines/thyroid.pdf

17. AIUM Practice Guideline for the Performance of Ultrasound Evaluation of the Prostate (and Surrounding Structures). Retrieved January 25, 2015 from http://www.aium.org/resources/guidelines/prostate.pdf

18. Kawamura D, Lunsford B. *Diagnostic Medical Sonography: Abdomen and Superficial Structures.* 3rd ed. Philadelphia, PA: Lippincott Williams & Wilkins; 2012.

19. ACR practice parameter for the performance of a breast ultrasound examination. Retrieved January 25, 2015 from http://www.acr.org/~/media/ACR/Documents/PGTS/guidelines/US_Breast.pdf

20. AIUM Practice Guideline for the Performance of Neurosonography in Neonates and Infants. Retrieved January 25, 2015 from http://www.aium.org/resources/guidelines/neurosonography.pdf

21. AIUM Practice Guidelines for the Performance of a Musculoskeletal Ultrasound Examination. Retrieved January 25, 2015 from http://www.aium.org/resources/guidelines/musculoskeletal.pdf

22. ARDMS Pediatric Sonography. Retrieved January 25, 2015 from http://www.ardms.org/credentials_examinations/pediatric-sonography

23. AIUM Practice Guidelines for the Performance of Ultrasound of the Female Pelvis. Retrieved January 25, 2015 from http://www.aium.org/resources/guidelines/femalePelvis.pdf

24. AIUM Practice Guidelines for the Performance of Sonohysterography. Retrieved January 25, 2015 from http://www.aium.org/resources/guidelines/sonohysterography.pdf

25. Orenstein BW. Current trends in OB/GYN sonography. *SDMS News Wave*, April 2010:1–4.

26. AIUM Practice Guidelines for the Performance of Obstetric Ultrasound Examinations. Retrieved January 25, 2015 from http://www.aium.org/resources/guidelines/obstetric.pdf

27. AIUM Practice Guidelines for the Performance of Fetal Echocardiography. Retrieved January 25, 2015 from http://www.aium.org/resources/guidelines/fetalEcho.pdf

28. Orenstein BW. Current trends in echocardiography. *SDMS News Wave*. February 2010: 1–4.

29. Cordeiro E, et al. High-intensity focused ultrasound (HIFU) for definitive treatment of prostate cancer. *BJU Int* [serial online]. 2012;110(9):1228–1242. Available from: Academic Search Complete, Ipswich, MA. Accessed May 20, 2014.

30. Warden S, et al. Ultrasound produced by a conventional therapeutic ultrasound unit accelerates fracture repair. *Phys Ther* [serial online] 2006;86(8):1118–1127. Available from: CINAHL with Full Text, Ipswich, MA. Accessed May 20, 2014.

31. ExAblate®2000 System – P040003. Retrieved January 25, 2015 from http://www.fda.gov/MedicalDevices/ProductsandMedicalProcedures/DeviceApprovalsandClearances/Recently-ApprovedDevices/ucm080704.htm

32. Kaneko OF, Willmann JK. Ultrasound for molecular imaging and therapy in cancer. *Quant Imaging Med Surg* 2012;2(2): 87–97.

33. Christensen A, et al. Three-dimensional endoluminal ultrasound-guided interstitial brachytherapy in patients with anal cancer. *Acta Radiol* [serial online]. 2008;49(2): 132–137. Available from: Academic Search Complete, Ipswich, MA. Accessed May 21, 2014.

34. irli R, et al. Liver elastography for the diagnosis of portal hypertension in patients with liver cirrhosis. *Med Ultrason* [serial online]. 2012;14(3): 225–230. Available from: Academic Search Complete, Ipswich, MA. Accessed May 21, 2014.

35. Sandulescu L, et al. Real-time elastography applications in liver pathology between expectations and results. *J Gastrointestin Liver Dis* [serial online]. 2013;22(2): 221–227. Available from: Academic Search Complete, Ipswich, MA. Accessed May 21, 2014.

36. Rim Y, et al. Volumetric three-dimensional intravascular ultrasound visualization using shape-based nonlinear interpolation. *Biomed Eng Online* [serial online]. 2013;12(1): 1–15. Available from: Academic Search Complete, Ipswich, MA. Accessed May 21, 2014.

37. Jung Min C, et al. Breast cancers initially detected by hand-held ultrasound: detection performance of radiologists using automated breast ultrasound data. *Acta Radiol* [serial online]. 2011;52(1): 8–14. Available from: Academic Search Complete, Ipswich, MA. Accessed May 21, 2014.

38. Espinoza J, et al. Does the use of automated fetal biometry improve clinical workflow efficiency? *J Ultrasound Med* 2013;32:847–850.

39. Siemens H. Siemens Showcases World's First Wireless Ultrasound System at RSNA 2012. *Business Wire (English)* [serial online]. November 2012; 11. Available from: Regional Business News, Ipswich, MA. Accessed May 21, 2014.

Thinking Critically

1. Research the advantages and disadvantages of the automated technique used in sonography.
2. Research new technologies in your specialty, and share your findings with your classmates.
3. Recall your early research and thoughts about your specialty before you entered sonography school. Was there any insight about your specialty that this chapter offered of which you were not aware? If so, discuss these with your classmates.
4. Is 3D sonography more advantageous than 2D for some applications? Research the use of 3D technology in your specialty, and share your findings with your classmates.
5. Research how Doppler technology is used in other fields. For example, how is Doppler used in meteorology? What other occupations use the Doppler effect?
6. Recall ultrasound transducers use lead zirconate titanate to create the piezoelectric effect. What is lead zirconate titanate? Does it naturally occur, or is it synthetic? Are there any other elements that produce the piezoelectric effect?

Chapter 3
Review Questions

1. **What instrument uses ultrasound to detect flaws in metals?**
   a. Hydrophone
   b. Doppler transducer
   c. Reflectoscope
   d. Continuous-wave transducer

2. **What instrument was designed to be used underwater for recording or listening to underwater sound?**
   a. Hydrophone
   b. Spectral transducer
   c. Reflectoscope
   d. Realtime scanner

3. **What mode displays the depth of the returning echo represented on the x-axis and the strength (amplitude) of the reflector represented along the y-axis?**
   a. B-mode
   b. A-mode
   c. C-mode
   d. M-mode

4. **What technology is used to analyze the relative stiffness of a mass?**
   a. Sonohysterography
   b. Plethysmography
   c. Photoplethysmography
   d. Elastography

5. **Triplex imaging includes which of the following?**
   a. A-mode, B-mode, and M-mode
   b. B-mode, spectral Doppler, and color Doppler
   c. M-mode, B-mode, and color Doppler
   d. Spectral Doppler, power Doppler, and B-mode

6. **Which testing method utilizes information gathered from one area of the body to predict disease in another part of the body?**
   a. Indirect
   b. Direct
   c. Coherent
   d. Incoherent

7. **A technology that uses a computer system to obtain measurement of images, such as fetal biometry, is said to be**
   a. superior.
   b. mechanical.
   c. automated.
   d. direct.

8. **What is an alteration in the normal structure or number of a chromosome?**
   a. Congenital defect
   b. Fetal aberration
   c. Chromosomal anomaly
   d. Congenital anomaly

9. **What mode captures the movement of structures along a single scan line represented over time?**
   a. B-mode
   b. C-mode
   c. A-mode
   d. M-mode

10. **Which of the following is not considered a medium through which sound can travel?**
    a. Vacuum
    b. Solid
    c. Liquid
    d. Gas

11. **Who has been referred to as the "father of ultrasound?"**
    a. Doppler
    b. Spallanzani
    c. Boethius
    d. da Vinci

12. **What is the most common element or crystal used within the ultrasound transducer?**
    a. Copper titanate
    b. Lead iron titanate
    c. Iron copper titanate
    d. Lead zirconate titanate

13. **Who established the pebble theory?**
    a. Doppler
    b. Spallanzani
    c. Boethius
    d. da Vinci

14. What technology does sonography assist in administering radioactive materials close to or within a cancerous tumor?
    a. Fusion imaging
    b. Hybrid imaging
    c. Ultrasound-guided brachytherapy
    d. Therapeutic ultrasound

15. Who first recognized the frequency shift that is created when sound impinges upon a moving object?
    a. Christian Doppler
    b. Robert Boyle
    c. Jacques Currie
    d. Charles Langevin

16. What is the term for an abnormality with which someone is born?
    a. Chromosomal retardation
    b. Congenital anomaly
    c. Chromosomal fluctuation
    d. Fetal karyotyping

17. Which of the following would not be an effective stand-off device?
    a. Gel pad
    b. Balloon
    c. Mound of gel
    d. Bag of saline

18. What ultrasound mode do we use today to acquire routine grayscale images?
    a. Doppler
    b. B-mode
    c. A-mode
    d. M-mode

19. What type of scanner allows for constant visual imaging of anatomy as if one were watching a movie?
    a. A-mode
    b. Continuous-wave
    c. Realtime
    d. M-mode

20. Who was the first to use diagnostic ultrasound in the United States?
    a. Christian Doppler
    b. Joan Baker
    c. Jeffrey W. Penny
    d. George Ludwig

4

Professional Environment, Leadership, and Career Establishment

CHAPTER OBJECTIVES

- Explore the professional environment of the sonographer, including academic accreditation, certification organizations, and professional membership societies.
- Determine the value of leadership, and appreciate that we are all leaders in some way.
- Assess various job opportunities for sonographers.
- Work toward career goals and career establishment.

KEY TERMS

360-degree feedback – form of professional feedback in which both the employee is evaluated by the leader and the leader is evaluated by the employee

Academic accreditation – an effort to assess the quality of institutions, programs, and services, measuring them against agreed-upon standards and thereby assuring that they meet those standards

Advanced cardiovascular sonographer – ASE-proposed cardiovascular sonographer; mid-level provider occupation

Advanced practice sonographer – SDMS-proposed medical sonographer; mid-level provider occupation

American Institute of Ultrasound in Medicine – multidisciplinary membership organization that includes all areas of sonographic practice involved in the establishment of standards and practices

American Society of Echocardiography – national membership organization for echocardiographers

Autocratic leadership style – leadership style in which the leader gives orders to followers and is the ultimate decision maker for the group

Cardiovascular Credentialing International – credential-granting organization for both cardiac and vascular specialists

Continuing medical education – educational credits required to maintain certification in a medical profession; can be obtained in various manners, including reading CME articles, attending lectures, and publishing

Followership – the act of following a leader

Invasive procedures – a diagnostic or therapeutic medical procedure that requires the use of a medical instrument that must either break the skin or be inserted into a body cavity

Laboratory accreditation – a method of measuring quality for imaging laboratories and specialties

Leadership – the ability to influence others to accomplish a specific goal

National certification – the initial recognition of an individual who satisfies certain standards within a profession

Nuchal translucency – a region in the posterior fetal neck that can be measured during a sonogram between 11 and 14 gestational weeks; thickening of this area has been linked with fetal heart and chromosomal defects

Online networking – the online exchange of information or services among individuals, groups, and institutions

Personal networking – the face-to-face exchange of information or services among individuals, groups, and institutions

Professional development – knowledge and additional skills gained by an employee for either professional or personal growth

Recertification – the process of maintaining certification in sonography by taking additional examinations on a scheduled basis

Research sonographer – a registered, experienced sonographer who is involved in medical research

Servant leadership – a leader who not only works collaboratively with employees to make the best decisions possible but furthermore places the needs of others before his or her own

Social networking – the face-to-face or electronic exchange of information or services among individuals, groups, and institutions

Society of Vascular Ultrasound – a national membership organization for physicians, vascular technologists, students, and other cardiac and vascular professionals

Sonography manager – a sonographer who is placed in a leadership position who has the power to make departmental decisions and who works closely with the administration of an institution

Specialties – areas of sonographic expertise (e.g., adult echocardiography, abdomen, vascular)

Staff sonographer – sonographers who work on the front lines serving patients and performing sonographic examinations on a daily basis

Stewardship – to help those served to grow as individuals, reach autonomy, and produce to their full potential

Transactional leader – a leader who guides and motivates followers to achieve the organizational goals and the specific goals of a department or an institution through a system of rewards and punishment

Transformational leader – a leader who exhibits charisma and offers inspiration for followers

Ultrasound practitioner – a proposed occupation for advanced sonographers in which the sonographer would both perform and interpret ultrasound procedures in a primary or specialty care setting

Ultrasound radiologist assistant – a proposed occupation for advanced sonographers that would allow sonographers to work as a link between the interpreting physician and sonographer to refine sonography reports and train residents

INTRODUCTION

In the previous chapters, the discussion was focused on the clinical functions of the sonographer and the primary concern of providing competent patient care. In this chapter, the focus will shift toward the professional environment in which a sonographer practices. There are many opportunities for you to make your mark on the profession and to leave a legacy of excellence behind for future generations. As you progress through the process of becoming a registered sonographer, try to remember that sonographers have to continually enhance their knowledge in order to adjust to an evolving healthcare field. This chapter will provide you with an overview of our strong professional community and solidify your enthusiasm about the career opportunities that exist within your chosen profession.

PROFESSIONAL ENVIRONMENT

Though the role for student sonographers is limited in the clinical setting, once you have graduated, a world of opportunity awaits you. The sonographer exists within a thriving community of enthusiastic healthcare professionals. It is a profession in which you can choose to make a personal difference and in which your career progression is up to you. The following sections will provide an overview of the professional environment for sonographers, including **academic accreditation**, professional organizations, **national certification**, and **laboratory accreditation**. Students, educators, and sonographers have the option to join many professional organizations, and membership is an invaluable means by which a sonographer maintains competence and can be prepared to adjust to the ever-changing healthcare environment and the subsequent demands of an evolving career.

Academic Accreditation (CAAHEP, JRC-DMS, JRC-CVT)

Academic accreditation is a significant identifier in education because it "is an effort to assess the quality of institutions, programs, and services, measuring them against agreed upon standards and thereby assuring that they meet those standards."[1] Consequently, the administration of an educational institution and those educators operating a sonography program within that institution could choose to pursue national accreditation in order to meet specific quality expectations of the sonography profession. The distinction of being accredited demonstrates the program's desire to maintain high standards and to graduate exceptional entry-level sonographers.

National accreditation is granted through the Commission on Accreditation of Allied Health Education Programs (CAAHEP). CAAHEP is the organization that establishes educational standards by which many different allied health programs are reviewed. The review process is exceedingly rigorous and undertaken by the Joint Review Committee on Education in Diagnostic Medical Sonography (JRC-DMS). Thus, CAAHEP accredits programs based upon the recommendation of the JRC-DMS. Staff members of the JRC-DMS, who are often other educators or professionals in sonography, review program-specific materials and personally visit the educational institutions before accreditation is granted or denied. As a student and eventually a sonographer, you may be asked questions by the JRC-DMS team during an accreditation site visit at your school or hospital. Accreditation can be obtained for either five or ten years, while a substantial fee and annual reporting are required to maintain accreditation.

Similar to the function of the JRC-DMS, the Joint Review Committee on Education in Cardiovascular Technology (JRC-CVT) makes accreditation recommendation for cardiovascular technology programs to CAAHEP.

Sound Off

The distinction of being accredited demonstrates the program's desire to maintain high standards and to graduate exceptional entry-level sonographers.

Professional Organizations (SDMS, SVU, ASE, SOPE, AIUM)

Professional organizations in sonography provide the sonographer with both a means by which the sonographer can receive the latest information about his or her occupation and the opportunity to make a personal impact on the profession. There are both state-level and national-level societies that sonographers may actively join. Some societies, like the North Carolina Ultrasound Society and the Midwest Society of Diagnostic Ultrasound, exist on a state or regional level. These smaller-membership societies offer continuing medical education (CME) opportunities for sonographers in resident and neighboring states.

Sound Off

Professional organizations in sonography provide the sonographer with both a means by which the sonographer can receive the latest information about his or her occupation and the opportunity to make a personal impact on the profession.

On a nationwide level, the Society of Diagnostic Medical Sonography (SDMS), founded in 1970, is a national membership organization for all **specialties** in sonography. It consists of students, sonographers, physicians, researchers, and other sonography-associated practitioners. The SDMS provides benefits to its members, including an annual national meeting where CME credits can be obtained. Additionally, the SDMS provides online resources for CME, and a professional journal—the *Journal of Diagnostic Medical Sonography* (*JDMS*)—that includes CME articles and other peer-reviewed manuscripts. The *JDMS* is published quarterly, and both sonographers and sonography students are encouraged to submit original materials for possible publication. There are multiple other benefits for SDMS members, including scholarships for students through the SDMS Foundation, optional professional liability insurance, medical insurance, educational resources, CME tracking, and legislative advocacy. Students can join the SDMS for a reduced membership fee.

Similar to the SDMS, the **Society of Vascular Ultrasound** (SVU) is a national membership organization for physicians, vascular technologists, students, and other cardiac and vascular professionals. The SVU provides multiple benefits to its members as well, including a professional journal, the *Journal of Vascular Ultrasound* (*JVU*). The *JVU* is published quarterly and includes CME articles and other peer-reviewed manuscripts related to vascular and cardiac imaging. There are local chapters of the SVU, and the society also offers monthly webinars, educational resources including a national annual meeting, scholarships, and legislative advocacy like the SDMS. Students can join the SVU for a reduced membership fee.

The **American Society of Echocardiography** (ASE) is a national membership organization with many of the same benefits for echocardiographers as the SDMS and the SVU. The ASE publishes a journal also, the *Journal of the American Society of Echocardiography* (*JASE*). The *JASE* plays a vital role in disseminating information to both sonographers and cardiologists, providing both peer-reviewed original research articles and CME articles for credits. The society offers online articles from the *JASE*, webinars, other educational resources including a national annual meeting, and scholarships through the ASE Foundation. Students can join the ASE for a reduced membership fee. Like the ASE, the Society of Pediatric Echocardiography (SOPE) provides CME through various means and clinical practice updates in pediatric and fetal echocardiography for its membership.

The **American Institute of Ultrasound in Medicine** (AIUM) is a multidisciplinary membership organization that includes all areas of sonographic practice. The AIUM primary goal is "advancing the safe and effective use of ultrasound in medicine through professional and public education, research, development of guidelines, and accreditation."[2] The AIUM is similar to the SDMS, SVU, and ASE, providing membership benefits. However, the AIUM also establishes practice guidelines for each specialty and makes official statements on behalf of the profession on a range of issues, including safe ultrasound practice techniques and reaffirming declarations regarding the safety and potential biologic effects of ultrasound. The AIUM has a national meeting, offers CME, and publishes the *Journal of Ultrasound in Medicine* (*JUM*). The *JUM* includes peer-reviewed professional journal articles and CME articles as well. Students are allowed to join the AIUM for reduced rates.

National Certification (ARDMS, CCI, ARRT)

Often recognized as the standard in national certification for sonographers, the American Registry of Diagnostic Medical Sonography (ARDMS) is an organization that offers certification examinations for all sonography specialties: registered diagnostic medical sonographer (RDMS), registered diagnostic cardiac sonographer (RDCS), and registered vascular technologist (RVT). The ARDMS is nationally recognized, so credentials are portable across state borders. For one to attempt the certification examinations, the ARDMS has established distinct pathways for candidates, which includes documented competence in both didactic and clinical training.

The pathways for each specialty are provided in Figure 4-1. It is important to note that the Sonography Principles and Instrumentation (SPI) examination only has to be passed once by qualified candidates and not for every specialty one chooses to pursue. That is to say, there is only one physics examination—the SPI. If you choose to become certified in additional areas, there is no need to take any other additional physics certification examination. At publication, the physics examination costed $200, while the specialty examinations costed $250. Of course, these prices can change at any time.

The ARDMS SPI examination can now be taken after one completes an approved physics class. Furthermore, students in accredited programs are allowed to take specialty examinations 60 days prior to graduation through the ARDMS, though graduation is required to receive credentials. Not included in chart format is the new musculoskeletal sonography (MSK) certification examination offered by the ARDMS. For the MSK exam, there are explicit clinical prerequisites that must also be accomplished before a candidate is eligible to take the examination, and for sonographers, the examination cost is currently $450. At publication, the ARDMS has established a pediatric sonography certification examination as well.

Sound Off

The SPI examination can now be taken after one completes a physics class. Furthermore, students in accredited programs are allowed to take specialty examinations 60 days prior to graduation through the ARDMS, though graduation is required to receive credentials.

Cardiovascular Credentialing International (CCI) is another credentialing organization for both cardiac and vascular specialists. CCI offers examinations aimed at cardiovascular technology with certifications including registered cardiac sonographer (RCS) and registered vascular specialist (RVS). Similar to the ARDMS, CCI has prerequisite requirement for examinations, a strict code of ethics, and high standards for candidates. However, CCI, unlike the ARDMS, provides one examination for each cardiac and vascular specialty, while the examinations include both specialty information and physics. CCI examinations costed $350 at publication.

The American Registry of Radiologic Technologists (ARRT) offers credentialing examinations for sonographers as well. The ARRT has long been the standard in certification for radiographers and other imaging modality specialists, such as CT, MRI, and nuclear medicine technologists. For sonography, the ARRT offers both primary and post-primary certification in sonography. The general sonography exam is formatted to include ultrasound physics, abdomen, small parts, obstetrics, and gynecology. Once passed, the individual obtains the credentials RT (S). The ARRT also offers certification in vascular sonography, RT (VS), and breast sonography, RT (BS).

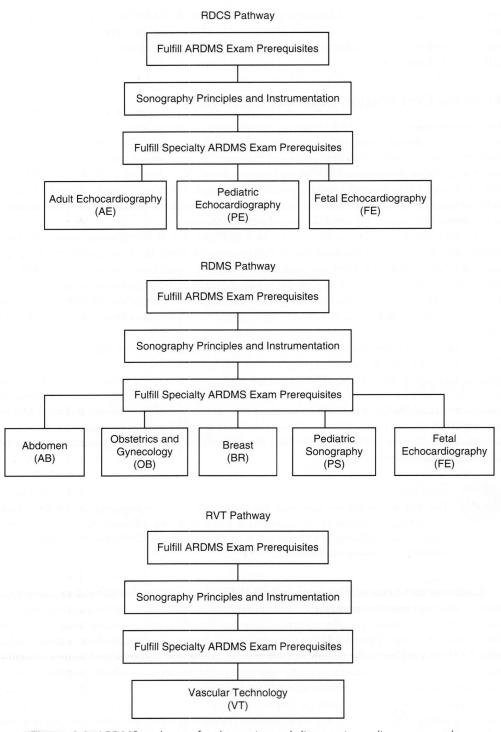

Figure 4-1. ARDMS pathways for the registered diagnostic cardiac sonographer (RDCS), registered diagnostic medical sonographer (RDMS), and registered vascular technologist (RVT).

Some states require licensure. For example, Oregon, New Mexico, West Virginia, and New Jersey currently require both national certification and state licensure. Legislation on the state level encourages standards and further emphasizes accountability. Find out if your state requires licensure, and if so, learn more about the process before you graduate. Additionally, there are other certifications, such as **nuchal translucency**, cervical assessment, and **invasive procedures** for obstetric sonographers through the Fetal Medicine Foundation (FMF).[3] FMF offers training modules and other resources for sonographers who would like to gain further explicit certifications in obstetrics.

Maintaining Certification

The process of maintaining certification is accomplished by obtaining **continuing medical education** (CME) credits. Though the requirements may differ between certification agencies, the ARDMS requires that sonographers obtain 30 ARDMS-accepted CME credits within a three-year period—triennium—following initial certification. Sonographers can obtain CMEs through various means including attending meetings, successfully passing additional certification exams, and publishing original academic papers.[4] There has been discussion in recent years regarding sonographer **recertification**. The ARDMS currently notes that credentials will be valid for 10 years, and recertification will be required for each specialty (AB, OB, AE, etc.). Currently, proposed recertification will be maintained by taking additional online examinations based on the number of current certifications of a sonographer. There is no recertification proposed for the physics examination. Thus, for every specialty that a sonographer has, he or she must recertify through additional testing on a scheduled basis—every 10 years. The recertification process begins in 2019.[5]

Laboratory Accreditation

Laboratory accreditation for vascular testing is through the Intersocietal Commission for the Accreditation of Vascular Laboratories (ICAVL), while echocardiography is granted through the Intersocietal Accreditation Commission (IAC) of Echocardiography. The American College of Radiology (ACR) and the AIUM are also involved with accreditation of ultrasound practices. The ICAVL, IAC, ACR, and AIUM accreditation processes are rigorous. However, like certification for individuals, accreditation for laboratories and sonography departments provides a standard of practice that enhances patient care and ensures a high level of uniformity between examinations.

LEADERSHIP ROLES IN SONOGRAPHY

The previous section highlights the need for appropriate **leadership** in our profession. But as a student, you may be looking at this section and wondering why an introductory book to sonography would include a section on leadership. It is simple; we are all leaders. You are a leader, whether you identify yourself as one or not. Anytime you seek to influence the thinking, behavior, or development of another person, you are embracing a leadership role.[6] Proper leadership is becoming more vital for those working in the patient care settings. In healthcare, well-informed leaders recognize that patients are customers and that as customers, our patients must be satisfied with their experience. In fact, healthcare delivery and Medicare reimbursement rates are now strongly associated with patient satisfaction surveys.[7]

Sound Off
Proper leadership is becoming more vital for those working in health professions as healthcare delivery and Medicare reimbursement rates are now strongly associated with patient satisfaction surveys.

Technically, leadership is defined as the ability to influence others to accomplish a specific goal.[8] But how does a sonographer lead? A sonographer who demonstrates ethical and appropriate patient care is engaging in an act of leadership, because first, the sonographer is influencing the patient in a positive manner, and second, the sonographer is making a personal choice about how and to what extent he or she will use his or her influence. The following sections will provide some details regarding leadership styles and then offer several career opportunities you can pursue after graduation.

Sound Off

A sonographer who demonstrates ethical and proper patient care is engaging in an act of leadership.

Leadership Styles and Followership

There are many different leadership styles, and in order to become an effective leader, you should evaluate different leadership styles and either discount or utilize these approaches as you interact with others daily. Some leaders may practice leadership in an autocratic manner, meaning they give orders to followers and are the ultimate decision maker for the group. Though the work is organized and certainly gets accomplished, the **autocratic leadership style** can dampen creativity and create an environment in which motivation dwindles.[9]

A **transactional leader** is one who guides and motivates followers to achieve the organizational goals and the specific goals of the sonography department, through a system of rewards and punishment.[8] This form of leadership is much more democratic in nature. But a **transformational leader** not only guides and motivates those he or she leads but also exhibits charisma and offers inspiration. Transformational leadership encourages the development of respectful relationships with the leader, resulting in a somewhat a collective devotion that unites both leader and follower. A charismatic, transformational leader has a defined vision for the organization or department, takes risks and makes changes, has confidence in his or her skills as a leader, effectively communicates, and has high emotional intelligence (EI).[8] Transformational leaders also provide rewards for good behavior and hard work.[9] This style of leadership has been proven to increase job satisfaction for both the leader and follower in the healthcare setting.[10]

Another form of leadership that would be suitable for healthcare workers is **servant leadership**. Robert Greenleaf first explored this concept. Servant leadership is one of the best options for leadership styles in any helping profession, especially in healthcare. A servant leader works collaboratively with employees to make the best decisions possible, but furthermore places the needs of others before his or her own. Greenleaf described his leadership model as "servant first," in that the leader chooses to serve the needs of others—**stewardship**—to help those served to grow as individuals, reach autonomy, and produce to their full potential.[11] In essence, the natural role of serving others first that should be accepted by all healthcare workers can ultimately be applied to leadership; both leader and follower work in an environment in which both can accomplish maximum job satisfaction and effectiveness.

Sound Off

A servant leader works collaboratively with employees to make the best decisions possible, but furthermore places the needs of others before his or her own.

Recall, EI has now been linked in this book (Chapter 2) with the reduction of stress in the workplace, effective decision making, job satisfaction, and now leadership as well. Great leaders tend to be in touch with their emotions and are able to identify the emotional needs of followers.[9] Those leaders with high EI gain follower trust, and trust is the foundation of the leader-follower relationship.

If one does not trust the leader, the leader will not be effective. Essentially, the emotionally intelligent leader listens attentively, perceives unspoken concerns, acknowledges and respects the work of others, unites employees, and points them toward a common, shared goal.[9] One manner of feedback that leaders with high EI cherish is **360-degree feedback**, in which the leader evaluates the employee, and the employee evaluates the leader.[12] Leaders with high EI relish feedback from subordinates because they have confidence in their abilities and respect for the feelings of others.[12] These leaders approach conflict with grace and strength, thinking about all involved—the patient, the employee, and the organization.

Sound Off

The emotionally intelligent leader listens attentively, perceives unspoken concerns, acknowledges and respects the work of others, unites employees, and points them toward a common, shared goal.

Effective leaders cannot be successful without effective followers. Therefore, equally important to your success as a sonographer is to know how to be an effective follower by demonstrating consistent **followership**, which is the act of following a leader. In turn, leaders recognize valuable followers, and you will be much more likely to have an opportunity for both occupational advancement and a longer, more fulfilling career if you prove yourself to be an effective and competent follower.

According to Satterlee,[8] there are 10 rules of followership:

1. Support your immediate leaders in organizational changes as it is most likely not in their control when unpopular decisions or policies are implemented.
2. Only argue with your leaders when it is necessary and always in private.
3. Use initiative and make your own decisions, but be sure to explain your reasons to your leaders when clarification is needed.
4. If you are asked to take a leadership role, take it.
5. Always tell the truth. A leader cannot lead without honesty from the follower.
6. Be ready for conflict, and anticipate necessary changes.
7. When you have a good idea, share it, but you should also be prepared to be the one to take the lead on it.
8. Openly share the successes of others to leaders, and do not dwell on problems over which you have no control.
9. If you see a problem, show initiative and fix it yourself.
10. Always do your best, and put in more than an honest day's work.[8]

Sound Off

Effective leaders cannot be successful without effective followers.

In summary, being an effective follower means being skilled, self-directed, and always active, and it requires investing one's time in group work, thinking critically, and advocating for new ideas.[9] Being a good follower does not mean agreeing with every decision that a supervisor makes. However, it is important to try to understand the reasoning behind a leader's actions, offer an honest opinion respectfully, and adjust to unexpected changes in the workplace. When a problem or issue arises at work that you feel negatively impacts the quality of your work, it is up to you to approach management. Leaders cannot help you if they do not know you are having difficulties. Remember, patient care and safety are your primary concerns, and your work should always be focused on providing consistent effective patient care. If anything inhibits your ability to do so, you should let your supervisor know immediately.

Staff Sonographer

The first role for most sonography graduates is that of a **staff sonographer**. We can think of the staff sonographer as those individuals who work on the front lines, serving patients, and performing sonographic examinations on a daily basis. As discussed in Chapter 1, sonographer salaries can differ considerably, and though many duties vary, staff sonographers are typically responsible for performing varying types of sonographic exams. Staff sonographers may be employed in hospital settings, medical offices, and clinics. Depending upon the place of employment, some staff sonographers may be required to take call—either at night, on the weekends, or both. A staff sonographer may also be involved in research studies and may be referred to as a **research sonographer**. These sonographers are part of teams of clinical researchers and may be involved in the writing and publishing process. It is true that the staff sonographer has essential core responsibilities. However, the staff sonographer still has the capacity to influence the profession in a positive manner through **professional development** (Table 4-1).

Sound Off

It is true that the staff sonographer has fundamental core responsibilities. However, the staff sonographer still has the capacity to influence the profession in a positive manner.

Advanced Practice Sonographer

Since 1996, the SDMS has been investigating and pursuing the creation of a mid-level sonographer provider position referred to as an **advanced practice sonographer** or **ultrasound practitioner**.[13] According to the proposals, these sonographers would both perform and interpret ultrasound procedures in primary or specialty care settings.[13] Like the SDMS, a similar position, the **advanced cardiovascular sonographer**, is a proposal of the ASE task force.[13] An additional opportunity, referred to as an **ultrasound radiologist assistant**, exists as well. These individuals work between the interpreting physician and sonographer to refine sonography reports and train residents.[13] There are several individuals within the United States working as advanced practice sonographers under the guidance of qualified physicians. And although there are no formal certification or didactic training programs at the time of publication, the potential for those in the near future certainly exist.

TABLE 4-1	Staff sonographer professional development
Learn new specialties	Do not stop with one specialty; expand your knowledge and get certified in different areas of sonography.
Publish journal articles	Sonographers have access to limitless interesting cases. A good case report is easy to write and beneficial for both the author and reader.
Lecture	Provide lectures and training for local sonographers.
Join societies	Join societies and apply for leadership roles on the local or national level.
Teach students	Everyone can help train the next generation by being a great leader, demonstrating skills, and teaching.
Get an advanced degree	If your current program of study is an associate degree, continue to seek your bachelor's or master's degree.

Management in Sonography

Many people think "management" and "leadership" are synonymous terms, but they instead have two distinct functions. A **sonography manager**, also referred to as the sonography director, is responsible for planning, controlling, directing, and organizing the day-to-day functions of the department. This type of manager may also be referred to as a lead sonographer, team manager, or head sonographer in some departments. These individuals may make rotation schedules for employees, order supplies, work with upper management, attend management meetings representing sonography, amend protocols, and work with the scheduling department and interpreting physicians to systematize sonographic examinations and procedures. Though management and leadership are not the same thing, a manager can be an effective leader.

An effective leader in sonography management would certainly have a better opportunity to progress toward upper management within an organization. Recall, an effective leader has the following qualities: integrity, courage, initiative, energy, optimism, perseverance, balance, the ability to cope with stress, and self-awareness.[9] Because we are all leaders in some way, perhaps it is worthwhile to learn more about leadership beyond the information provided earlier in this chapter, primarily because you will improve your interactions with others, and secondarily because someday you may undertake a more defined leadership role in a healthcare setting.

Sound Off

Because we are all leaders in some way, perhaps it is worthwhile to learn more about leadership beyond the information provided earlier in this chapter, primarily because you will improve your interactions with others, and secondarily because someday you may undertake a more defined leadership role in a healthcare setting.

Sonography Educators

Working in education in sonography can be personally and professionally rewarding. Sonographers working in education can be involved in training many generations of sonographers in both the classroom and clinical environments. For most educator positions, prior clinical experience as a sonographer is mandatory, as clinically based knowledge enhances the classroom instructor's ability to communicate information. Furthermore, accreditation guidelines require classroom instructors to be certified in the areas in which they teach.[14]

Didactic sonography instructor pay varies, though most educators earn slightly less than their clinically based counterparts at around $70,000 per year as of 2012.[15] Therefore, it is clear that some sonographers choose a career in education for other reasons than monetary reward. For example, educators are often encouraged to pursue advanced degrees; make writing ventures; provide lectures to local, state, or national societies; and stay abreast of all the newest technology and studies related to ultrasound in medicine. Those who pursue a career in sonography education should have a thirst for knowledge, a love of sonography, and the passion to make a positive difference in the sonography profession by educating the next generation of sonographers.

Sound Off

Those who pursue a career in sonography education should have a thirst for knowledge, a love of sonography, and the passion to make a positive difference in the sonography profession by educating the next generation of sonographers.

Travel Sonographers

Sonographers may be employed by temporary staffing agencies and may be required to travel to different areas of the United States or even all over the world to perform sonography. Most travel companies pay much better than hospital or outpatient-based employers. They may even provide funds for residence, food, and possibly a company or rental car. However, though the pay may be better, temporary staffing agencies may not provide benefits like healthcare or retirement savings plans. There may not be much time for orientation to new departments either, so your skills will have to be finely tuned. For this reason, some temporary agencies may require you to practice sonography for a number of years before applying for a travel job. They may also ask that you be credentialed in multiple specialties as well. However, some sonographers truly enjoy traveling, and for those people, this job provides both adventure and professional satisfaction.

Consultants or Technical Advisors

An ultrasound consultant is someone who among other things assists organizations and hospitals in the process of ultrasound lab accreditation processes. They may also advise organizations concerning changes in ultrasound practices and assist with specific training for sonographers. Ultrasound consultants tend to be sonographers with extensive experience in accreditation processes, and they stay updated on healthcare legal issues.

Sales/Application Specialist

Ultrasound manufacturers may employ sonographers as part of the sales force for ultrasound equipment. Depending upon the company, the sonographer may be required to have a certain number of years of clinical experience, multiple credentials, and some may even require advanced education. The sonographer employed by sales organizations must undergo extensive training on machines and equipment marketed by the company. These jobs almost certainly require state travel and occasionally national travel.

Sonography Entrepreneur

A sonography entrepreneur is someone who owns part or all of a business related to sonography sales or training. Opportunities exist in the establishment of sonography training schools, creating and implementing CME programs, and writing. These individuals tend to have many years of experience in the profession, are highly motivated, and have a thorough understanding of business practices.

CAREER ESTABLISHMENT

Before pursuing a job in sonography, you should work on creating or enhancing your resume. Allied health profession resumes should consist of all applicable patient care work completed, including clinical internships, specialty training, and experience in routine sonographic examinations, interventional techniques, and invasive procedures. This section will provide you with some helpful tips on creating your resume, job searching, and interview tips in preparation for your first job in sonography. As you read this section, it is important to note that there may be resume writing and job interviewing resources—even supportive classes offered—at your educational institution or at a local college in your area. Also, libraries and the internet are full of valuable resources concerning these topics. Utilize the resources available so that you not only distinguish yourself from others but you have the greatest opportunity to get the job that you desire. And though extensive coaching suggestions for interviews and resumes lies beyond the scope of this book, it would be wise to be prepared for the job market long before you graduate.

Sound Off

It would be wise to be prepared for the job market long before you graduate.

As stated earlier in this chapter, the ARDMS allows students from accredited institutions to attempt specialty certifications 60 days prior to graduation.[4] Though you will not receive your certification until graduation, having already qualified for certification is a huge accomplishment and one that can certainly distinguish you from other job candidates. The success rate for the certification examinations is likely to be inversely proportional to the time at which you take it following graduation. In other words, the sooner you take the examination after or before graduation, the more likely you are to be successful. Therefore, you should take your examinations as soon as possible as long as you feel fully prepared. Table 4-2 shows the pass rates for some ARDMS specialty examinations.

Sound Off

The success rate for the certification examinations is likely to be inversely proportional to the time at which you take it following graduation. In other words, the sooner you take the examination after or before graduation, the more likely you are to be successful.

Searching and Applying for Jobs

An important truth concerning the process of looking for a job after school is to first understand the reality that the perfect job does not always exist at the perfect time. You may want a 9-to-5, no-call, no-weekend job, but that job may not be available once you graduate. Also, a job may not be available in the surrounding area where you live, so you may have to travel or move to obtain a job. Sometimes one must simply obtain a job to gain experience before a better job comes along.

Sound Off

An important truth concerning the process of looking for a job after school is to first understand the reality that the perfect job does not always exist at the perfect time. You may want a 9-to-5, no-call, no-weekend job, but that job may not be available once you graduate.

The internet provides a wealth of information pertaining to job searching. Online job search sites, such as Indeed.com, UltrasoundJobs.com, and CareerOneStop.org, exist for rapid and convenient job searching. Also, many organization websites have human resources department pages that list opportunities listed for both internal and external job candidates. Your educational institution may

TABLE 4-2	ARDMS examination pass rates in 2012
ARDMS Examination	**Overall Pass Rate**
Abdomen	60%
Adult Echocardiography	59%
Fetal Echocardiography	74%
Obstetrics and Gynecology	72%
Pediatric Echocardiography	64%
Sonography Principles and Instrumentation	70%
Vascular Technology	58%

From Yate M. *Knock 'em Dead: Secrets & Strategies for Success in an Uncertain World.* Avon, MA: Adams Media; 2011.[16]

have additional resources available to you as well. One of the best ways to know about jobs is by word of mouth, and for that reason, forming good relationships with clinical sonographers and managers is invaluable in your job pursuit.

Resume Writing and Social Networking

It is difficult to know exactly what an employer wants to see on a resume. You certainly do not want to minimize your experience, but providing too much information can overwhelm the reader, resulting in a loss of interest. Therefore, the first challenge is to get an opportunity for an interview and having an effective resume is the way to get there.

Table 4-3 provides seven basic steps to creating an effective resume. However, the first thing to remember for creating an effective resume is to adapt the resume to the specific position for which you are applying. This means you must look at what the employer is asking for within the job description component of the job posting and tailor your resume and cover letter to match the job description; your resume and cover letter should be adaptable and job-specific. A free online assessment tool that grades your uploaded resume can be found at rezscore.com.

Social networking has two vastly different components: **personal networking** and **online networking**. Both of these have advantages. Personal networking is accomplished through developing individual face-to-face relationships with others. One author suggests that the best way to find a job is to talk to people face to face.[18] As stated earlier, the best way to increase your opportunity to get a job is to get to the interview process, and you can further your cause by getting into conversations

TABLE 4-3	Seven basic steps for resume writing
Steps	**Explanation**
1. Identify your resume format.	For sonography, you may want to use the functional format or a combination of functional and chronological.
2. Evaluate yourself.	Take some time and write down your past jobs, job tasks, personal attributes, skills, and strengths. This does not have to be a well-ordered document; you will organize it later. Write down the clinical experience that you have, including all clinical rotations and sonography specialties and certifications that you have or will have before or shortly after you graduate.
3. Identify the specific job requirements for the position.	Match your attributes, skills, strengths, and experience to the job position and use action verbs (e.g., "accomplished," "administered," and "implemented"). Use bullet points that begin with action verbs to get the reader's attention.
4. Identify your achievements.	If you have obtained any distinguishing rewards for personal or professional achievements, make sure that you include that information in your resume.
5. Create a first draft.	Do not worry about neatness, just compile and organize all of your information.
6. Make a bulleted list of your information.	Using action verbs, put your information in bullet point format using logical sentences under headings (e.g., education, internships, job experience).
7. Create your final draft.	Create your final draft. If you have access, take it to a human resources individual for proofing.

From Mackay H. *Use Your Head to Get Your Foot in the Door: Job Search Secrets No One Else Will Tell You.* New York, NY: Penguin Group; 2010.[17]

with people who may want to hire you.[18] Therefore, you may want to call department managers or sonographers whom you have met through your clinical rotations expressing your interest and asking questions about the department and potential job opportunities.

Sound Off
The best way to find a job is to talk to people face to face.

Online networking is accomplished through social media websites like Facebook, Twitter, LinkedIn, and others. Online networking is a bit more impersonal. However, you can also reach many more people at one time, therefore increasing your network capacity. Be cautious of what you share on the internet, however; employers look closely at the internet footprint of potential hires, and you leave footprints every time you post something on the internet. Employers tend to act more favorably if you are strategic and not haphazard about what you put on the internet.[19] Resources like Google, Facebook, and LinkedIn are increasingly important in the employee selection process.[19]

Sound Off
Resources like Google, Facebook, and LinkedIn are increasingly important in the vetting process. Be cautious of what you share on the internet.

Interview Tips

Going to an interview for a job can be highly stressful, especially if you are not prepared adequately (Table 4-4). Most likely, you were selected for an interview because you at least met the minimum requirements. Remember to know your resume. If you do not know what is on your resume, you will appear unprepared. Of course, knowing ahead of time what questions an interviewer is going to ask is difficult, though there are a few common interview questions for which you should be prepared. One of the first prompts many face is "Tell me about yourself." Adding chronology to your answer can help focus your mind. In order, describe your work history with pertinent duties that relate to the job at hand.[18] Other questions often concern strengths and weaknesses. Return to Chapter 2 in which you attempted a personal inventory of strengths and weaknesses. If you do not remember the results, complete the process again.

TABLE 4-4	Steps to take before an interview

1. Research the company and the sonography department. Learn more about the company because they will often ask why you would like to work there.
2. Know what is on your resume.
3. Make copies of your resume to hand to the interviewer(s) when you leave. They may already have them, but this shows you are prepared.
4. Make copies of references.
5. Have a note pad and a pencil to take notes. This shows you are attentive.
6. Have a list of questions ready to ask the interviewers.
7. Wear a professional outfit—nothing too flashy. If you are a man, wear at least a tie, and if you are a woman, wear business casual attire.
8. Get a haircut if you need one.
9. Don't wear too much perfume or cologne.
10. Get adequate sleep the night before.
11. Don't be late.

Everyone likes to talk about their strengths, but few of us relish talking about our weaknesses. However, everyone has weaknesses, both personal and professional, that can be discussed during an interview. An unwillingness to admit to weaknesses may be interpreted as an unwillingness to learn and improve. Yate suggests identifying a weakness that you can ultimately describe as strength.[18] The best thing you can do is know yourself, be confident, and give it your best shot. During the interview, always seem interested, sit intently, and take your time answering questions. Leave your cell phone in your car. After you have the interview, send a thank you note for the opportunity. Many interview tips are available online.

SUMMARY

This chapter has provided an overview of the environment in which the sonographer practices. Though your priority in school is to become clinically competent, you should work toward developing professional relationships with sonographers and managers in the clinical facilities in which you study. The sonography profession is replete with organizations that allow one to grow as a professional. Once you have established a career in sonography, you will recognize the need to expand your education, a service that professional organizations readily provide.

REFERENCES

1. Joint Review Committee on Education in Diagnostic Medical Sonography. Retrieved on February 1, 2015 from http://www.jrcdms.org/

2. The American Institute of Ultrasound in Medicine. Retrieved on February 1, 2015 from http://www.aium.org/

3. The Fetal Medicine Centre. Retrieved on February 1, 2015 from http://www.fetalmedicine.com/

4. ARDMS CME General Information. American Registry of Diagnostic Medical Sonography. Retrieved on February 1, 2015 from http://www.ardms.org/registrant_resources/cme_general_information/

5. ARDMS Recertification General Information. Retrieved on February 1, 2015 from http://www.ardms.org/registrant_resources/recertification_general_information

6. Blanchard K, Hodges P. *Lead Like Jesus*. Nashville, TN: Thomas Nelson; 2005.

7. Center for Medicare and Medicaid Services. Retrieved on February 1, 2015 from http://cms.gov/Medicare/Quality-Initiatives-Patient-Assessment-Instruments/HospitalQualityInits/HospitalOutpatientQuality ReportingProgram.html

8. Satterlee A. *Organizational Management and Leadership: A Christian perspective*. Roanoke, VA: Synergistics; 2009.

9. Whitehead DK, Weiss SA, Tappen RM. *Essentials of Nursing Leadership and Management*. 5th ed. Philadelphia, PA: F.A. Davis Company; 2010.

10. Wang X, Chontawan R, Nantsupawat R. Transformational leadership: effect on the job satisfaction of Registered Nurses in a hospital in China. *J Adv Nurs* 2010;68:444–451. doi: 10.1111/j.1365-2648.2011.05762.x.

11. Frick DM, Spears LC, eds. *On Becoming a Servant Leader: The Private Writings of Robert K. Greenleaf*. San Francisco, CA: Jossey-Bass; 1996.

12. Dye CF. *Leadership in Healthcare: Values at the Top*. Chicago, IL: Health Administration Press; 2000.

13. News Wave (October 2011). Society of Diagnostic Medical Sonography. Retrieved on February 1, 2015 from http://www.sdms.org/members/news/NewsWave/NW-October-2011.pdf

14. JRCDMS Standards and Guidelines. Retrieved on February 1, 2015 from http://www.jrcdms.org/pdf/Standards 2011.pdf

15. News Wave (January 2013). Society of Diagnostic Medical Sonography. Retrieved on February 1, 2015 from http://www.sdms.org/members/news/NewsWave/NW-January-2013.pdf

16. Yate M. *Knock 'em Dead: Secrets & Strategies for Success in an Uncertain World*. Avon, MA: Adams Media; 2011.

17. Mackay H. *Use Your Head to Get Your Foot in the Door: Job Search Secrets No One Else Will Tell You*. New York, NY: Penguin Group; 2010.

18. ARDMS Global Exam Summary Report 2012. Retrieved on February 1, 2015 from http://www.ardms.org/files/downloads/ExamPerform_Summary2012.pdf

19. Salvador EU. *Step-by-Step Resumes*. 2nd ed. Indianapolis, IN: JITs Works; 2011.

Thinking Critically

1. List some ways in which students can make a positive difference in the sonography profession.
2. Considering the different occupational pathways you can take after you graduate, which of the jobs listed in this chapter most interests you and why? Which of the jobs least interests you and why?
3. Reflect upon your goals of becoming a registered sonographer. Which specialty examination would you want to attempt first? Will you try to take the examination before you graduate or after?
4. Among the list of professional membership organizations, is there one that you think would most benefit students in your specialty? Would you consider joining one of these societies while you are in school? If so, why? If not, why not?

Chapter 4
Review Questions

1. **Which of the following is not a certification-granting organization?**
   a. ARDMS
   b. CCI
   c. ARRT
   d. AIUM

2. **Which of the following is considered the best way to get a job?**
   a. Face-to-face meeting
   b. Online networking
   c. Social networking
   d. Online searching

3. **Which of the following membership organizations publishes the *Journal of Diagnostic Medical Sonography*?**
   a. AIUM
   b. SDMS
   c. SVU
   d. JUM

4. **Which of the following is not a quality of an effective leader?**
   a. Courageous
   b. Oppressive
   c. Optimistic
   d. Honest

5. **To maintain certification through the ARDMS, how many credits must a sonographer obtain in three years?**
   a. 40
   b. 24
   c. 16
   d. 30

6. The organization that offers the RVS certification is
   a. ARDMS.
   b. ARRT.
   c. CCI.
   d. SVU.

7. Which form of leadership places the concerns of others before the self?
   a. Transformational leadership
   b. Servant leadership
   c. Autocratic leadership
   d. Transactional leadership

8. How many days before graduation can a student of an accredited sonography program take the specialty examinations offered by the ARDMS?
   a. 30
   b. 45
   c. 50
   d. 60

9. What type of leadership not only guides and motivates employees but exhibits charisma and offers inspiration?
   a. Servant leadership
   b. Transformational leadership
   c. Transactional leadership
   d. Autocratic leadership

10. Which of the following establishes practice guidelines for each specialty and makes official statements on behalf of the profession on a range of issues, including safe ultrasound practice techniques?
    a. SDMS
    b. ASE
    c. AIUM
    d. FFE

11. Which national membership organization publishes the *Journal of Ultrasound in Medicine*?
    a. AIUM
    b. ARRT
    c. SDMS
    d. ASE

12. What organization is the national organization for echocardiographers?
    a. ARRT
    b. ASE
    c. SDRS
    d. SVU

13. What organization establishes standards by which many different allied health programs are reviewed?
    a. AIUM
    b. JRC-DMS
    c. ACR
    d. CAAHEP

14. **Which of the following is the national membership organization for physicians, vascular technologists, students, and other cardiac and vascular professionals?**
    a. ARRT
    b. ASE
    c. SDRS
    d. SVU

15. **To become a registered sonographer through the ARDMS, one must do which of the following?**
    a. Pass the SPI examination
    b. Pass the SPI examination and a specialty examination
    c. Pass a single specialty examination
    d. Pass two specialty examinations

16. **If a RDMS would like to become certified in an additional certification, he or she would have to do which of the following?**
    a. Pass the SPI examination
    b. Pass the SPI examination and a specialty examination
    c. Pass a single specialty examination
    d. Pass two specialty examinations

17. **In what year does recertification begin through the ARDMS?**
    a. 2016
    b. 2017
    c. 2018
    d. 2019

18. **Which of the following is *not* a true statement about good followership?**
    a. You should offer your honest opinion respectfully, and adjust to unexpected changes in the workplace.
    b. Openly share the successes of others to leaders, and do not dwell on problems over which you have no control.
    c. Being a good follower means you have to agree with every decision your supervisor makes.
    d. Use initiative and make your own decisions, but be sure to explain your reasons to your leaders when clarification is needed.

19. **What is defined as the ability to influence others to accomplish a specific goal?**
    a. Followership
    b. 360-degree feedback
    c. Leadership
    d. Emotional intelligence

20. **In 2019, registered sonographers will be required to take additional examinations to maintain qualifications. This process is referred to as**
    a. national certification.
    b. continuing medical education.
    c. professional development.
    d. recertification.

5

Ergonomics and the Prevention of Work-Related Musculoskeletal Disorders

CHAPTER OBJECTIVES

- Understand the importance of the use of proper posture and body mechanics in sonography.
- Gain an appreciation for the basic causes of work-related musculoskeletal disorders in sonography.
- Assess the most likely locations of work-related musculoskeletal disorders in sonography.
- Explain the ways in which work-related musculoskeletal disorders can be prevented.

KEY TERMS

Abduction – when part of the body, such as the arm, is moved away from the midline of the body

Adduction – when part of the body, such as the arm, is moved toward the midline of the body

Ambidextrous scanning – the ability to use the right or left arm to manipulate the transducer during scanning while the other arm is used for keyboarding

Body habitus – the general body type of a person

Bursa – a closed, fluid-filled sac that contains synovial fluid

Bursitis – inflammation of the bursa

Cable support brace – a device which is placed on the arm to hold the cord of the transducer in place while the transducer is maneuvered during scanning

Carpal tunnel syndrome – a repetitive strain disorder characterized by the median nerve becoming compressed or aggravated within the carpal tunnel of the wrist

Constriction – tightening

Cubital tunnel syndrome – a repetitive strain disorder characterized by the ulnar nerve becoming compressed or aggravated within the cubital tunnel of the elbow

Cumulative trauma disorder – see work-related musculoskeletal disorder

De Quervain disease – a repetitive motion injury that is characterized by tenosynovitis of the thumb side of the wrist

Epicondylitis – the inflammation of the periosteum in the area of insertion of the biceps tendon into the distal humerus; lateral epicondylitis is referred to as tennis elbow

Ergonomic interventions – processes used to improve a worker's comfort, safety, and productivity

Ergonomics – the scientific study of creating tools and equipment that help the human body adapt to the work environment

Force – relates to how much pressure is applied by one object (transducer) to the surface of another object (the patient)

Ganglion cysts – palpable, painful cysts located within the tendons or joints of the hands, wrists, ankles, or feet

Kyphosis – a hump-shaped curvature of the spine

Muscle spasm – involuntarily contraction of a muscle

Musculoskeletal system – system of the body that consists of muscles, joints, tendons, ligaments, cartilage, and bones

Nerve entrapment – see pinched nerve

Occupational injuries – physical injury acquired carrying out one's job duties

Orthotic devices – medical instruments used to promote the use of proper body mechanics by aligning, immobilizing, or supporting parts of the musculoskeletal system

Overuse syndrome – see work-related musculoskeletal disorder

Pinched nerve – a disorder that results from the compression, abnormal stretching, or the constriction of a nerve or group of nerves

Plantar fasciitis – inflammation of the ligament on the bottom of the foot

Posture – a position of the body or part of the body

Proper body mechanics – technique that ensures that the spine is in appropriate alignment for virtually any position required to function in one's daily tasks, such as moving, sitting, standing, and lifting

Repetitive motion injuries – see work-related musculoskeletal disorder

Repetitive motions – similar movements that may be required to perform a task

Repetitive strain injuries – see work-related musculoskeletal disorders

Static muscle loading – maintained muscle work over a long period of time, which is thought to result in the gradual damage to muscles due to abnormal contraction and consequent buildup of fibrous tissue within the muscles

Support cushion – a device used to support the scanning arm of the sonographer

Synovial fluid – the lubricating and nourishing fluid located within joints

Tarsal tunnel syndrome – a nerve entrapment disorder that results in the inflammation or irritation of the tibial nerve located within the tarsal tunnel in the foot

Tendinitis – inflammation of a tendon

Tennis elbow – lateral epicondylitis of the elbow

Tenosynovitis – inflammation of the sheath around a tendon

Thoracic outlet syndrome – the compression of the nerves and blood vessels of the neck and shoulder due to repetitive strain

Tinel sign – test used to diagnose cubital tunnel syndrome; if tapping over the cubital tunnel produces a tingling sensation down the ulnar nerve into the forearm and hand, then the test is positive for cubital tunnel syndrome

Trigger finger – form of tenosynovitis that is caused by repetitive gripping actions and can result in a finger that becomes locked in a position and then must be popped to be freed again

Work-related musculoskeletal disorders – occupationally acquired or occupationally aggravated injuries to an individual's muscles, tendons, ligaments, or cartilage that results from repetitive use

INTRODUCTION

As a sonography student, you should be enthusiastically preparing for a long-lasting and fulfilling career as a sonographer. In Chapter 2, we discussed the overarching demands placed upon the sonographer as related to some physical and mental health issues, job duties, and workplace stress. This chapter will focus primarily on the physical aspects of the occupation of sonographer—the act of conducting the sonographic examination.

There are two main reasons why this chapter will chiefly address the prevention of **work-related musculoskeletal disorders** for sonographers. First, though our work is strongly linked with the development of these disorders, their etiologies and manifestations are not entirely understood, making treatment options difficult and usually case-specific. Secondly, because you are now only beginning your career, it is best at this time to recognize the potential for work-related musculoskeletal disorders in the sonography profession and to provide techniques to prevent them from happening to you by offering some helpful **ergonomic interventions** and prescribed best practices. It is evident from the research that the prevention of work-related musculoskeletal disorders is a crucial step in your journey of pursuing a long, satisfying career as a diagnostic sonographer.

WHAT ARE WORK-RELATED MUSCULOSKELETAL DISORDERS?

Occupational injuries, or physical injury acquired carrying out one's job duties, are the main reasons for long-term absences among healthcare workers. The cost for treating these occupational injuries is astounding. According to Hagen-Ansert, these injuries cost businesses $60 billion per year, mostly in workers' compensation claims.[1] For example, on average, it costs $13,263 per claim to treat the common workplace injury of **carpal tunnel syndrome**.[1]

A study conducted in 2009 of more than 600 vascular sonographers found that perceived pain while scanning and the eventual quality of sonographic examinations were inversely related.[2] Furthermore, there appears to be a small window—only an average of five years—before a sonographer starts to experience pain associated with his or her job duties.[3] Several studies suggest that between 80% and 90% of sonographers scan in pain, and as a result of the persistence of pain, 20% of sonographers either retire early or decide to change careers.[4,5] Pain experienced by the sonographer during an examination is a significant distraction that counteracts the successful and accurate completion of job duties, and it may ultimately affect the ability of the sonographer to execute adequate patient care.

Our **musculoskeletal system** consists of muscles, joints, tendons, ligaments, cartilage, and bones. Sonography is indeed a job that consists of tasks that require the use of our musculoskeletal system to perform manual labor. One subcategory of occupational injuries is referred to as work-related musculoskeletal disorders (WRMSDs), previously mentioned. WRMSDs are essentially either occupationally acquired or occupationally aggravated injuries to an individual's muscles, tendons, ligaments, or cartilage that results from repetitive use.[6] As you will see in this chapter, WRMSDs can lead to pain, swelling, inflammation, spine degeneration, and the gradual deterioration of tendons and ligaments.[7] These injuries acquired during the everyday work of the sonographer may also be referred to as **repetitive strain injuries**, **repetitive motion injuries**, **overuse syndrome**, and **cumulative trauma disorder**.[1,6]

In sonographic practice, WRMDs manifest as a wide range of chronic musculoskeletal and nerve disorders that affect the sonographer's hands, wrists, arms, shoulders, neck, and back (Table 5-1).[8] As stated earlier, these are mostly repetitive use injuries. In other words, these injuries are the result of stress or tension applied to particular groups of muscles, nerves, tendons, and ligaments in *cycles*. For example, often, abdominal sonographers are required to scan patients of large **body habitus**. The sonographer may feel that because the patient is large, there is an obligation to apply increased pressure with the transducer against the patient's abdomen to obtain better images. Applied repetitively, the pressure must be maintained for only a few seconds to several minutes at a time. At the time of the exam, the sonographer may experience a small amount of pain, burning, or discomfort in a focal

TABLE 5-1	Most common areas of work-related injury for sonographers
Shoulder (84%)	
Neck (83%)	
Wrist (61%)	
Back (58%)	
Hands (56%)	

From Coffin C, Baker J. Ultrasound clinics. Preventing work-related injuries among sonographers and sonologists. *Contemporary OB/GYN* [serial online] 2007;52(7):78. Available from: CINAHL with Full Text, Ipswich, MA. Accessed June 9, 2014.

area of his or her body as a result of miniscule connective tissue damage. The pain may subside when the examination is over. However, the damage to the soft tissue accumulates with time, and pain can become persistent. Initially, the sonographer may take over-the-counter pain medications that seem to alleviate the pain. But in due course, the repetition of these and other uncomfortable motions can result in lasting injuries to muscles, joints, tendon, and ligaments. Consequently, the pain resulting from these repetitive injuries tends to gradually worsen, culminating in a nagging pain that is consistently evident, unavoidable, and seemingly untreatable without further medical and/or surgical intervention.

ERGONOMICS

The practice of sonography is fundamentally an individual skills-driven modality, relying almost exclusively on the aptitude of the sonographer's intellect and physical well-being. This means that the accuracy of the examination is highly dependent upon how practiced, mentally discerning, and physically prepared the sonographer is at the time the study occurs. Unfortunately, there are many environmental and personal stressors in the workplace that may interrupt the ultimate goal of providing the correct diagnosis.

Ergonomics is the scientific study of creating tools and equipment that help the human body adapt to the work environment.[9] An understanding of ergonomics helps reduce the influence of stressors thereby increasing the efficiency of the sonographer and accuracy of the examination. The National Institute for Occupational Safety and Health requires that employers comply with certain ergonomic recommendations (Table 5-2).

TABLE 5-2	Several ergonomic requirements of the National Institute for Occupational Safety and Health

- Always use assistive devices to move heavy items or patients.
- Use alternative equipment for tasks that require **repetitive motions**.
- Position equipment no more than 20–30 degrees away or about arm's length to avoid reaching or twisting the trunk or neck.
- Use chairs that have good back support. The chair should be high but only high enough so that you can still rest both feet flat on the ground.
- When working on a computer, keep your elbows flexed no more than 100 to 110 degrees, and keep your wrists in a neutral position.
- Work under non-glare lighting.

From Timby BK. *Fundamental Nursing Skills and Concepts*. 10th ed. Philadelphia, PA: Lippincott Williams & Wilkins; 2013.

BODY MECHANICS

As we explore the common locations of musculoskeletal injuries for sonographers, keep in mind that the use of **proper body mechanics** and merely making it a habit to think about using correct **posture** before acting can save you from both immediate pain and cumulative pain in the future. For instance, it is important to know that when a person is standing, the center of gravity is located at the center of the pelvis.[10] Simply maintaining the correct center of gravity during your workday can save you from pain and increase your longevity in the profession (Fig. 5-1). Postural support devices, which serve the purpose of reducing **kyphosis** and back strain, can be purchased by sonographers to encourage the use of correct posture throughout the work day (Figs. 5-2 and 5-3).

Proper body mechanics ensure that the spine is in appropriate alignment for virtually any position required to function in one's daily tasks as a sonographer, such as moving, sitting, standing, and lifting (Table 5-3). Though the correct position is always optimal, you may encounter situations in which the patient's physical state suggests that you must deviate from the use of correct posture. At these critical times, never hesitate to ask for assistance. The effectiveness of the provided ergonomic interventions for WRMSDs in the upcoming sections should always be preceded and supplemented with the use of proper body mechanics. This chapter will provide some beginning steps toward the use of proper body mechanics in patient care, and more specific patient care assistance skills and steps will also be discussed again in a later chapter.

PERSONAL AND ENVIRONMENTAL RISK FACTORS

While the research behind the causes of WRMSDs is ongoing, in general, there are a few risk factors that have been linked with the development of WRMSDs that are relevant to the sonographer: posture and body positioning, repetitive motions and **force**, room and equipment design, job design, and some other threatening physical predisposing factors.[9] Though there are minimal fundamental differences in scanning techniques between sonographic specialties, some specialties lend themselves to certain risks. Research has confirmed that the main ergonomic factors that have been identified as primary concerns for echocardiographers are posture, repetition, force, and equipment design.[3]

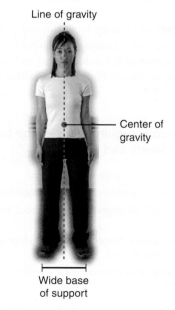

Line of gravity

Center of gravity

Wide base of support

Figure 5-1. Try using a wide stable base of support. A strong base of support promotes good posture and keeps the body aligned.

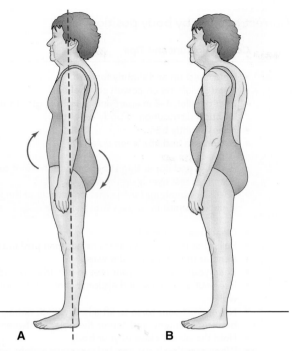

Figure 5-2. A. Contraction of the abdomen and gluteal muscles results in a good standing posture. **B.** Relaxation of the abdominal muscles often results in a poor standing posture.

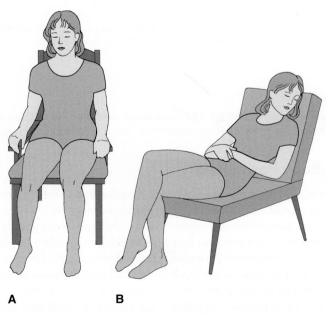

Figure 5-3. A. Good sitting posture. **B.** Poor sitting posture.

TABLE 5-3	Correct posture by body position
Position	**Correct Posture and Tips**
Standing	• Hold chest up and slightly forward. • Head should be erect with chin held in. • Feet parallel, 4–8 in apart and at right angles to the lower legs with identical distribution of body weight • Knees slightly bent • Buttocks in and abdomen up and in
Sitting	• Buttocks and upper thighs become the base of support. • Both feet rest evenly on the floor. • Knees are bent, and the posterior aspects of the knees (popliteal surface) are not in contact with the chair.
Lifting and moving (Fig. 5-4)	• Clear area of obstacles. • Pulling or rolling heavy items rather than pushing them is better. • Bend at the knees, not the waist. • Keep your body over your feet to provide a broad base of support. • Use your arms, legs, and abdominal muscles—not your back—to do the work. • Never twist your torso to lift a heavy load; rather, move your feet to get better placement, and center the object between your feet. • Hold the object close to your body. • When assisting a patient, balance your weight over both feet and stand close to the patient. Bend your knees to provide support, and use your arm and leg muscles to help move the patient (also ask the patient to perform as much work as possible if they appear physically capable). • Rest between heaving lifting periods. • Avoid reaching across structures and holding objects awkwardly and for an extended amount of time in a fixed position.

From Timby BK. *Fundamental Nursing Skills and Concepts*. 10th ed. Philadelphia, PA: Lippincott Williams & Wilkins; 2013; Dutton AG, et al. *Torres' Patient Care in Imaging Technology*. 8th ed. Philadelphia, PA: Lippincott Williams & Wilkins; 2013.

Sound Off

The main ergonomic factors that have been identified as primary concerns for cardiac sonographers are posture, repetition, force, and equipment design.

Posture and Body Positioning

Posture is the manner in which the body is held, or the position of the body.[11] Correct posture means that all body parts are aligned and balanced.[10] Unfortunately, maintaining correct posture is a struggle for most people, because poor posture is often more comfortable than correct posture. This conundrum is a direct result of how we have trained our ligaments, muscles, and tendons to relax while in certain positions, though most of these positions would be classified as examples of poor posture. Performing work while in a poor posture position can result in a painful **muscle spasm**, as strained muscles are forced to work beyond their normal ability, thus resulting in involuntarily contraction.[11]

Besides the torso, correct posture also includes the manner in which your extremities are held. For example, a common manner in which an echocardiographer performs examinations requires that the sonographer hold his or her scanning arm in **abduction** and unsupported while reaching across the patient (Fig. 5-5).[3] Abduction of the arm requires that the arm be moved away from the

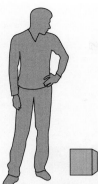
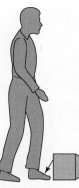
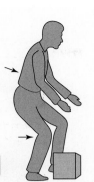

Plan your lift and ask for help if you need it.

Stand close to the object and widen your base of support.

Bend your knees and keep your back straight.

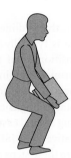
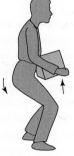
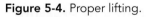

Tighten your abdominal muscles.

Lift with your leg muscles.

Figure 5-4. Proper lifting.

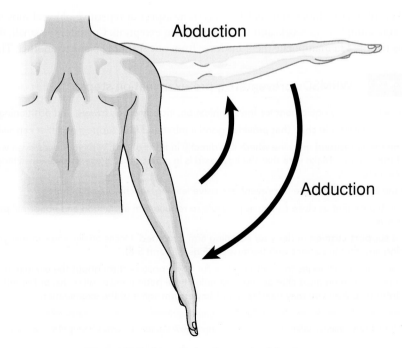

Abduction

Adduction

Figure 5-5. Arm abduction and adduction.

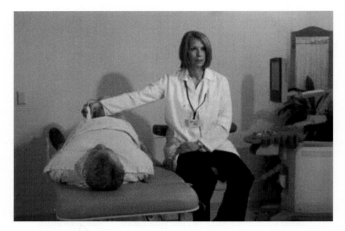

Figure 5-6. Extreme arm abduction. Notice the sonographer's awkward shoulder position. (With permission from Sound Ergonomics.)

midline of the body, while **adduction** is moving the arm closer to the midline. In a position that requires extreme arm abduction, the sonographer's cervical spine is typically flexed forward and rotated as well (Fig. 5-6).[3] The repeated use of such awkward positioning of the extremities and torso can result in the development of WRMSDs. Consequently, a proper scanning technique, equipment adjustments, and work station variability among sonographers are vital to reduce WRMSDs. For the sonography student, utilizing proper body position and establishing correct posture during early scanning experiences are crucial and can be done by completing several easy preventative steps. Though these will be discussed throughout this chapter, preventative WRMSDs pre-examination actions are summarized in Table 5-4. Eventually, the more you utilize these steps and other preventative measures, the more routine they will become.

Repetitive Motions and Force or Pressure

Almost every job that includes manual labor has some aspect of repetitive physical movements that are required to complete the work, and sonography is no exception. Consider the small, finer motor movements required to manipulate the transducer from one scanning plane to another. These subtle,

TABLE 5-4	WRMSDs preventative pre-examination steps

1. Obtain all necessary equipment for the examination, including gel, towels, and positioning devices.
2. Choose a comfortable chair that provides good lumbar and foot support and that can swivel.
3. Position the ultrasound machine where it is directly in front of you, with your eyes even with the top of the monitor. Make sure that the keyboard is in a place that prevents over-stretching of your non-scanning arm.
4. Raise the examination table to prevent excessive leaning, reaching, and bending.
5. Position the patient as close to you as possible to reduce arm abduction and abnormal posturing of the wrist.
6. Place a **support cushion** under your scanning arm if needed. Occasionally, you can rest your scanning arm on the patient with permission (Figs. 5-7 and 5-8).
7. Make appropriate changes to accommodate for good posture throughout the examination when the patient's position must change. For example, if the patient must roll on his or her left side away from you, then you may need to stand to perform some of the examination.

From Top 10 list for sonographer safety. Retrieved from http://www.soundergonomics.com/pdf/topten.pdf.[12]

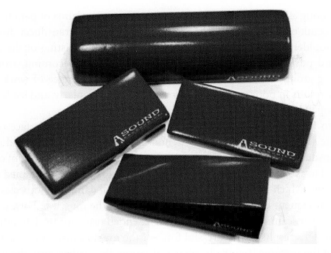

Figure 5-7. Example of support cushion that can be used during scanning. (With permission from Sound Ergonomics.)

delicate movements require the use of many coordinated muscles, tendons, and ligaments within the elbow, forearm, hand, wrist, and fingers. At the same time, the sonographer must apply recurring force with the transducer on the patient to achieve optimal images. The more repetitive the task, the more muscles needed to perform the work, and the more time needed to rest when the work is complete.[9]

The physiology behind muscle fatigue is logical. Basically, the more force required to perform a job, the more muscle effort is necessary, and this results in an actual decrease in the blood supply to the working tissues.[9] The decrease in the blood supply to the tissue is recognized by the worker as

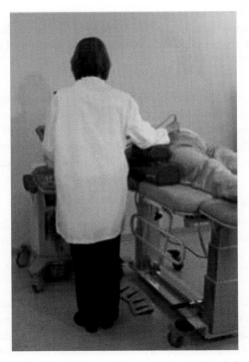

Figure 5-8. Example of how support cushions can be utilized during scanning. (With permission from Sound Ergonomics.)

muscle fatigue. Among all experience levels of sonographers, complaints of pain have been shown to be persistent as a result of the application of pressure applied by the transducer during the examination, sustained shoulder abduction, and from repetitive or static twisting of the trunk and neck.[13] Sustained awkward postures can lead to overused muscle groups becoming stronger and shorter, while the opposing group becomes weaker and longer.[1] This imbalance of work between muscles groups ultimately results in poor posture, strains the muscles irregularly, and leads to the disproportion of strength capabilities between the muscles.

Force relates to how much pressure is applied by one object to the surface of another object. In sonography, the second object is the patient, and the first object is the transducer. The pressure applied with a transducer while sustaining a static posture for an extended amount of time can lead to something referred to as **static muscle loading**. Static muscle loading is maintained muscle work over a long period of time, which is thought to result in the gradual damage to muscles due to abnormal contraction and consequent buildup of fibrous tissue within the muscles.[9] For example, a sonographer may use his or her scanning arm to perform an extended reach for the left kidney using forceful muscular exertion. This results in the stressful force of the muscles that comprise the shoulder joint and many parts of the upper extremity. In such a situation, the farther away the patient is from the sonographer, the greater the pressure needed by the shoulder muscles to apply the necessary force.[14]

Duration relates to the length of a task that must be performed. Sonographic examinations can vary from only minutes to hours in length. The longer you perform a specific activity without taking a break, the more likely you are to suffer from injury as a result of that activity.[9] Human physiology requires that while we are awake, we move and vary our body positions on a regular basis. Moving results in an increase in blood supply to the structures that are required to perform movements, thereby increasing oxygen levels and toxin removal from those regions.[1] Essentially, moving ensures that all muscle groups are supplied with an appropriate amount of nutrients to consistently perform when called upon.

Sound Off

Human physiology requires that we move on a regular basis. Moving ensures that all muscle groups are supplied with an appropriate amount of nutrients to consistently perform when called upon.

To counteract the force needed to obtain better images, Jakes suggests that periods of exertion should be quickly followed by similar-length periods of rest.[15] For instance, if applied pressure to the abdomen of a patient is required to be sustained for 10 seconds, then 10 seconds of rest is recommended to counter the effects of the duration of force. Varying tasks throughout the day is another way to reduce the duration of tasks and ensure the use of more muscle groups while performing work.

Sound Off

To counteract the force needed to obtain better images, Jakes suggests that periods of exertion should be quickly followed by similar-length periods of rest.[15]

Room Design

First, consider that most sonography rooms for a single specialty are arranged in a similar manner; this can be referred to as room design. In other words, an ultrasound room used for abdominal, gynecologic, and obstetrics in one hospital is most likely arranged in a similar manner to a sonography room in most other hospitals. Secondly, consider that the majority of these examinations are performed from the left side of the bed with the use of the sonographer's right arm. Therefore, there will be some physical movements that mandate repetition simply because of the room design.

Consequently, poor room design inherently provides some physical restraints that ultimately encourage tedious physical movements, increasing the likelihood of repetitive strain injuries.

Varying the room design to accommodate **ambidextrous scanning** in the department could prevent some repetitive injuries. For example, for general imaging departments that perform abdominal and small parts studies, arranging one room to be used for left-handed scanning could help reduce the likelihood of injuries. Initially, the room could be used for sonographic examinations that included the larger structures in the abdomen since an adjustment period for minute transducer manipulations would undeniably be warranted for individuals accustomed to right-handed scanning. Though this model would take much practice and commitment on the part of the staff sonographers, eventually there may be a significant reduction in cumulative strain. In fact, studies have shown that ambidextrous scanning benefits both experienced and inexperienced sonographers without increasing risk factors for WRMSDs.[16]

Room design also includes the lighting used within the room, air quality, and comfortable flooring. Eye strain can result from poorly lit rooms. A dimmer switch may be helpful for a quick adjustment to be made if eye strain occurs. One author suggests that the walls of the sonography room be painted in light colors and that the sonographers should wear light-colored lab coats as well to reduce eye strain.[3] Furthermore, the sonographer should occasionally look away from the monitor and refocus his or her eyes to reduce eye fatigue.

Good air quality should be maintained as well. Sterilization equipment for transducers that contain glutaraldehyde should not be in the sonography examination rooms, as the fumes could cause poor air quality resulting in headaches and other complications. Also, foot support pads on the floors adjacent to the machine can help to prevent strain while standing.

Poor room design can negatively affect student learning as well. Students are often required to stand for an extended amount of time to observe sonographic examinations. Standing in one place too long can cause you to feel tired, and your legs may begin to ache causing a lack of concentration, which is a distraction to your educational experience.[9] Over time, this manner of static muscle loading can cause significant discomfort as well and possibly even physical injury.[9] Therefore, it may be best to vary your observations from sitting to standing. Unfortunately, some rooms may not be designed to accommodate extra seating for students. In this situation, try to take breaks and short walks between observed examinations. Comfortable shoes should be worn to clinical as well. Table 5-5 provides some tips for you to try if you are feeling any physical pain during clinical observations.

TABLE 5-5	Helpful tips for physical aches during clinical observations

- Make sure you are fully rested before clinical.
- Make sure that you wear comfortable clothing and shoes.
- Try to vary your observational body positions; stand for one, and sit for one.
- Try to maintain good posture in any body position.
- Vary the examinations that you observe if you can. Some examinations take longer than others. Observe a long exam, and follow it with a short one.
- Ask to scan after or before the sonographer, if only for a few minutes, to vary your body positions and practice good posture.
- Stretch between observed examinations.
- Take a short walk between observed examinations.
- Leave the department during your breaks, especially lunch break. Go outside for some fresh air; sit in your car; go to the snack shop; get away just for a few minutes. Rest and clear your mind, and often, your body will begin to feel better.
- Inform your clinical supervisor and/or sonography program staff if you are experiencing persistent pain in clinical as a result of observations.

Try to avoid the use of pain medications, as these are often only a temporary cure. Instead, make minor alterations to your routine, and always inform your immediate clinical supervisor and/or sonography program administrators when you are experiencing persistent pain in clinical as a result of observations, as they may be able to offer additional suggestions. As discussed in the previous chapters, maintaining good mental and physical health will improve your capacity to learn and ultimately make you a better sonographer.

Sound Off

Always inform your immediate clinical supervisor and/or sonography program staff when you are experiencing persistent pain in clinical as a result of observations, as they may be able to offer additional remediation suggestions.

Equipment Design

Equipment design relates to how tables, chairs, ultrasound machines, and other accessories needed for the sonographer are fashioned. As you may expect, the long-term costs of poor ergonomic design exceed the short-term costs of quality design; "an ergonomically state-of-art ultrasound system, table, chair, and accessories can be purchased for $188,200. In contrast, failure to address ergonomics in the workplace setting can result in $580,000 in revenue loss, medical bills, the average cost of a workers' compensation claim, and new staff recruitment."[17] Therefore, room design and equipment design must be coordinated.

In the past, ultrasound machines were bulky, difficult to maneuver, and certainly not user-friendly. The transducers were heavy as well, providing an added challenge for the sonographer. Over the past few decades, the trend has fortunately progressed toward offering more ergonomically correct ultrasound machines, which are lighter in weight and have larger, high-definition monitors that swivel, keyboards that can be tucked away, and touch screens that make the task of changing machine functions nearly intuitive (Fig. 5-9). Transducers have also become lighter and easier to manipulate. Many machines now even come equipped with voice recognition capabilities, allowing the sonographer to freeze images, store images, and perform other routine functions with the spoken word.

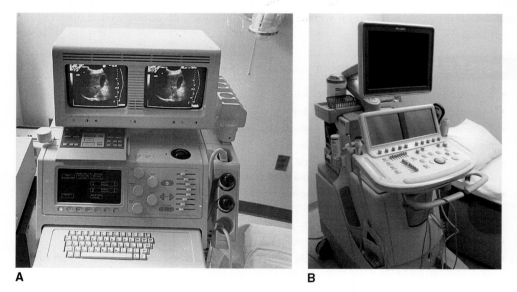

A   **B**

Figure 5-9. A. Older ultrasound machines had small monitors and were bulky. **B.** Newer display screen and control panel of a Philips ie33 ultrasound machine. This machine is much lighter, ergonomically correct, and user-friendly.

Some of the newest technologies mentioned in Chapter 4 permit automated measurement gathering as well. However, although automated uses may expand in use in our future, currently, the ultrasound machine should still be viewed as medical equipment that is a "tool in the hands of an experienced and educated professional."[18] This view maintains that ultrasound equipment should be designed according to the needs of the user (the sonographer), and therefore, it should provide convenience, preventing unnecessary challenges. Ultimately, the equipment should be designed to ensure job safety and work in a manner that prevents WRMSDs and other occupational hazards.[18]

Many ultrasound machines currently in use offer a sense of personalization.[18] For example, text buttons may be customized to fit the purpose of the individual sonographer. Multifunctional labeling buttons can reduce the amount of typing needed and ultimately the length of the examination. The machine height can also be adjusted for the sonographer as well. As a result, if a sonographer alters his or her scanning position from standing to sitting, the height of the ultrasound machine can be adjusted to maintain proper posture while scanning. Machines that do not allow such maneuverability of the ultrasound system controls have been shown to contribute to WRMSDs.[14] Specifically, studies have shown that machines that allow keyboard and control panel adjustments in height, rotation, and movement toward the sonographer, as well as height-adjustable chairs, help maintain a more neutral left arm position thereby reducing muscle strain.[14]

One of the most vital aspects of equipment design is the ultrasound transducer. While performing a sonographic examination, the sonographer must maintain transducer pressure applied to the patient's body. Consequently, the ultrasound transducer has been identified as a significant contributor to hand and wrist strain in sonographers.[16] Indeed, studies have proven that patient body habitus and required transducer pressure are directly related.[16] In other words, the more overweight the patient, the more applied pressure is needed to obtain quality sonographic images. One small-scale study used a pressure-sensing device to analyze the amount of grip pressure, also referred to as grip and pinch strength, applied to the transducer by the sonographer during scanning. The results revealed that maximum pressure and average force exerted were higher when scanning with a small transducer compared to a large transducer and that the thumb exerted the greater pressure and force.[16] Transducer sizes are highly variable and specific to machines. Furthermore, sonographers differ in their reasoning for choosing a specific transducer. They typically site the transducer's handling comfort, image quality, and maneuverability as the main reasons for selecting a particular transducer.[16] Therefore, it is vital for each of us to be aware of transducers that cause us individual discomfort and to make adjustments accordingly. As you scan more, you will discover which transducer works best for you. However, it should be noted that some examination and/or departmental protocols require the use of a specific transducer.

Lastly, sonographers play a vital role in the selection of ultrasound equipment, and manufacturers know this fact. For this reason, ultrasound machines are marketed to the end users, the physician and the sonographer.[18] Someday, it may be your job to offer input into the selection of an ultrasound machine for your department. Although you should strive to update your department with more modern ultrasound equipment, you should also consider the ergonomics of the machine as part of the selection process. To accomplish this task, it would be wise to work with the equipment for several days or weeks before making a final decision and reflect upon the alterations in the equipment that can be made in order to provide a balance between diagnostic capabilities and the ease of exercising proper ergonomics.

Job Design

As we recognized in Chapter 2, the stress from intellectual strain is evident in the job duties of the sonographer. Therefore, if an individual is provided with a supportive framework from which to perform his or her essential job duties, then many unnecessary workplace stressors can be alleviated.

TABLE 5-6	Top 10 job tasks that aggravate musculoskeletal symptoms

1. Scanning obese patients
2. Sustained shoulder abduction
3. Applying sustained transducer pressure
4. Sustained twisting of the neck and trunk
5. Repetitive twisting of the neck and trunk
6. Scanning with outdated equipment
7. Maneuvering of equipment in the examination room
8. Performing portable examinations
9. Holding the transducer
10. Control panel manipulation

From Muir M, et al. The nature, cause, and extent of occupational musculoskeletal injuries among sonographers: Recommendations for treatment and prevention. *J Diagn Med Sonogr* 2004;20:317–325.

One characteristic of removing workplace stressors is establishing an effective **job design** for an employee. If we look closely at the job design for sonographers, we can see specific, unique challenges. One study listed the top 10 activities that a sonographer performs during the day that tend to aggravate musculoskeletal symptoms (Table 5-6).[19]

One 2010 study found that the average workload for sonographers was between nine and 11 examinations per day, with each examination lasting between 20 to 25 minutes.[20] With an aging population, this workload will most likely increase. If the examinations are also complicated by the scanning challenges of obese patients, portable examinations, taking calls, and subsequent reduction in the time for breaks, then job design changes may be warranted. In fact, the option of taking frequent breaks seems to be a key to prevention in much of the research. Horkey and King suggest sonographers take recurrent breaks—at least 15 minutes every two hours—and that simply rotating the examination type could make a significant impact on job design.[3]

Underlying Predisposing Conditions

There are a few underlying health risks that could predispose one to developing a WRMSD, including having previous trauma to the body, diabetes, chronic fatigue, obesity, smoking, excessive alcohol consumption, rheumatoid arthritis, and Lyme disease.[9] Also, it appears that any condition that is associated with excessive fluid retention, such as hypothyroidism and pregnancy, can predispose someone to a WRMSD.[9] In general, simply having an unhealthy lifestyle can increase the likelihood of developing a WRMSD.[9] Creating an exercise plan and eating healthy can help you prevent WRMSDs.[9] The exercise plan should target flexibility, core stabilization, strength building, stretching, muscle relaxation, and postural restoration.[19]

INFLAMMATORY DISEASES LINKED TO WORK-RELATED MUSCULOSKELETAL DISORDERS

WRMSD symptoms include inflammation and swelling, numbness, muscle spasm, burning, a "pins and needles" feeling, stabbing pain, tingling, or the loss of sensation.[6] Unfortunately, many people suffering from WRMSDs may not present for treatment until the symptoms are severe, perhaps because the damage that occurs is intermittent damage in many WRMSDs it may only result in intermittent pain in the early days of the disorder.[21] For that reason, early recognition and intervention is vital. Along with the diseases mentioned in the following sections, there are a few common

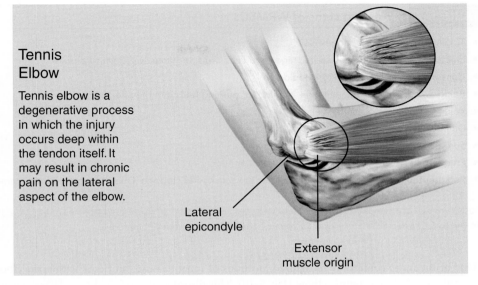

Tennis Elbow

Tennis elbow is a degenerative process in which the injury occurs deep within the tendon itself. It may result in chronic pain on the lateral aspect of the elbow.

Lateral epicondyle

Extensor muscle origin

Figure 5-10. Tennis elbow.

universal complications that result from repetitive strain, such as **tendinitis, tenosynovitis, epicondylitis, bursitis,** and **pinched nerves**.

Tendinitis is the inflammation of a tendon, while tenosynovitis is the inflammation of the sheath around the tendon. Tendons are a form of soft tissues that attach the ends of muscles to bones. Normally, tendons can handle stress for the purposes of routine, varied work. However, tendinitis is the result of microscopic tears in the tendon caused by repetitive motion or sustained irregular posturing of the tendon. Eventually, these tiny tears accumulate, and the damage becomes perceptible in the form of pain in the region. Though pain is common, some describe the discomfort as burning or tightening within the joint.

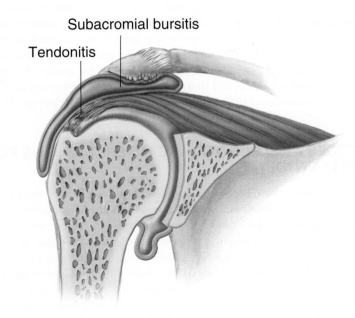

Subacromial bursitis

Tendonitis

Figure 5-11. Shoulder bursitis and tendinitis.

TABLE 5-7	Warning signs of WRMSDs

- Tingling in the hands or fingertips
- Frequently feeling the need to massage shoulders, arms, or hands to relieve tension
- Constant aching of the neck or shoulders
- Being awakened at night with pain, tingling, or burning feeling in the affected region
- Weak-feeling arms or hands
- Difficulty gripping objects
- Sore hands and arms, even after work is over
- Frequent headaches and tension in shoulders or neck
- Persistent pain for more than 24 hours after the activity has stopped (Does it hurt even away from work or on vacation?)

From Peddie S. *The Repetitive Strain Injury Sourcebook.* Los Angeles, CA: Lowell House; 1998.

One of the more commonly recognized locations of repetitive use injuries is within the elbow, commonly referred to as **tennis elbow** (Fig. 5-10). This disorder, also referred to as lateral epicondylitis, results from the repeated twisting of the forearm. Epicondylitis is the inflammation of the periosteum in the area of insertion of the biceps tendon on the distal humerus.[1] It results from tiny microtears in the muscles and tendons of the elbow as a result of strain placed on that joint.[9] However, one does not have to be an avid tennis player to develop tennis elbow, because many of those muscles and tendons may be placed in similar straining positions in everyday work. Common locations for tendinitis in the sonographer are the shoulder, elbow, and wrist.

Bursitis is inflammation of the **bursa** within a joint. A bursa is a closed, fluid-filled sac that contains **synovial fluid**. Bursas are located within joints throughout the body, and they provide lubrication between structures allowing for a decrease in friction and an increase in motion. Bursitis may present with symptoms similar to tendinitis and can even be found in the presence of tendinitis. Most often, bursitis is an ailment that can affect the sonographer's shoulder joint in his or her scanning arm (Fig. 5-11).

Pinched nerve, also referred to as **nerve entrapment** or nerve compression, is a disorder that results from the compression, abnormal stretching, or the **constriction** of a nerve or group of nerves. Pinched nerves lead to pain or discomfort, tingling, numbness, and general muscle weakness anywhere along the course of the nerve. Common locations for pinched nerves for the sonographer are the elbow, wrist, and neck. Some examples of nerve entrapment syndrome that affect the sonographer are carpal tunnel syndrome, **cubital tunnel syndrome**, and **thoracic outlet syndrome**.[6] Though all of these will be discussed in this chapter, a summary of the warning signs for many WRMSDs are provided in Table 5-7.

BEST PRACTICES AND ERGONOMIC INTERVENTIONS FOR THE SONOGRAPHY STUDENT

Prevention is the best treatment for WRMSDs.[22] As noted, there are several anatomic locations where a sonographer may suffer from pain as a result of WRMSDs. As a result, ergonomic interventions, which are processes used to improve a worker's comfort, safety, and productivity, have been recommended.[23] Preventative measures, such as conditioning and stretching exercises, have also shown evidence of yielding promising results in some studies.[24] Sonographer stretches can be found on the website of the Society of Diagnostic Medical Sonography (SDMS) (Table 5-8). The SDMS suggests the practice of various stretches throughout the workday, which includes shoulder abduction, shoulder extension, and scapular protraction.[25] A video link of stretches for sonographers is also provided in Table 5-8.

The best practices to reduce the likelihood of developing a WRMSD were approved by the 2011 Consensus Conference on Work-Related Musculoskeletal Disorders in Sonography, and

TABLE 5-8	Web links for sonographer stretches
Society of Diagnostic Medical Sonography	http://www.sdms.org/msi/exercise.asp
Medical Positioning Incorporated	http://info-etudiants.com/videos/?v=−IM5eX4sahY

these are provided for you in Table 5-9.[26] By combining preventative measures such as stretching, exercise, and workplace best practice techniques, you may be capable of preventing WRMSDs and extending your career. The following section will explain some of the causes and suggest some specific ergonomic interventions for the most common locations of pain and WRMSDs in sonography.

Shoulder and Elbow

Craig first described the disorder of "sonographer's shoulder" in 1985.[6] The shoulder is the most common source of pain for sonographers.[7] In fact, shoulder pain is experienced by 75% of diagnostic and vascular sonographers.[27] WRMSDs specific to the sonographer's shoulder include rotator cuff tears, tendinitis, and bursitis.[6] Work that requires an individual to hold his or her shoulder higher than the other or to extend an arm away from the body for an extended amount of time can contribute to the development of these WRMDs.[9] In fact, the degree of forward shoulder flexion (reach) increases the amount of muscle fatigue, and an increase in horizontal distance causes that fatigue to manifest more rapidly.[14] The optimal position for the shoulder is in a neutral position with the goal of the shoulders in a horizontal line while avoiding the lifting of the shoulders toward the ears or hunching the shoulders forward (Fig. 5-12).

TABLE 5-9	Summary of best practices as prescribed by the Consensus Conference on Work-Related Musculoskeletal Disorders

- Minimize sustained bending, twisting, reaching, lifting, pressure, and awkward postures; alternate sitting and standing, and vary scanning techniques and transducer grips.
- Adjust all equipment to suit user's size, and have accessories on hand before beginning to scan.
- Use measures to reduce arm abduction and forward and backward reach to include instructing the patient to move as close to the user as possible, adjusting the table and chair, and using arm supports.
- Relax muscles periodically throughout the day.
- Stretch hand, wrist, shoulder muscles, and spine.
- Take small breaks during procedures.
- Take meal breaks separate from work-related tasks.
- Refocus eyes onto distant objects.
- Vary procedures, tasks, and skills as much as reasonably possible.
- Use correct body mechanics when moving patients, wheelchairs, beds, stretchers, and ultrasound equipment.
- Report and document any persistent pain to your employer, and seek competent medical advice.
- Maintain a good level of physical fitness in order to perform the demanding work tasks required.
- Collaborate with employers on staffing solutions that allow sufficient time away from work.

From Roll S, et al. An analysis of occupational factors related to shoulder discomfort in diagnostic medical sonographers and vascular technologists. *Work* [serial online] 2012;42(3):355–365. Available from: CINAHL with Full Text, Ipswich, MA. Accessed June 9, 2014.

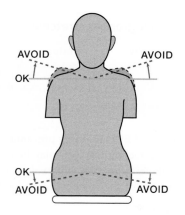

Figure 5-12. Neutral shoulder position. The goal is to have the shoulder in a horizontal line, with the weight evenly balanced when seated. Try to avoid lifting the shoulders toward the ears, hunching your shoulders forward, and sitting with most of your weight on one hip.

Though a neutral shoulder position is optimal, sonographers must utilize their shoulders to obtain sonographic images. Muscle fatigue increases dramatically when the shoulder is abducted greater than 30 degrees.[14] Therefore, the suggested position of the scanning arm is no more than a 30-degree angle of abduction.[14] This position can be improved with the use of positioning cushions, foam blocks placed under the scanning arm in the appropriate position, and/or altering the height of the examination table to achieve such an angle. It is important to note that some sonographers who are short in stature may have to stand for many examinations.

Ergonomic interventions for upper extremity discomfort also include positioning the patient as near to you as possible, utilizing some form of arm support device (whether it be the patient, roll of towels, or a foam block), utilizing a **cable support brace**, adjusting the monitor and control panel to a more comfortable position, and utilizing proper foot support (Table 5-8, Fig. 5-13).[22] A cable support brace is similar to an armband. It is used to hold the cord in place while the transducer is maneuvered. Additionally, there is also a specialized device referred to as the shoulder assist, which can be used to support the entire upper extremity while scanning.[7]

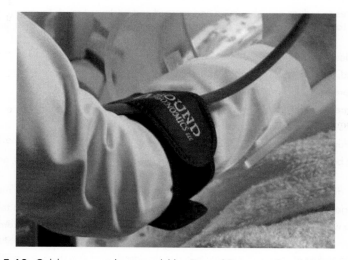

Figure 5-13. Cable support brace sold by Sound Ergonomics. (With permission from Sound Ergonomics.)

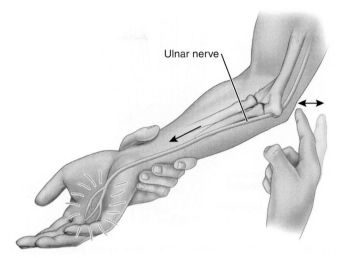

Ulnar nerve

Figure 5-14. The Tinel sign is revealed by tapping over the cubital tunnel. A positive Tinel sign will produce a tingling sensation down the ulnar nerve into the forearm and hand, which indicates nerve entrapment.

The elbow can be another region where pain can manifest while scanning. In sonography, the most common cause of pain within the elbow is from static forceful scanning.[15] However, WRMSDs may also be caused by holding the elbow straight while extending the arm or resting the elbows on a hard surface.[9] Even continual pressure applied to the ulnar nerve while awkwardly resting the elbow on the examination table can lead to a disorder called cubital tunnel syndrome.[6] Cubital tunnel syndrome can be diagnosed using the **Tinel sign**—when simply tapping over the cubital tunnel produces a tingling sensation down the ulnar nerve into the forearm and hand (Fig. 5-14).

While Table 5-10 offers mostly ergonomic interventions for the elbow and shoulder of the scanning arm, one must also be concerned about the position of the non-scanning arm as well. The non-scanning arm, or the typing arm of the sonographer, should be held at a position that allows the elbow to be at a 90-degree angle, thus allowing the upper arm to hang freely by the side.[3,15] With the consistent use of adjustable ultrasound equipment, ergonomic accessories, and patient positioning devices, both of the sonographer's shoulders and elbows can be protected from injury.

TABLE 5-10	Steps to prevent shoulder and elbow discomfort

1. Position the patient near to you.
2. Position ultrasound equipment to reduce awkward postures and promote back, neck, shoulder, and arm comfort.
3. Use a foam block support, extra towels, or the patient's body to support your elbow and rest your arm scanning upon.
4. Use a transducer cord stabilization device such as a cable support brace.
5. Use good foot support.
6. Stand for scanning if needed.
7. If pain or discomfort manifests, take a short break, and change your position immediately.

From Coffin C, Baker J. Preventing work-related injuries among sonographers and sonologists. *Contemporary OB/GYN* [serial online] 2007;52(7):78. Available from: Publisher Provided Full Text Searching File, Ipswich, MA. Accessed July 13, 2014.

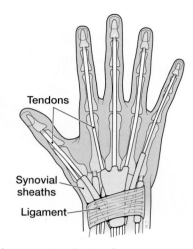

Tendons

Synovial
sheaths

Ligament

Figure 5-15. Tendinitis of the wrist. Tendinitis of the wrist is the painful inflammation of the tendons of the wrist resulting from repetitive strain. It is caused by repeatedly extending the hand up or down at the wrist. The symptoms include pain in the wrist, especially on the outer edges of the hand.

Wrist and Hand

According to one study, 65% of the sonographers complain of pain in the wrist, while 61% complain of pain in the hand or fingers secondary to transducer manipulation.[13] Indeed, there is a range of tissue damage that can result from the manipulation of the transducer, and this is referred to as "transducer use syndrome."[28] Transducer design was found to be the most likely cause of hand and wrist complaints among sonographers.[3] Complaints of hand and wrist pain vary per specialty, and some may stem from tendinitis (Fig. 5-15). For echocardiographers, discomfort is most often experienced in the left wrist and hand, while all other specialty groups indicated more pain in the right wrist and hand.[13] As the sonographer continues to work, the numbness and weakness in the wrists and hands tend to increase.[13] Some of these symptoms can even lead to muscle strength loss to the point where the transducer becomes difficult to manipulate, and it may even be painful to hold in certain positions.[6] Any movement that requires that the wrist be taken out of a neutral position (similar to that of a routine handshake) reduces the strength of the wrist.[9] These non-neutral positions include bending the wrist up, back, and sideways (Figs. 5-16 through 5-18).

There are several WRMSDs that can affect the wrists and hands of the sonographer. One condition that results from sustained awkward wrist positions is carpal tunnel syndrome. Carpal tunnel syndrome is an example of nerve entrapment or a pinched nerve. It is characterized by the median nerve becoming compressed or aggravated within the carpal tunnel (Fig. 5-19). In one study, the diagnosis of carpal tunnel syndrome markedly increased in proportion to the number of years a

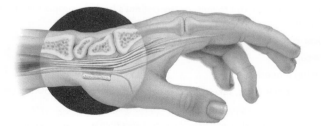

Figure 5-16. A neutral wrist position is the optimal position to reduce wrist strain.

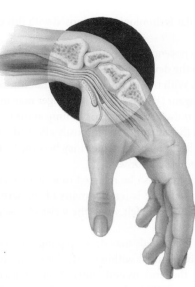

Figure 5-17. The median nerve becomes compressed in the carpal tunnel with flexion of the wrist.

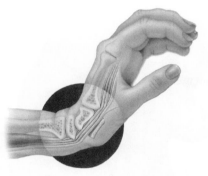

Figure 5-18. The median nerve in the wrist is stretched during extension.

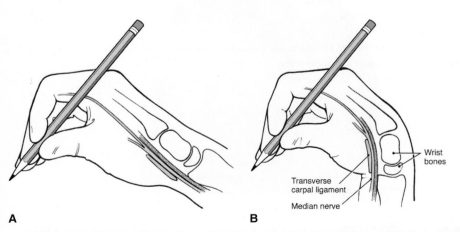

A   B

Figure 5-19. Abnormal wrist positioning can lead to carpal tunnel syndrome. **A.** Wrist in neutral position in straight line with forearm is appropriate. **B.** A bent wrist causes cramping of median nerve in the carpal tunnel of the wrist. Repeated pressure on the median nerve can cause carpal tunnel syndrome.

sonographer worked, with vascular technologists diagnosed with this disorder more often than those in other specialties.[13]

Trigger finger is a form of tenosynovitis, another WRMSD that is caused by repetitive gripping actions. A trigger finger leads to the development of a painless nodule in a flexor tendon in the palm near the head of the metacarpal. With trigger finger, the finger becomes locked in a position and then must be popped to be released again (Fig. 5-20). Trigger finger may initially present with stiffness in the finger, a popping or clicking noise in the finger, or a bump at the base of the finger.[29] This disorder is typically more pronounced in the morning, and it mostly affects the thumb, ring finger, and middle finger of the dominant hand.[29] Eventually, the finger may become locked in a bent position. Trigger finger can accompany carpal tunnel syndrome.

De Quervain disease, which may also be referred to as gamer's thumb or BlackBerry thumb, is another repetitive motion injury that is tenosynovitis of the wrist on the thumb (lateral) side of the wrist (Fig. 5-21). Pain is typically felt when the wrist is twisted or gripping of an object is required.

Also within the wrist, some individuals may develop **ganglion cysts** (Fig. 5-22). These cysts are often recognized as palpable, painful lumps within the tendons or joints of the hands or wrist, though they may also be located within the tendons and joints of the ankles and feet.[30] Ganglion cysts may also be referred to as Bible bumps or Bible thumper cysts, because in the past, people would take a large book like a Bible and rupture the cyst by hitting it with the book. However, this is quite painful

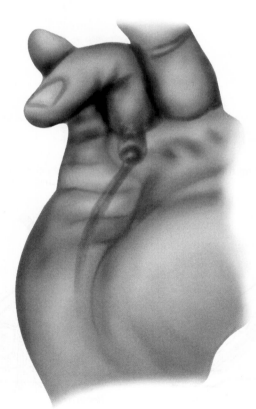

Figure 5-20. A trigger finger results from the development of a painless nodule in a flexor tendon in the palm, near the head of the metacarpal. The nodule eventually becomes too large to enter easily into the tendon sheath when the person tries to extend the fingers from a flexed position. With extra effort or assistance, the finger extends with a palpable and audible snap as the nodule pops into the tendon sheath.

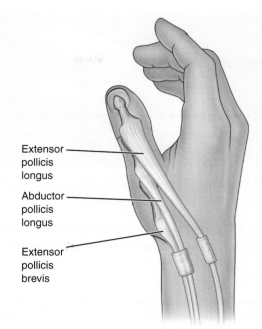

Extensor
pollicis
longus

Abductor
pollicis
longus

Extensor
pollicis
brevis

Figure 5-21. De Quervain tenosynovitis. Excessive friction among the tendons, sheath, and bony process leads to tenosynovitis of the tendons with the thumb. Pain is typically felt when the wrist is twisted or gripping of an object is required.

and not suggested because the cyst will typically return. To properly treat painful ganglion cysts, it is recommended that they either be drained or surgically removed.[30] In an occupation that heavily depends upon the flexibility and use of the wrist, it would not be wise for a sonographer to hit his or her wrist with a heavy book, possibly causing even more significant damage to soft tissue or bone.

One common challenge for sonographers is how to manage the transducer cord. The cord tends to pull against the transducer, resulting in strain from awkward hand and wrist positions. To prevent the discomfort caused by the cord, some sonographers tend to drape the cord around their necks. Or sonographers may place the cord next to the stretcher while holding it firmly in place with a leg.[22] However, these positions are not encouraged and can place unwarranted strain on the cervical and lumbar spine.[22] Draping an unclean cord around the neck could contribute to the spread of microorganisms to the sonographer's neck. To prevent wrist strain and to manage the cord, a cable support brace can provide some much needed support. A wrist brace may also be used to alleviate

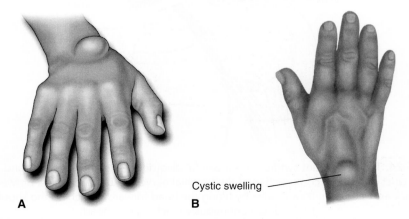

Cystic swelling

A   **B**

Figure 5-22. A large ganglion cyst in the wrist **(A and B)** may be referred to as a Bible bump.

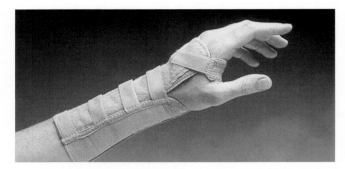

Figure 5-23. The Norco wrist brace is used to treat carpal tunnel and other forms of tendinitis in the wrist.

exaggerated flexion of the wrist (Fig. 5-23). In the future, further development of the cordless transducer may provide some relief from the challenges of the transducer and its cord.

Sound Off

Draping the transducer cord around the neck and holding the cord against the stretcher with your leg are not recommended. These two habits may cause unnecessary strain to your neck and back.

Neck and Back

In conjunction with the upper extremity strains placed upon the sonographer, the neck and back are often areas in which pain can manifest. In fact, the neck and back were cited as having the highest diagnosed frequency of pain in one study.[13] This study revealed that sustained and repetitive twisting of the neck and body aggravated discomfort.[13] One of the WRMSDs that can result from repetitive use is thoracic outlet syndrome. Thoracic outlet syndrome is a term used to describe the compression of the nerves and blood vessels of the neck and shoulder (Fig. 5-24). This disorder can cause pain and tingling in the neck, shoulder, arm, and hand.[9] It is often misdiagnosed as carpal tunnel syndrome.

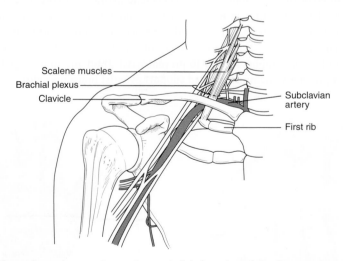

Scalene muscles
Brachial plexus
Clavicle
Subclavian artery
First rib

Figure 5-24. Thoracic outlet syndrome is a painful disorder of the fingers, hand, and possibly the wrist due to the compression of the brachial nerve plexus and vessels between the neck and shoulder. It can cause by tilting the head forward, hunching the shoulders forward, or continuously reaching overhead.

Neck and back pain can manifest because of repetitive twisting of the neck and trunk and can ultimately lead to spinal dysfunction. Spinal dysfunction manifests as neck, upper back, and scapula pain. The most vulnerable area in the back is in the thoracic spine, especially between T3 and T5.[31] However, according to one study, 28% of those surveyed cited the lower back as a source of pain as well.[31] Altering your position and taking occasional short breaks can alleviate some of the strain placed on specific muscle groups in the neck and back. To prevent twisting, you should place the ultrasound machine as close as possible to the examination table and manipulate the ultrasound monitor to reduce neck twisting. If standing, keep your spine straight with your weight evenly distributed between both legs.[1] As mentioned earlier, postural support devices, which serve the purpose of reducing kyphosis and back strain, can be purchased by sonographers as well to reduce neck and back strain.

Lower Extremities

To a lesser extent, the lower half of the body can be a source of WRMSDs. Though others may occur, two WRMSDs that can affect the sonographer are **plantar fasciitis** and **tarsal tunnel syndrome**. Plantar fasciitis is the inflammation of the ligament on the bottom of the foot (Fig. 5-25). It often results in heel pain or a stabbing pain within the foot.[32] Plantar fasciitis is most often caused by continual pressure applied to the ligaments of the foot by standing, but it may be felt after a long period of sitting followed by standing as well. There are personal **orthotic devices** that can be worn on the foot and ankle to prevent the pain associated with plantar fasciitis by providing adequate arch support. Switching to more comfortable or orthotic shoes may remedy the issue as well.

Tarsal tunnel syndrome, like carpal tunnel syndrome, is a nerve entrapment disorder. The tarsal tunnel contains the tibial nerve in the foot. Inflammation or irritation of the nerve can lead to a feeling of burning, stinging, or numbness of the foot and can result from extended periods of standing, walking, or running.[33] Treatment can be accomplished with simple orthotic devices, pain medicine, or injections. Again, switching to more comfortable or orthotic shoes may remedy the issue as well, but recurring or continual pain should be reported to your supervisor.

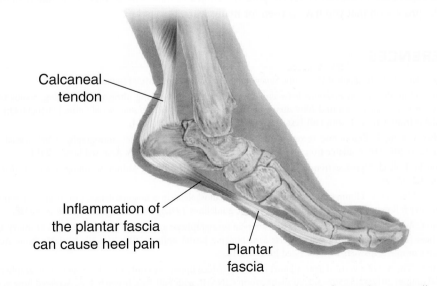

Calcaneal tendon

Inflammation of the plantar fascia can cause heel pain

Plantar fascia

Figure 5-25. Plantar fasciitis is inflammation of the plantar fascia that typically results in heel pain.

GENERAL TREATMENT OF WRMSDs AND LIFESTYLE IMPACT

Though the focus of this chapter has been on prevention, there are many treatment options for WRMSDs. The most common treatment is typically rest and antiinflammatory medications, though some individuals do require more extensive occupational therapies.[13] Other options include chiropractics, massage therapy, acupuncture, fitness programs, athletic programs, trigger point injections, herbal treatments, and physiotherapy.[19] All of these have varying degrees of effectiveness and may work for some and not others.[19] To choose the best option, you should work closely with a qualified physician who has experience treating WRMSDs, because early recognition and treatment is crucial.

Though the overall economic impact has been previously mentioned, one must also consider the personal lifestyle impact caused by the development of WRMSDs as well. As we have discovered, the manifestation of these disorders will certainly affect your ability to perform your job, but they can also negatively affect your lifestyle and even your relationships with others. Being able to perform normal physical exercise is important to our emotional well-being, and our emotional state helps maintain our ability to adjust to everyday challenges. For this reason, if at any time in your career you feel that you may be developing a WRMSD, take immediate action to prevent any further damage, notify your doctor, and notify your employer, so that you can fulfill your dream of maintaining a long-lasting and healthy career in sonography.

SUMMARY

WRMSDs are either occupationally acquired or occupationally aggravated injuries to an individual's muscles, tendons, ligaments, and cartilage that results from repetitive use. The most common locations of WRMSDs for sonographers are the shoulder, neck, wrist, back, and hands. This chapter provided an overview of the most frequently encountered WRMSDs for the practicing sonographer. Though the symptoms of each disorder were provided, the main focus has been on the steps you can take in order to prevent the development of these disorders. By being aware that your new chosen profession could offer some physical challenges for you in the future, you can mediate and try to prevent these challenges early in your career by making it routine to practice the aforementioned guidelines and best practices offered in this chapter throughout your workday. Be cognizant of pain that you experience in the initial days of your training, and make alterations immediately in order to enjoy the profession that you have chosen for many years.

REFERENCES

1. Hagen-Ansert SL. *Textbook of Diagnostic Sonography*. 7th ed. St. Louis, MO: Elsevier; 2012.

2. Polak J, et al. Possible associations between scan quality and pain during ultrasound scanning: results from the Society for Vascular Ultrasound 2009 survey on ergonomics. *J Vasc Ultrasound* [serial online] 2010;34(4):171–174. Available from: CINAHL with Full Text, Ipswich, MA. Accessed June 9, 2014.

3. Horkey J, King P. Ergonomic recommendations and their role in cardiac sonography. *Work* [serial online] 2004;22(3):207–218. Available from: Business Source Complete, Ipswich, MA. Accessed June 9, 2014.

4. Pocratsky J, et al. Upper extremity kinematics in sonographers during kidney scanning. *J Diagn Med Sonogr* 2014;30(2):67–76.

5. Euler E, Meadow V. Elimination of sonographer musculoskeletal in a hospital-based cardiovascular sonography laboratory following implementation of ergonomic guidelines. *J Diagn Med Sonogr* 2012;28(6):325–328.

6. Coffin C. Work-related musculoskeletal disorders in sonographers: a review of causes and types of injury and best practices for reducing injury risk. *Reports Med Imaging* [serial online] 2014;7:15–26. Available from: Academic Search Complete, Ipswich, MA. Accessed June 9, 2014.

7. Coffin C. The use of a vertical arm support device to reduce upper extremity muscle firing in sonographers. *Work* [serial online] 2012;42(3):367–371. Available from: CINAHL with Full Text, Ipswich, MA. Accessed June 9, 2014.

8. Coffin C, Baker J. Ultrasound clinics. Preventing work-related injuries among sonographers and sonologists. *Contemporary OB/GYN* [serial online] 2007;52(7):78. Available from: CINAHL with Full Text, Ipswich, MA. Accessed June 9, 2014.

9. Peddie S. *The Repetitive Strain Injury Sourcebook*. Los Angeles, CA: Lowell House; 1998.

10. Dutton AG, et al. *Torres' Patient Care in Imaging Technology*. 8th ed. Philadelphia, PA: Lippincott Williams & Wilkins; 2013.

11. Timby BK. *Fundamental Nursing Skills and Concepts*. 10th ed. Philadelphia, PA: Lippincott Williams & Wilkins; 2013.

12. Top 10 list for sonographer safety. Retrieved from http://www.soundergonomics.com/pdf/topten.pdf

13. Evans K, et al. Factors that contribute to wrist-hand-finger discomfort in diagnostic medical sonographers and vascular technologists. *J Diagn Med Sonogr* [serial online] 2010;26(3):121–129. Available from: CINAHL with Full Text, Ipswich, MA. Accessed July 13, 2014.

14. Murphey S, Milkowski A. Surface EMG evaluation of sonographer scanning postures. *J Diagn Med Sonogr* [serial online] 2006;22(5):298–307. Available from: CINAHL with Full Text, Ipswich, MA. Accessed July 13, 2014.

15. Jakes C. Sonographers and occupational overuse syndrome: cause, effect, and solutions. *J Diagn Med Sonogr* [serial online] 2001;17(6):312–322. Available from: CINAHL with Full Text, Ipswich, MA. Accessed July 13, 2014.

16. Vetter L, et al. Variation of pinch and grip force between different size transducers: a preliminary study. *J Diagn Med Sonogr* [serial online] 2013;29(6):245–252. Available from: CINAHL with Full Text, Ipswich, MA. Accessed July 13, 2014.

17. Industry standards for the prevention of work-related musculoskeletal disorders in sonography: consensus conference on work-related musculoskeletal disorders in sonography. *J Diagn Med Sonogr* [serial online] 2011;27(1):14–18. Available from: CINAHL with Full Text, Ipswich, MA. Accessed July 13, 2014.

18. Evans K. Focusing on the issues. The interface between sonographer and the sonographic machine: a post-postmodern perspective. *J Diagn Med Sonogr* [serial online] 2007;23(1):38–43. Available from: CINAHL with Full Text, Ipswich, MA. Accessed July 13, 2014.

19. Muir M, et al. The nature, cause, and extent of occupational musculoskeletal injuries among sonographers: recommendations for treatment and prevention. *J Diagn Med Sonogr* 2004;20:317–325.

20. Evans K, et al. Factors that contribute to wrist-hand-finger discomfort in diagnostic medical sonographers and vascular technologists. *J Diagn Med Sonogr* [serial online] 2010;26(3):121–129. Available from: CINAHL with Full Text, Ipswich, MA. Accessed July 13, 2014.

21. Wilkinson M, Grimmer K. Sonographic analysis: normal variability of muscle and tendon of the shoulder in response to daily activity and exercise. *J Diagn Med Sonogr* [serial online] 2004;20(1):25–36. Available from: CINAHL with Full Text, Ipswich, MA. Accessed July 13, 2014.

22. Coffin C, Baker J. Preventing work-related injuries among sonographers and sonologists. *Contemporary OB/GYN* [serial online] 2007;52(7):78. Available from: Publisher Provided Full Text Searching File, Ipswich, MA. Accessed July 13, 2014.

23. Leyshon R, et al. Ergonomic interventions for office workers with musculoskeletal disorders: a systematic review. *Work* [serial online]. 2010;35(3):335–348. Available from: Business Source Complete, Ipswich, MA. Accessed June 9, 2014.

24. Alaniz J, Veale B. Stretching for sonographers: a literature review of sonographer-reported musculoskeletal injuries. *J Diagn Med Sonogr* [serial online] 2013;29(4):188–190. Available from: CINAHL with Full Text, Ipswich, MA. Accessed July 13, 2014. SDMS website http://www.sdms.org/msi/exercise.asp

25. Industry standards for the prevention of work-related musculoskeletal disorders in sonography: consensus conference on work-related musculoskeletal disorders in sonography. *J Diagn Med Sonogr* [serial online] 2011;27(1):14–18. Available from: CINAHL with Full Text, Ipswich, MA. Accessed July 14, 2014.

26. Roll S, et al. An analysis of occupational factors related to shoulder discomfort in diagnostic medical sonographers and vascular technologists. *Work* [serial online] 2012;42(3):355–365. Available from: CINAHL with Full Text, Ipswich, MA. Accessed June 9, 2014.

27. Hill JJ, et al. Anthropometric measurements, job strain, and prevalence of musculoskeletal symptoms in female medical sonographers. *Work* 2009;33:181–189.

28. Trigger finger. Retrieved from http://www.mayoclinic.org/diseases-conditions/trigger-finger/basics/definition/con-20043819

29. Ganglion cyst. Retrieved from http://www.mayoclinic.org/diseases-conditions/ganglion-cyst/basics/definition/con-20023936

30. Brown G, Baker J. Work-related musculoskeletal disorders in sonographers. *J Diagn Med Sonogr* 2004;20(2):85–93.

31. Bastian E, et al. Effects of work experience, patient size, and hand preference on the performance of sonography studies. *J Diagn Med Sonogr* [serial online] 2009;25(1):25–37. Available from: CINAHL with Full Text, Ipswich, MA. Accessed July 13, 2014.

32. Plantar fasciitis. Retrieved from http://www.mayoclinic.org/diseases-conditions/plantar-fasciitis/basics/definition/con-20025664

33. Tarsal tunnel syndrome. Retrieved from http://www.hopkinsmedicine.org/neurology_neurosurgery/centers_clinics/peripheral_nerve_surgery/conditions/tarsal-tunnel-syndrome.html

Thinking Critically

1. Observe the sonographers during your clinical rotations, and document and discuss with your classmates the occupational stressors that you see during the workday of the staff sonographer.
2. Evaluate the room design in the sonography department at your clinical facility. What changes could be made in an effort to prevent WRMSDs?
3. Interview a staff sonographer, and inquire about his or her awareness of WRMSDs. Is he or she scanning in pain? If so, offer some insight about how to prevent further damage.
4. Evaluate the equipment design (machines, transducer, stretchers, chairs, etc.) in the sonography department at your clinical facility. What changes could be made in an effort to prevent WRMSDs?
5. Do you have any of the predisposing conditions to WRMSDs? If so, make a plan to discuss any concerns you may have with your doctor and your sonography program faculty and administration. Prevention is the key!

Chapter 5
Review Questions

1. **Which of the following locations would be the most likely location for a sonographer to suffer a WRMSD?**
   a. Neck
   b. Back
   c. Hand
   d. Shoulder

2. **Which of the following is not a nerve entrapment disorder?**
   a. Carpal tunnel syndrome
   b. Thoracic outlet syndrome
   c. Tarsal tunnel syndrome
   d. Trigger finger syndrome

3. **What disorder is described as a repetitive motion injury that is characterized by tenosynovitis of the thumb side of the wrist?**
   a. Carpal tunnel syndrome
   b. De Quervain disease
   c. Plantar fasciitis
   d. Cubital tunnel syndrome

4. **Moving the arm away from the body is referred to as**
   a. abduction.
   b. adduction.
   c. flexion.
   d. extension.

5. **What percentage of sonographers reports scanning in pain?**
   a. Between 80% and 90%
   b. Between 40% and 50%
   c. Between 95% and 99%
   d. Between 20% and 35%

6. What is defined as the scientific study of creating tools and equipment that help the human body adapt to the work environment?
   a. Body mechanics
   b. Posture science
   c. Ergonomics
   d. Work-related musculoskeletal discipline

7. Which of the following would be least likely to increase an individual's likelihood of developing a WRMSD?
   a. Previous trauma to the body
   b. Exercise
   c. Smoking
   d. Excessive alcohol consumption

8. The suggested position of the scanning arm is no more than a __-degree angle of abduction?
   a. 45
   b. 40
   c. 30
   d. 15

9. To prevent repetitive trauma and strain placed upon the sonographer's wrist and elbow, what device should be worn on the arm?
   a. Thoracic outlet sling
   b. Cable support brace
   c. Baker device
   d. Support cushion

10. Which of the following is not another name for work-related musculoskeletal disorders?
    a. Abduction injuries
    b. Repetitive strain injuries
    c. Cumulative trauma disorders
    d. Overuse syndrome

11. The main ergonomic factors that have been identified as primary concerns for cardiac sonographers are posture, repetition, force, and
    a. overall health.
    b. work schedule.
    c. equipment design.
    d. room design.

12. What is described as maintaining muscle work over a long period of time that results in the gradual damage to muscles due to abnormal contraction and consequent buildup of fibrous tissue within the muscles?
    a. Abduction
    b. Muscular atrophy
    c. Muscle spasm
    d. Static muscle loading

13. Which of the following would be the least helpful practice to prevent WRMDs?
    a. Stretch hand, wrist, and shoulder muscles.
    b. Take small breaks during procedures.
    c. Take meal breaks separate from work-related tasks.
    d. Dim the monitor to help strengthen the eye muscles.

14. **The patient position should be adjusted so that the patient is**
    a. as close as possible to the sonographer.
    b. at arm's length from the sonographer.
    c. at 30 degrees from the sonographer's elbow.
    d. at 45 degrees from the sonographer's elbow.

15. **Which of the following is another name for lateral epicondylitis?**
    a. Trigger finger
    b. Tennis elbow
    c. Carpal tunnel syndrome
    d. Plantar fasciitis

16. **The most vulnerable area for pain in the sonographer's back is between**
    a. T1 and T3.
    b. L1 and L5.
    c. L3 and L5.
    d. T3 and T5.

17. **Ganglion cysts are most likely found in the**
    a. neck.
    b. back.
    c. wrist.
    d. finger.

18. **Trigger finger is a form of**
    a. tendinitis.
    b. tenosynovitis.
    c. epicondylitis.
    d. bursitis.

19. **Which of the following is described as the compression of the nerves and blood vessels of the neck and shoulder due to repetitive strain?**
    a. Thoracic outlet syndrome
    b. Plantar fasciitis
    c. Rotator cuff tear
    d. Epicondylitis

20. **What structure is most affected by plantar fasciitis?**
    a. Ligament in the bottom of the foot
    b. Tendon sheath in the top of the foot
    c. Lateral epicondyle in the knee
    d. Medial epicondyle in the ankle

6

Ethics and Professionalism

CHAPTER OBJECTIVES

- Understand the ethical standards of the sonography profession.
- Discuss ethical issues in diagnostic medical sonography.
- Comprehend the importance of professionalism.

KEY TERMS

Altruism – actions aimed at increasing the welfare of others, particularly those in need

Codes of ethics – the statements of acceptable and unacceptable behavior of a profession

Conflicts of interest – exist when there are inappropriate relationships between personal interests and professional obligations

Consequentialism – ethical theory that seeks to find out the end result in decision making, and it is based on the consequences of the decision being made to benefit the largest amount of people

Deontologic theory – ethical theory based on duty; thus, one makes the decision out of obligation that the rules must be followed at all times regardless of the consequences

Duty – the open recognition of a commitment to service

Entertainment ultrasound – non-diagnostic sonography performed to provide video amusement for the obstetric patient, family, and friends

Ethical decision making – a process that we use to make choices based on our moral principles and personal values

Ethics – a set of morals and a code of behavior that helps inform a person or group of people as to what is right (moral) and what is wrong (immoral)

Excellence – demanding one's very best

Fetal keepsake imaging – non-diagnostic sonography performed to provide the obstetric patient with keepsake photos and videos of the fetus

Golden rule – do to others what you would have them do to you

Humanism – concept that involves selfless behavior and the act of crediting others when credit is due to them; also includes admitting wrong doing

Informed consent – process of gaining permission before a medical procedure is conducted

Medical ethics – the application of our moral principles in interactions with others in the medical profession, including our coworkers, patients, and the community

Moral compass – internal compass that helps guide us as we face daily challenges that involve instances that require ethical decision making

Moral principles – accepted rules of conduct, including integrity, compassion, honesty, and respectfulness

Morals – generally accepted customs of right living and behavior within our society

Nonconsequentialism – see deontologic theory

Norms – group-held beliefs or standards that are agreed upon by individuals or groups of individuals

Patient confidentiality – refers to the concept of privacy; no personal patient information

should be shared with anyone uninvolved with the patient's care

Personal values – things that someone holds in high regard and that are highly desirable and worthy of esteem

Professional ethics – publicly displayed ethical conduct of a profession or a particular group

Professional etiquette – the everyday practice of good manners and being agreeable within the exercise of one's occupation

Professionalism – an awareness of conduct, aims, and qualities that define a profession

Teleologic theory – see consequentialism

Virtue ethics – ethical theory that focuses on the use of practical wisdom and moral character, providing elements of both teleologic and deontologic thinking

INTRODUCTION

Throughout the previous chapters, there have been multiple references to ethics and professionalism. Specifically, early in Chapter 1, within a brief discussion on professionalism in the clinical setting, the professional code of ethics for sonographers was mentioned. In Chapter 2, the importance of work ethic was discussed in sonography. This chapter takes a more in-depth look at professional ethics and professionalism. Pursuing a career in sonography requires that you appraise your own personal motives behind your choices. Ultimately, however, regardless of the reasoning behind your intentions for becoming a sonographer, we all share in the same obligation to provide ethical and professional care to each patient equitably, regardless of the patient's condition.

ETHICS AND PERSONAL VALUES

Ethics is a set of **morals** and a code of behavior that helps inform a person or group of people as to what is right (moral) and what is wrong (immoral).[1] Morals are generally accepted customs of right living and behavior within our society.[2] Ethics is not just about how you feel, but rather how we treat others "face to face, person to person, day in and day out, over a prolonged period of time."[3] Ethics should be grounded in reason and fact.[4] For example, most people know that cheating is wrong. Ethics is not just making the claim that cheating is wrong. Rather, ethics is providing a reason why cheating is wrong—because it gives an unfair advantage to the cheater.[4] Ultimately, our ethics enlightens us as to how to interact with others, personally, professionally, and within society.[1,5]

Most of us are guided by moral standards or **moral principles**, which are accepted rules of conduct, including integrity, compassion, honesty, and respectfulness. Moral principles are acquired throughout our lives, with the initial principles being established early in our youth. Most of us learned from our parents the basics of right and wrong behavior. As we age and have more interactions with society, we learn how to interact appropriately by openly expressing our moral principles, either in words or by our actions. Many moral principles like honesty and compassion have a dual purpose. Honesty both protects us from legal concerns in society and it enhances the trust that others have in us, while compassion improves our lives and the lives of others. Conversely, immoral behavior, like theft, lying, or purposely harming another person, negatively affects both our lives and the lives of others.

In Chapter 2, we learned that personal values are things that someone holds in high regard, and these are highly desirable and worthy of respect. We also learned that a person's character comprises how he or she thinks, feels, and acts. One's moral character is defined by what one values. People with strong moral character value honesty, integrity, and fairness.[3] As a result, people with strong moral character also have a natural inclination to care for the well-being of others.[3]

Personal values include family, financial resources, friends, health and fitness, home and place, leadership, leisure pursuits, personal growth, public service, spirituality, and work satisfaction.[6] As a result, our personal values can be ranked according to priority. A life value assessment tool can be found at http://www.whatsnext.com/content/life-values-self-assessment-test. If you choose to complete the life value assessment tool, it is important to note that because our life conditions change, the ranking of our personal values change as well. That is to say, just because you value financial stability greatly at this time in your life, your personal values could change as you become more financially established.

Ethical Theories

There are several ethical theories or schools of thought. The following section discusses three: **teleologic theory**, **deontologic theory**, and **virtue ethics**. Teleologic theory, or **consequentialism**, seeks to find out the end result in decision making, and it is based on the consequences of the decision being made to benefit the largest amount of people; the result is the highest amount of benefits for the most people.[7] Deontologic theory, or **nonconsequentialism**, is based on **duty**, and thus, one makes the decision out of obligation that the rules must be followed at all times regardless of the consequences.[7] Here, duty is defined as the open recognition of a commitment to service.

For example, a consequentialist sonographer may lie to a patient if he or she felt the patient would benefit from that lie. A nonconsequentialist sonographer would never lie to a patient because lying is wrong. Sonographers do have a duty to be honest (deontologic theory) with patients in the performance of their occupation, but they must also do so with the consequences of their decisions in mind (teleologic theory). Virtue ethics focuses on the use of practical wisdom and moral character, providing elements of both teleologic and deontologic thinking.[8] Instead of just analyzing the duty and possible end result of the decision, virtue ethics takes into account how decisions affect everyone involved, including the patient, the patient's family, and even how society might be impacted.[7]

The **golden rule**—"Do to others what you would have them do to you"—is not "old school."[9] It is not obsolete or old-fashioned. There may be no other elementary yet concrete ethical truism upon which proper patient care can be based. The golden rule is not just a religious mandate for a few, but rather, it is a maxim advocated by many people of many different religions all over the world. It is a fundamental rule upon which many base their lives. Fortunately, treating every patient fairly with respect and compassion is quite easily accomplished. All one has to do is consistently place oneself in the patient's situation and follow the golden rule.

Patients come to us when they are in need of care. Many of them are at fragile moments in life. Always treat them fairly. If you lose this tendency at any time in your career, it would most certainly benefit your future patients if you were to reflect upon the reasons why this has happened. In many ways, the ethical theories of Immanuel Kant are in agreement with the golden rule. Kant thought that a truly moral act is never influenced by self-interest; rather, a moral person sees the act as duty.[10] Kant's theory can be divided into three parts, all of which pertain to actions that are morally founded upon the principle of treating everyone equitably (Table 6-1).

To help you avoid the legal concerns in the following chapter, you must continually ask yourself as you work with others, "How would I want to be treated in this situation?" You may also imagine

TABLE 6-1	Immanuel Kant's ethical theory

1. If you wish to act morally, act as if your action in each circumstance is to become law for everyone, yourself included, in the future.
2. If you wish to act morally, always treat other human beings as "ends in themselves" and never merely as "means." (In other words, never use people as a means to get what you want.)
3. If you wish to act morally, always act as a member of a community in which all the other members of that community are "ends" just as you are. (Treat people equally.)

From Seedhouse D. *Ethics: The Heart of Health Care.* 3rd ed. Chichester, GBR, UK: John Wiley & Sons; 2009. ProQuest ebrary. Web. 17 July 2014.

your closest loved one in the patient's situation—perhaps your mother, father, child, or sibling. How would you want him or her to be treated? This may seem to be a primitive assignment, but it is valuable, and it will guarantee that you continually consider your patient's circumstances and hopefully be mindful of treating all patients equitably and fairly.

Sound Off

Treating every patient fairly with respect and compassion is quite easily accomplished. All one has to do is to consistently place oneself in the patient's situation and follow the golden rule.

Ethics in Action

Ethical decision making is a process that we use to make choices based on our moral principles and personal values. We each have a **moral compass** that helps guide us as we face daily challenges that involve instances that require ethical decision making. We use our moral compass frequently, often subconsciously. In his book, *Winners Never Cheat*, Jon Huntsman claims that no one is raised in a "moral vacuum" and that regardless of our different religious upbringings, we are all taught from an early age that cheating and lying are wrong.[11] You may create ways to bend the truth and even get away with it, but deep down, you know what is really true.

Life consists of a constant bombardment of choices. Most of our choices are benign and seemingly inconsequential, like choosing what to eat for breakfast. But some can be critical. For example, what if a sonographer who must leave a sleeping patient alone for only a few minutes disregards extending the bedrails in order to save time? Certainly, the patient might stay asleep, not change position, and therefore not roll off of the bed. But the patient could potentially roll off the bed and become badly injured. Ultimately, it is the sonographer's choice to put up the bedrails. But is this situation the result of an ethical decision or rather a routine job duty that has been neglected? Indeed, this situation provides an example of negligence, which will be discussed in the next chapter. However, if we recall that ethical decision making is the process that we use to make choices based on our moral principles and personal values, then we must recognize that ethical decision making should *always* include being mindful of the patient's safety (regardless of time saved). Our compassion for others should outweigh the need to get something done quickly; thus, taking the minimal time that it takes to raise the bedrails to prevent a fall could save the patient from unnecessary pain, and at the same time, it avoids legal consequences.

Like the example provided in the previous paragraph, though there is a process for ethical decision making, our choices are typically made in "the moment," with the final decision being based on the situation and our emotional state at that particular time (Table 6-2).[10] Unfortunately, when caught off guard, some of these impulsive choices can make us deviate from our moral principles. For example, early in your academic experience, you may have made the ethical decision to never cheat on a test. However, when you are faced with the spontaneous opportunity to cheat on a test for which you did not fully prepare for without apparent ramifications, you are again faced with an impulsive ethical choice to make. What will you choose? This is a question of your integrity.

TABLE 6-2	Ethical decision-making process

1. Define the problem
2. Know the principles, standards, and laws that relate to the problem
3. Develop a possible course of action
4. Analyze the possible course of action
5. Choose the best course of action that represents your values
6. Review the results of your actions
7. Learn from your actions

From U.S. Army. Ethical Decisions and the Decision Making Process. Retrieved from http://www.acsap.army.mil/programs/pccert/ethicsonline/Decisionmaking.asp

Integrity, which was defined in Chapter 2 as thinking with honesty and choosing the best path to follow based on high standards, can be observed by others on a daily basis in the manner in which you interact with others. However, as a sonographer, you will make countless decisions that are not readily observed by others that impact the well-being of your patients. Like the choice of cheating on a test, there may be no obvious consequences that results from mistreating or disrespecting patients. Always remember, the true test of integrity occurs when no one is watching.[13]

Sound Off
The true test of integrity occurs when no one is watching.

Medical Ethics and Codes of Ethics

Medical ethics refers to the application of our moral principles in interactions with others in the medical profession, including our coworkers, patients, and the community.[4] Many of these ethical interactions relate to everyday patient care, but they are also concerned with critical topics associated with legal matters, such as end-of-life decisions, **informed consent**, **patient confidentiality**, and patient rights, all of which will be discussed in the next chapter.[14] However, there are several principles contained within medical ethics that can help guide you when confronted with ethical dilemmas in the practice of patient care (Table 6-3).[4]

The Sonographer Code of Ethics

Professional ethics is defined as publicly displayed ethical conduct of a profession or a particular group.[2] As a profession becomes more established, that profession eventually institutes **codes of ethics**, which are statements of acceptable and unacceptable behavior of a profession, including accepted principles and expectations that help guide the individual professional in the standard ethical practice of his or her occupation. Codes provide the professional with an operational blueprint of **norms** that one should follow. Norms are group-held beliefs or standards that are agreed upon by individuals or groups of individuals.[2] Codes of ethics increase the level of competence within a profession and promote a certain level of **professionalism**.[15]

The Society of Diagnostic Medical Sonography (SDMS) offers a code of ethics for the sonographer (Table 6-4). According to the SDMS, the objectives of the code of ethics include the following: to create and encourage an environment in which professional and ethical issues are discussed and addressed, to help the individual diagnostic medical sonographer identify ethical issues, and to provide guidelines for individual diagnostic medical sonographers regarding ethical behavior.[16] The initial framework for many codes of ethics is based on duties and principles, but the modern approach to medical ethics must recognize the need for professional regulation and law.[17] For this reason, the following chapter returns to many of these codes and provides you further with an overview of legal matters as they relate to the sonography profession.

TABLE 6-3	Guiding ethical principles of medical ethics
Principle	**Explanation**
Principle of autonomy	People have the right to make decisions about their lives.
Principle of beneficence	To "do good." To act in a manner that will benefit others.
Principle of nonmaleficence	To "do no harm." While on your quest to do good, do no harm to the patient.
Principle of justice	Treat all patients equally, no matter what their economic, physical, or mental conditions.
Principle of confidentiality	Refers to the concept of privacy. No personal patient information should be shared with anyone uninvolved with the patient's care.
Principle of fidelity	The duty to fulfill one's commitments; applies to keeping promises. Never promise results you cannot deliver.
Principle of paternalism	The approach that prompts healthcare workers to make decisions about the care of a patient without the patient's direct input. Always acting in instances to prevent harm to a patient, even if the patient has no input in the decision.
Principle of the sanctity of life	One cannot make life and death decisions for patients based on personal values. Nobody has the right to conclude that another person's life is not of value and should be terminated.
Principle of veracity	Refers to the honesty in all aspects of one's life.
Principle of respect of property	Refers to keeping the patients' belongings safe and taking care to not damage it.

From Fremgen BF. *Medical Law and Ethics*. 3rd ed. Upper Saddle River, NJ: Pearson Prentice Hall; 2009; and Dutton AG, Linn-Watson TA, Torres LS. *Torres' Patient Care in Imaging Technology*. 8th ed. Philadelphia, PA: Lippincott, Williams, & Wilkins; 2013.

Ethical Issues in Diagnostic Medical Sonography

Ethical issues abound in healthcare. There are several ethical dilemmas that are at the forefront of medicine and sonography in the United States. Some of them have been resolved, if only temporarily by laws that have been created by the people's representatives. However, just because a consensus has been established and thereby laws enacted, strong ethical views exist on both sides of most arguments. Some views are simply based on emotions, some are founded on scientific research and facts, and some combine both emotions and science. The following section is not offered to provide biased opinion about ethical topics but rather to initiate your own reflection on these topics by offering both sides of the argument in the hopes that you will do your own research and form your own conclusions.

Non-Diagnostic Use of Ultrasound

Although the topic may be seen by some as both an ethical and legal issue, the question of the non-diagnostic use of ultrasound is still an unresolved argument in our society. If ultrasound is said to be biologically safe at diagnostic ranges, then why can we not employ this imaging tool for non-diagnostic purposes? Examples of the non-diagnostic use of ultrasound include **entertainment ultrasound** and three-dimensional/four-dimensional (3D/4D) **fetal keepsake imaging**.

TABLE 6-4	SDMS principles of the *Code of Ethics for the Profession of Diagnostic Medical Sonography*

Principle I: In order to promote patient well-being, the diagnostic medical sonographer shall:

A. Provide information to the patient about the purpose of the sonography procedure and respond to the patient's questions and concerns.

B. Respect the patient's autonomy and the right to refuse the procedure.

C. Recognize the patient's individuality and provide care in a nonjudgmental and nondiscriminatory manner.

D. Promote the privacy, dignity, and comfort of the patient by thoroughly explaining the examination, patient positioning, and implementing proper draping techniques.

E. Maintain confidentiality of acquired patient information, and follow national patient privacy regulations as required by the "Health Insurance Portability and Accountability Act of 1996 (HIPAA)."

F. Promote patient safety during the provision of sonography procedures and while the patient is in the care of the diagnostic medical sonographer.

Principle II: To promote the highest level of competent practice, diagnostic medical sonographers shall:

A. Obtain appropriate diagnostic medical sonography education and clinical skills to ensure competence.

B. Achieve and maintain specialty specific sonography credentials. Sonography credentials must be awarded by a national sonography credentialing body that is accredited by a national organization, which accredits credentialing bodies, i.e., the National Commission for Certifying Agencies (NCCA); http://www.noca.org/ncca/ncca.htm or the International Organization for Standardization (ISO); http://www.iso.org/iso/en/ISOOnline.frontpage.

C. Uphold professional standards by adhering to defined technical protocols and diagnostic criteria established by peer review.

D. Acknowledge personal and legal limits, practice within the defined scope of practice, and assume responsibility for his/her actions.

E. Maintain continued competence through lifelong learning, which includes continuing education, acquisition of specialty specific credentials and recredentialing.

F. Perform medically indicated ultrasound studies, ordered by a licensed physician or their designated healthcare provider.

G. Protect patients and/or study subjects by adhering to oversight and approval of investigational procedures, including documented informed consent.

H. Refrain from the use of any substances that may alter judgment or skill and thereby compromise patient care.

I. Be accountable and participate in regular assessment and review of equipment, procedures, protocols, and results. This can be accomplished through facility accreditation.

Principle III: To promote professional integrity and public trust, the diagnostic medical sonographer shall:

A. Be truthful and promote appropriate communications with patients and colleagues.

B. Respect the rights of patients, colleagues, and yourself.

C. Avoid conflicts of interest and situations that exploit others or misrepresent information.

D. Accurately represent his or her experience, education, and credentialing.

E. Promote equitable access to care.

F. Collaborate with professional colleagues to create an environment that promotes communication and respect.

G. Communicate and collaborate with others to promote ethical practice.

H. Engage in ethical billing practices.

I. Engage only in legal arrangements in the medical industry.

J. Report deviations from the Code of Ethics to institutional leadership for internal sanctions, local intervention and/or criminal prosecution. The Code of Ethics can serve as a valuable tool to develop local policies and procedures.

From SDMS Code of Ethics for the Profession of Diagnostic Medical Sonography. Retrieved from http://www.sdms.org/about/codeofethics.asp

Our professional organizations are clear about their stance concerning the non-diagnostic use of ultrasound in medicine. The official statement of the American Institute of Ultrasound in Medicine (AIUM) is that the organization "advocates the responsible use of diagnostic ultrasound and strongly discourages the non-medical use of ultrasound for entertainment purposes. The use of ultrasound without a medical indication to view the fetus, obtain images of the fetus, or determine the fetal gender is inappropriate and contrary to responsible medical practice."[18]

However, on the other side of the argument, some may point to another official statement by the AIUM regarding the clinical use of ultrasound that in part states "No independently confirmed adverse effects caused by exposure from present diagnostic ultrasound instruments have been reported in human patients in the absence of contrast agents. Biological effects (such as localized pulmonary bleeding) have been reported in mammalian systems at diagnostically relevant exposures, but the clinical significance of such effects is not yet known."[18] Some may argue that since there are no proven "adverse effects" that ultrasound is safe for anyone to use. However, the AIUM statement continues to read: "Ultrasound should be used by qualified health professionals to provide medical benefit to the patient" and that "ultrasound exposure during examinations should be as low as reasonably achievable."[18]

It appears that the "clinical use" of ultrasound in medicine is the key to the professional argument. The AIUM offers a clear distinction for the clinical use of ultrasound to "provide medical benefit to the patient." Alternatively, the entertainment argument would claim that the AIUM suggests that ultrasound is safe, as "no independently confirmed adverse effects caused by exposure from present diagnostic ultrasound instruments have been reported in human patients in the absence of contrast agents," and therefore, elective studies should be permitted.

Entertainment ultrasound in obstetrics is the use of ultrasound to provide additional viewing of the fetus for the family and for the amusement of other onlookers. There are businesses that offer "sonogram parties" for prospective parents, family, and friends to view the fetus. The main arguments for entertainment ultrasound include the following: (1) there are no proven biologic effects of ultrasound on the fetus, (2) the sonogram is not for diagnostic purposes, and (3) the sonogram is performed after an official diagnostic sonogram has been completed.

Fetal keepsake imaging sonograms, which often include both 3D or 4D imaging of the fetus, can be performed as an adjunct to a diagnostic sonographic examination, or as a separate elective examination. While the adjunct images to the diagnostic exams are often performed under a physician's guidance in an office or hospital setting, some freestanding facilities may provide the 3D or 4D images for the patients without providing diagnostic information. These may be referred to as elective sonograms. In the physician's office setting, the supplementary 3D or 4D images may be included in the obstetric examination cost, or there may be an additional cost to the patient. In the freestanding facility, the patient is typically required to pay out of pocket.

Regarding fetal keepsake videos, the Food and Drug Administration (FDA) claims that "Persons who promote, sell, or lease ultrasound equipment for making 'keepsake' fetal videos should know that FDA views this as an unapproved use of a medical device. In addition, those who subject individuals to ultrasound exposure using a diagnostic ultrasound device (a prescription device) without a physician's order may be in violation of state or local laws or regulations regarding use of a prescription medical device."[19] In a 2015 update, the FDA further warned that "there is no control on how long a single imaging session will last, how many sessions will take place, or whether the ultrasound systems will be operated properly," and for this reason, the FDA advises expectant mothers to avoid fetal keepsake imaging.[19]

Ultrasound Screening for Vascular Disease

Ultrasound screening companies provide their customers with pay-out-of-pocket ultrasound exams like abdominal aortic aneurysm screening, carotid artery screening, and peripheral arterial disease screening. These examinations are not ordered by physicians. That is to say, patients who undergo these elective screening sonograms are often asymptomatic for disease. The AIUM claims that "there is no evidence in the peer-reviewed medical literature suggesting the value for duplex carotid artery screening using ultrasound in asymptomatic patients without clinical risk factors. Therefore, the AIUM states that at this time, the use of ultrasound in carotid artery screening in these patients has no proven clinical benefit"[20] However, the AIUM admits that "duplex carotid ultrasound screening of selected high-risk subpopulations may be of some benefit in cases where the prevalence of stenosis is expected to be high (greater than 18%) and the patient's surgical risk is low (less than 3%), particularly prior to major cardiovascular surgery."[20]

Though screening companies may perform their work in community centers, they may also partner with insurance companies and area hospitals to provide their services. Companies such as these should be thoroughly researched. Ultimately, it must be concluded that the company is accredited, that it provides useful diagnostic information, and that the patient care is performed by competent, certified sonographers and interpreted by licensed, qualified physicians. It should be noted that when perceptible disease is recognized on an unofficial diagnostic examination provided by these screening companies that an additional official sonographic examination is required by the patient's physician. These examinations, especially if found to be false positives, may result in unnecessary medical charges, while at the same time needlessly increasing patient anxiety.

The Role of the Sonographer in the Abortion Debate

Since its inception, sonography has probably made the most significant impact in obstetrics. Indeed, Taylor claims that "ultrasound technology has brought the fetuses of today 'to life' in a different way, and far earlier, than in decades past. The women who carry today's fetuses would, back when they were fetuses themselves, not have seemed 'alive' to their own mothers at the same stage of pregnancy, nor in quite the same way."[21] Sonography has the ability to demonstrate movement of the fetal heart and movement of the fetus itself long before the mother can feel it move within her. Though the elective abortion debate is certainly beyond the scope of this book, we will briefly analyze both sides of the argument for the use of sonography in the care of obstetric patients. Even if your chosen specialty is echocardiography or vascular sonography, the topic is still one that will interest you as a sonographer.

If you decide to work as a sonographer practicing obstetric sonography, you will most likely encounter patients who have had elective abortions or are thinking about having an elective abortion. Sonographers are people, and people carry strongly held ethical beliefs. That is to say, we cannot practice sonography in a vacuum. The pro-life sonographer considers the act of abortion, in most cases other than rape or incest, the destruction of an innocent life. On the other hand, the pro-choice sonographer considers abortion a woman's reproductive health issue and thus a personal choice that every woman has the right to make on her own behalf.

In most cases, prior to an elective abortion, a sonogram is performed to confirm and date the pregnancy. During an obstetric sonogram, a patient may request that the sonographer provide some visual display of the fetus, including demonstrating the fetal anatomy and the beating heart. Sonography is a powerful medical instrument in that it has been shown to change the mind of the mother from having an abortion to not having an abortion. There are even independent non-profit companies that provide patients with free obstetric sonograms and counseling with the ultimate goals of educating patients and preventing abortions. These facilities may employ registered sonographers and often have physician administrators.

In North Carolina and Oklahoma, laws were passed in which patients were not only forced to have a sonogram prior to an elective abortion but the sonogram had to include imaging of the fetus in clear view of the patient with a thorough demonstration and explanation of fetal anatomy. The laws have since been deemed unconstitutional, with the Oklahoma law nearly making it all the way to the Supreme Court. The Supreme Court decided against hearing the arguments.

Patients may decide to have an elective abortion for many personal reasons. The rationale behind having an abortion may be based on economics, emotions, or a combination of other personal motives. But as a diagnostic medical sonographer, how should you interact with patients contemplating an elective abortion? There is at least one documented case of a sonographer being fired for expressing his or her personal feelings about or moral objections to abortion in front of a patient. In 2002, a sonographer admittedly tried to dissuade a patient from having an abortion because of his or her religious beliefs. The hospital at which the sonographer was employed was informed by the patient. The sonographer was then told that it was beyond the scope of his or her professional duties to "proselytize or provide pastoral counseling."[22] However, the hospital told the sonographer that he or she did not have to perform any more studies on women who were contemplating having an abortion based on their religious beliefs. The sonographer then responded that "his or her belief required him or her to try to dissuade a woman from having an abortion, even if that meant losing his or her job."[22] The sonographer was fired and then chose to sue the hospital for religious discrimination based on Title VII of the Civil Rights Act of 1964. The lawsuit was eventually dismissed. The judge stated that "Title VII does not require employers to allow employees to impose their religious views on others."[22]

There are other instances in which elective abortion may be offered to a patient. Occasionally, patients may be offered choices that relate to the early termination of a pregnancy that is complicated by devastating chromosomal or nonviable fetal abnormalities as well. For example, as a sonographer, you may perform a sonogram on a fetus that is shown to have anencephaly. Anencephaly is a disorder in which the fetal skull is not fully developed, thus leaving varying amounts of brain tissue exposed to the elements. Although the fetus may survive in the womb, anencephalic fetuses rarely live long after birth. In this situation, the patient may be offered the option of aborting the pregnancy.

Obstetric patients who are undergoing fertility treatment, such as in vitro fertilization, have an increased risk for multiple gestations. In some cases, numerous gestations can be present within the uterus. The more gestations that are present, the more likely it is that complications will be encountered during and after the pregnancy to the mother and fetuses. Thus, to improve the likelihood of a good postnatal outcome for each fetus, selective reduction may be advised. Selective reduction is the reduction of multiple gestations from, for example, quadruplets to twins. With selective reduction, the chosen excessive gestations are eliminated. Selective reduction may also be offered to a patient with twins, in which case one fetus is normal while the other has some fatal chromosomal abnormality or defect that is not compatible with life outside of the womb.

These situations are emotionally charged, and you should provide your patient with compassion, regardless of her choice. If we return to the previous topic of professional ethics in this chapter, treating patients fairly and equally is an obligation of the sonographer. Some suggest that if one holds such strong beliefs against abortion, then working in a facility that offers abortion may not be the best option.[23] It may be wise, simply based on legal concerns, to maintain a professional distance without offering your personal opinions about the topic to patients. Be informed, make good decisions concerning employment, and be aware of the elective abortion laws in the state in which you become employed.

PROFESSIONALISM

Professionalism is an awareness of conduct, aims, and qualities that define a profession.[8] Therefore, professionalism must have a foundation built on clinical competence, communication skills, and ethical and legal understanding.[24] The principles of professionalism, according to the American Board of Internal Medicine are **excellence**, **humanism**, accountability, **altruism**, duty, honor and integrity, and respect for others.[12]

Excellence may be defined as demanding your best. As a sonography student, you should strive for excellence in all that you attempt, not just to obtain good academic standing, but because your future patients deserve only your best. Consequently, if you learn to strive for excellence now in school, you will have an easier transition into employment, where excellence is demanded of you by others.

Humanism involves selfless behavior and the act of crediting others when credit is due to them. It also includes admitting when you have done wrong. In this regard, accountability relates to humanism. Recall from Chapter 2 that accountability was defined as being responsible for one's own actions. As a sonographer, you will be accountable to procedures and processes of the profession and the duties assigned by the organization where you are employed. You will also be responsible for meeting a certain quality of care and for reporting any **conflicts of interest**. A conflict of interest exists when there are inappropriate relationships between personal interests and professional obligations.[25]

In this regard, accountability implies both personal responsibility for one's actions and consistently acting in a manner that is unselfish, avoiding putting your own needs above others.

Altruism is defined as actions aimed at increasing the welfare of others, particularly those in need.[24] However, some include the act of self-sacrifice in the definition of altruism as well.[26] Many see the altruistic maxim of placing others before oneself as a duty. Duty was previously defined as the free acceptance of a commitment to service.[26] The service mentioned in the definition is indeed frequently thought of as a duty to patients, and sonographers certainly have a duty to perform proper patient care. However, sonographers also have a duty to the profession of sonography. One can accomplish the functions of this obligation by serving in a variety of capacities in professional organizations, speaking, writing, or simply being a mentor in the clinical setting for future sonographers.

Another important principle of professionalism, which was also mentioned in the ethics portion of this chapter, is integrity. Recall, integrity was defined as thinking with honesty and choosing the best paths to follow based on high standards. Integrity and honor work together in professionalism. Combined, they involve being fair and truthful, keeping one's word, and being straightforward.[24]

The final principle of professionalism involves respect for others. Respect in professionalism includes respect for peers and for patient autonomy. Autonomy refers to the principle that a patient has final authority over his or her medical treatment and that he or she should be provided with informed consent in every situation, except for those that are narrowly defined as emergencies.[8] Though physicians offer patients with choices and information regarding their healthcare, it is the patient who makes the final decision for treatment. For the sonographer, we must accept the practice of autonomy and never perform procedures of which the patient is not adequately informed or those that the patient refuses.

Sound Off

If you place the demand upon yourself now to be your best, you will have an easier transition into employment, where excellence is demanded of you by others.

Professional Etiquette

Professionalism should not be confused with **professional etiquette**, which is the everyday practice of good manners and being agreeable within the exercise of one's occupation.[15] However, professional etiquette is part of being a professional, and it is exceedingly important for obtaining and maintaining good relationships at work. While etiquette is imperative, professionalism includes being agreeable while simultaneously maintaining competence and strictly adhering to the established code of ethics. Table 6-5 provides some professional etiquette best practices.

TABLE 6-5	Best practices for professional etiquette

- Shake hands with a firm hand grip.
- Refer to patients or superiors using proper salutations unless informed otherwise by that person (e.g., "Ms." and "Mr.").
- Do not waste other people's time by being late.
- Do not check your e-mail, text messages, or phone during conversations or meetings with others.
- Maintain eye contact when speaking with people.
- Provide help when you identify that someone needs your help.
- Hold doors open for people.
- Always say "please" and "thank you."
- Acknowledge people when they walk into a room.
- Clean up after yourself.
- Listen when other people are talking, and do not interrupt to insert your opinion or comment until they are finished speaking.

From Makely S. *Professionalism in health care.* 3rd ed. Upper Saddle River, NJ: Pearson Prentice Hall; 2009.

First Impressions for the Sonography Student

Recall that in Chapter 2 we learned that reputation is how others view us. Perception *is* everything. As a sonography student, one of the most important parts of your current endeavor is the reputation that you form based on the perceptions that others have of you, especially those with whom you work every day. In the clinical setting, at least initially, perception is based solely on observation. If you are perceived in school or clinical as someone who is a "minimalist" or someone who "just wants to get by," then unfortunately, you will be perceived as remaining to be that person until you change the minds of those who hold those opinions about you.

   If one is initially perceived as lazy, regardless of if the perception is fair, that perception will most likely hinder his or her ability to obtain a job if that person does not work to remove such a perception. On the other hand, the perception of being someone who is a hard worker is nearly priceless. But being a professional in a health occupation involves more than just showing up and putting in the work for class or clinical. The professional attitude that you display now as a student is important to your future success as a sonographer. You should view every encounter as a job interview. Table 6-6 provides some tips for improving how you are perceived by others.

TABLE 6-6	Tips for improving how you are perceived by others in the workplace
Tips	**Explanation**
Be on time	If you have an obligation, be on time, or perhaps be a little early. People notice tardiness. This is a direct reflection upon your dependability.
Develop a professional attitude	Be enthusiastic and optimistic about the task at hand. Leave your negativity at home. Be thankful for your job. Focus on the good aspects of the job.
Respect yourself	Take care of your health, and make sure that your dress is professional at all times. Your clothes should be clean, neat, and not wrinkled. You should feel good about your decisions and acknowledge your successes. If you cannot respect yourself, you will not respect others.
Respect others	Recognize the fact that we are all different and that we all inherently deserve respect from others. It is acceptable to socialize with others, but be careful what you say.
Be a team player	Be ready to contribute, be responsible for your own actions, be dependable, and step up and take leadership if needed.
Respect the chain of command	Accept the fact that you will be working for someone else in most situations. Even people who own their own businesses must work to satisfy the needs of their customers. Understand that leadership will dictate work, your schedule, and your priorities in your sonography program and at work.
Beware of politics	Playing politics can damage your career. Try to avoid camps, cliques, and eternal pessimists.
Develop good work habits	Manage your time efficiently, be organized, always do your best, maintain your enthusiasm, and accept new challenges by viewing them as opportunities to learn.

From Manning M, *Patricia H. Developing As a Professional: 50 Tips for Getting Ahead*. Menlo Park, CA: Course Technology/Cengage Learning; 2003. ProQuest ebrary. Web. 14 August 2014.

TABLE 6-7	Topics to avoid to maintain professional decorum

Religion

Politics

Sex

Personal problems at home

Alcoholic drinking habits

Health problems (not related to your current duties)

Career aspirations (not related to your current duties)

Sound Off

The professional attitude that you display now as a student is important to your future success as a sonographer. You should view every encounter as a job interview.

Remember, first impressions are important. Acting like a professional also includes the following: demonstrating an appreciation for others and recognize other's accomplishments; expressing your gratitude; responding to people graciously and promptly; being considerate and listening to others (instead of only voicing your opinion); apologizing when needed; never using harsh language or profanity; treating everyone fairly; making others feel comfortable; and respecting others' opinions.[27] Just because you respect others' opinions does not mean you have to agree with them. To prevent conflict about strongly held opinions in everyday conversation with others, Table 6-7 provides some topics that you would most likely want to avoid at work, school, or clinical in order to maintain professional decorum (Table 6-7).

SUMMARY

Hopefully, as you examined this chapter, you recognized that ethics and professionalism are closely related concepts and that they are vital for the sonographer. While our ethics help guide us in the practice of our occupation, it is ultimately professionalism that helps display those ethics in the workplace. This chapter provided an explanation of terms like honor, duty, and integrity, and how these concepts are applied in a professional environment. Being a professional sonographer is much more than simply showing up for work and doing the job. A sonographer has an obligation to continually strive for excellence in all that he or she attempts.

REFERENCES

1. Lawrence AT, Weber J. *Business and Society: Stakeholders, Ethics, Public Policy.* 13th ed. New York, NY: McGraw-Hill; 2011.
2. Adler AM, Carlton RR. *Introduction to Radiologic Sciences and Patient Care.* 4th ed. St. Louis, MO: Saunders Elsevier; 2007.
3. Gini Al, Green RM. *Foundations of Business Ethics: Ten Virtues of Outstanding: Leaders Leadership and Character.* Somerset, NJ: John Wiley & Sons; 2013. ProQuest ebrary. Web. 21 July 2014.
4. Fremgen BF. *Medical Law and Ethics.* 3rd ed. Upper Saddle River, NJ: Pearson Prentice Hall; 2009.
5. Lewis MA, Tamparo CD. *Medical Law Ethics and Bioethics: For Health Professions.* 6th ed. Philadelphia, PA: F.A. Davis Company; 2007.
6. Life Value Assessment Tool. Retrieved from http://www.whatsnext.com/content/life-values-self-assessment-test
7. Dutton AG, Linn-Watson TA, Torres LS. *Torres' Patient Care in Imaging Technology.* 8th ed. Philadelphia, PA: Lippincott, Williams, & Wilkins; 2013.
8. Towsley-Cook DM, Young TA. *Ethical and Legal Issues for Imaging Professionals.* 2nd ed. St. Louis, MO: Mosby; 2007.

9. *The Bible*, NIV. Luke 6:31.

10. Seedhouse D. *Ethics: The Heart of Health Care*. 3rd ed. Chichester, GBR, UK: John Wiley & Sons; 2009. ProQuest ebrary. Web. 17 July 2014.

11. Huntsman JM. *Winners Never Cheat: Everyday Values We Learned as Children (But May Have Forgotten)*. Upper Saddle River, NJ: Pearson Education; 2005.

12. U.S. Army. Ethical Decisions and the Decision Making Process. Retrieved from http://www.acsap.army.mil/programs/pccert/ethicsonline/Decisionmaking.asp

13. Satterlee A. *Organizational Management and Leadership: A Christian Perspective*. Roanoke, VA: Synergistics; 2009.

14. Weber LJ. *Business Ethics in Healthcare: Beyond Compliance*. Bloomington, IN: Indiana University Press; 2001. ProQuest ebrary. Web. 16 July 2014.

15. Judson K, Hicks S. *Glencoe Law and Ethics for Medical Careers*. 3rd ed. New York, NY: McGraw Hill; 2002.

16. SDMS Code of Ethics for the Profession of Diagnostic Medical Sonography. Retrieved from http://www.sdms.org/about/codeofethics.asp

17. Wiley. *Everyday Medical Ethics and Law*. New York, NY: John Wiley & Sons; 2013. ProQuest ebrary. Web. 16 July 2014.

18. AIUM. Prudent Use in Pregnancy. Retrieved from http://www.aium.org/officialStatements/33

19. FDA. Fetal Keepsake Videos. Retrieved from http://www.fda.gov/MedicalDevices/Safety/AlertsandNotices/PatientAlerts/ucm064756.htm and http://www.fda.gov/ForConsumers/ConsumerUpdates/ucm095508.htm

20. AIUM. Carotid Screening in Asymptomatic Patients. Retrieved from http://www.aium.org/officialStatements/28

21. Taylor JS. *Public Life of the Fetal Sonogram: Technology, Consumption, and the Politics of Reproduction*. New Brunswick, NJ: Rutgers University Press; 2008. ProQuest ebrary. Web. 9 August 2014.

22. Law Room. No Need to Tolerate Sharing. Retrieved from http://www.lawroom.com/story.aspx?STID=1012 (*Grant v. Fairview* (MN 2004) no. 02–4232).

23. Craig M. *Essentials of Sonography and Patient Care*. 2nd ed. St. Louis, MO: Elsevier; 2006.

24. Thomas DS. *Measuring Medical Professionalism*. Cary, NC: Oxford University Press, USA; 2005. ProQuest ebrary. Web. 14 August 2014. Copyright © 2005. Oxford University Press, USA. All rights reserved.

25. Makely S. *Professionalism in Health Care*. 3rd ed. Upper Saddle River, NJ: Pearson Prentice Hall; 2009.

26. Mook WN, et al. Training and learning professionalism in the medical school curriculum: current considerations. *European Journal of Internal Medicine* 2009;20:96–100.

27. Manning M, Patricia H. *Developing As a Professional: 50 Tips for Getting Ahead*. Menlo Park, CA: Course Technology/Cengage Learning; 2003. ProQuest ebrary. Web. 14 August 2014.

Thinking Critically

1. What would you do if your boss asks you to do something that violated your professional standards?
2. What would you do if a patient asked you if she should have an abortion?
3. What would you do if a coworker used a racially offensive term in front of you?
4. What would you do if a coworker was rude in front of a patient who was unresponsive?
5. What should you do if a patient offers you money?

Chapter 6
Review Questions

1. **What is the process that we use to make choices based on our moral principles and personal values?**
   a. Ethical decision making
   b. Medical ethics
   c. Deontologic theory
   d. Consequentialism

2. **Which of the following is defined as accepted rules of conduct?**
   a. Norms
   b. Personal values
   c. Moral principles
   d. Virtue ethics

3. **Which ethical theory may also be referred to as consequentialism?**
   a. Virtue ethics
   b. Deontologic theory
   c. Teleologic theory
   d. The golden rule

4. **Which of the following refers to the application of our moral principles with others in the medical profession, including our coworkers, patients, and community?**
   a. Professional ethics
   b. Individual ethics
   c. Personal ethics
   d. Medical ethics

5. **Which medical ethics principle relates to honesty in all aspects of life?**
   a. Principle of veracity
   b. Principle of confidentiality
   c. Principle of justice
   d. Principle of nonmaleficence

6. **Which of the following are group-held beliefs that are agreed upon by individuals or groups of individuals?**
   a. Values
   b. Norms
   c. Ethics
   d. Professional values

7. **Which medical ethics principle would relate to never making promises that you cannot keep?**
   a. Principle of veracity
   b. Principle of fidelity
   c. Principle of confidentiality
   d. Principle of beneficence

8. **If a patient refuses to have a sonographic procedure, you should**
   a. talk to a close family member and discuss the importance of the procedure.
   b. talk the patient into having the procedure.
   c. perform the procedure.
   d. not perform the procedure.

9. **What medical ethics principle relates to treating all patients equally, no matter what their economic, physical, or mental condition?**
   a. Principle of justice
   b. Principle of paternalism
   c. Principle of beneficence
   d. Principle of autonomy

10. **If a pregnant patient asked you if she should have an abortion, you should**
    a. tell her you are pro-life.
    b. tell her you are pro-choice.
    c. tell her that you do not have an opinion.
    d. tell her to seek professional medical guidance concerning abortion.

11. **Regarding keepsake sonography, the American Institute of Ultrasound in Medicine states that**
    a. the procedure is inappropriate if it is not medically indicated and ordered by a physician.
    b. the procedure is appropriate, as long as it is performed by a registered diagnostic medical sonographer.
    c. the procedure is always appropriate.
    d. the procedure should never be performed, even as an adjunct to a medically indicated procedure.

12. **Which of the following is defined as actions aimed at increasing the welfare of others?**
    a. Beneficence
    b. Altruism
    c. Fidelity
    d. Ethics

13. **Which of the following is not a principle of professionalism according to the American Board of Internal Medicine?**
    a. Duty
    b. Atheism
    c. Humanism
    d. Altruism

14. **What term is defined as the everyday practice of good manners and being agreeable within the exercise of one's occupation?**
    a. Niceties
    b. Professionalism
    c. Excellence
    d. Professional etiquette

15. **Which of the following would not be considered appropriate professional etiquette?**
    a. Holding doors open for people
    b. Referring to patients by their first names
    c. Cleaning up after yourself
    d. Maintaining eye contact when someone is talking to you

16. **What is defined as demanding your very best?**
    a. Altruism
    b. Honesty
    c. Excellence
    d. Accountability

17. **Who makes the final decisions about a patient's care?**
    a. The closest family member
    b. The patient
    c. The ordering physician
    d. The interpreting physician

18. **"Do to others what you would have them do to you" describes**
    a. the golden rule.
    b. deontologic theory.
    c. teleologic theory.
    d. virtue ethics.

19. **Which of the following would be an appropriate topic to discuss at work?**
    a. Politics
    b. Religion
    c. Movies
    d. Career aspirations

20. **Which of the following would not be a good way to improve the manner in which others perceive you?**
    a. Keep to yourself
    b. Be on time
    c. Be a team player
    d. Respect the chain of command

Legal Essentials and Patient Rights

CHAPTER OBJECTIVES

■ Provide a brief overview of law and legal concerns in medicine.

■ Gain an appreciation of the legal environment in which sonographers practice.

■ Offer an analysis of the sonographer's scope of practice.

■ Examine patient's rights.

KEY TERMS

Administrative law – addresses statutes that are enacted regarding the power of agencies

Advance directives – legal documents that are created by a competent person to provide written information concerning his or her desires for treatment if for some reason the patient is unable to make decisions on his or her own

Assault – a deliberate act wherein one person threatens to harm another person, and the victim feels that the attacker has the ability to actually carry out the threat

Battery – the unlawful touching of a person without their consent, even if the act is performed for their benefit

Civil law – involves crime against an individual, and it includes such crimes as slander, libel, trespassing, and contract violation

Common law – the oldest form of law, many of which were initially established in England and France and then practiced in the American colonies

Consent – the voluntary agreement or permission that a patient gives a medical professional to allow that professional to touch, examine, and/or perform treatment or a procedure on them

Criminal law – involves crimes against the state or society as a whole

Defamation of character – exists when someone makes false or malicious statements about someone else

Diagnostician – a physician who provides a patient with a diagnosis

Do not resuscitate – a written physician's order instructing healthcare workers to not perform lifesaving cardiopulmonary resuscitation

Durable power of attorney for healthcare – legal document that appoints an agent to act on behalf of the patient to make decisions about that patient's care should the patient lose the ability make his or her own decisions; also referred to as a healthcare proxy

Embezzlement – the illegal appropriation of money or funds by someone who is typically entrusted with its care

False imprisonment – occurs in healthcare when a medical professional confines a patient in some way or when a patient is held against his or her will without justification or consent

Felonies – crimes that are either punishable by death or by imprisonment in a state or federal institution for more than one year

Fraud – any attempt to deceive someone deliberately in order to secure unjust or unlawful gain

Good Samaritan laws – laws that include protection for persons who provide emergency care to a stranger from civil or criminal liability

Healthcare advance directive – legal document that combines a living will and a durable power of attorney for healthcare

Immobilization devices – any device used to restrain a patient; requires a physician's order

Implied consent – consent offered when a patient demonstrates the acceptance of a procedure simply by his or her nonverbal actions

Infliction of emotional distress – results from intentionally causing emotional or mental suffering

Informed consent – the act of providing a patient with a proposed procedure or course of treatment, explaining the risks and benefits, and ultimately gaining permission to perform the procedure or treatment

Informed consent form – legal document signed by a patient that is used to obtain informed consent

Intentional torts – results in actions that are done in order to cause harm to another person

Invasion of privacy – the interference of a person's right to be left alone

Laws – mandatory rules to which all citizens must adhere or risk the consequences of civil or criminal liability

Libel – publishing information in a written form that is injurious to a person's reputation

Litigious – excessively prone to use legal means to settle a dispute

Living will – legal document that expresses a patient's wishes concerning his or her future medical care

Medicaid – U.S. health assistance program funded by the federal, state, and local government to help benefit low-income individuals

Medicare – U.S. health assistance program funded by the federal government to help the elderly (over 65) and some disabled individuals under the age of 65

Misdemeanors – crimes that are punishable by fines or imprisonment (other than in a jail) for less than one year

Negligence – occurs when someone has a duty to provide reasonable care and fails to do so regardless of intentions

Occupational Safety and Health Administration (OSHA) – administrative agency of the United States that establishes and enforces employee health and safety standards

Patient confidentiality – the protection of health-related information and maintaining patient privacy

Patient Protection and Affordable Care Act of 2010 – expansive federal law, which among many things, seeks to lower medical costs, while at the same time providing options for the uninsured to receive healthcare insurance; also referred to as "Obamacare"

Patient rights – the legal rights of the patient related to the patient-medical caregiver relationship

Patient Self-Determination Act of 1990 – established guidelines concerning the end-of-life desires of patients confronted with serious illnesses

Professional liability insurance – individual insurance purchased by a sonographer to guard against malpractice claims when employer coverage is ambiguous and to protect against personal loss

Res ipsa loquitur – doctrine of negligence, which means "the thing speaks for itself"

Respondeat superior – doctrine of medical malpractice, which means "let the master answer"

Rights – an individual's just claim or entitlement

Scope of practice – defines the role of a professional in the practice of his or her occupation

Slander – speaking potentially damaging malicious words about someone that could hinder his or her reputation

Standard of care – the care a reasonable and prudent person would provide in a given circumstance

Standards – statements of the minimal behavioral or performance levels that are acceptable. Something established by authority as a rule for the measure of quantity or quality

Stare decision – legal doctrine, which means "let the decision stand;" the basis for decisions that look upon the results of similar past case decisions for a resolution

Statutory duty to report – the obligation of health professionals to follow state public health laws to report medical conditions or incidents

Statutory law – includes laws, referred to as statutes, which are enacted by federal, state, or local governments

Tort – a wrong committed against a person or property, which may result in physical injury, damage to personal property, or deprivation of someone's personal liberty or freedom

Unintentional torts – acts that are not intentionally committed but result in an injury to a person

INTRODUCTION

The legal aspects of the sonography profession are discussed in this chapter. Therefore, the primary goal of this chapter is to provide you with an overview of the essentials of law as it pertains to sonographic practice. Although you must be mindful that we live in a society governed by law, combining an adequate appreciation of medical law with the everyday practice of professional ethics discussed in Chapter 6 will nearly guarantee that you provide patient care in a prudent and consistent manner to all patients, regardless of their mental or physical condition. There will be no need to fear the repercussions of legal actions in the workplace if you take measures now to understand medical law and practice sonography within the sonographer's official scope of practice.

LAW BASICS

We live in a **litigious** society. In fact, physicians often choose to practice a form of medicine referred to as "defensive medicine" as a result of the fear of being sued by patients. However, defensive medicine results in numerous unnecessary tests and procedures ordered to protect the physician from lawsuit claims that propose that he or she could have done more for a patient.[1] On the other hand, as the result of the fear that a patient may have a poor outcome resulting in a lawsuit claim, a physician may choose to not order an effective test because that test carries a high risk of complications. Reportedly, the practice of defensive medicine costs the U.S. economy $200 billion per year.[2]

Though they occasionally overlap, the difference between law and ethics is clear. While ethics are standards of conduct that we *should* follow, **laws** are rules of society that we *must* follow.[3] Laws are described as mandatory rules to which all citizens must adhere or risk the consequences of civil or criminal liability.[4] Basically, society agrees upon laws to solve some of the ethical dilemmas that people encounter. For example, there are laws against stealing because most rational, moral people agree that stealing is wrong. There are also actions that occur, such as lying and adultery, which most agree are immoral, though specific laws have not been written.

Constitutional law pertains to both the U.S. Constitution and the constitutions of the individual states. The founders of the United States established the constitution to provide a framework for the national government, and they created a checks-and-balances system to protect the entire nation from government overreach by separating and limiting the power of the federal government. The Constitution also provides for some basic **rights**, such as those to free speech and privacy, which are included in the Bill of Rights. Rights are an individual's just claims or entitlements.[5,6] Many laws are created to protect the rights of people in our society. There are two basic types of law: **common law** and **statutory law**.

Sound Off
Society agrees upon laws to solve some of the ethical dilemmas that people encounter.

TYPES OF LAW
Common Law

Current law involves common law and statutory law.[6] Common law is the oldest form of law. These laws were initially established in England and France and then practiced in the American colonies. Though many of the early case decisions were based on the sharing of knowledge between judges, eventually the case decisions were written down and then used as legal precedents. In many cases, the principle of *stare decision*, or "let the decision stand," is the basis for decisions that look upon the results of similar past case decisions for a resolution. This form of law is ever-evolving as new cases arise, and thus, it may also be referred to as judge-made law or case law. These judicial decisions are based on common law principles that are adapted to meet the needs of an ever-changing society. Should legal concerns not be resolved in the lower courts, the ultimate decision may be made by a state supreme court, or on the federal level, the Supreme Court of the United States.

Sound Off
The principle of *stare decision*, or "let the decision stand," is the basis for decisions that look upon the results of similar past case decisions for a resolution.

Statutory Law

Statutory law includes laws, referred to as statutes, which are enacted by federal, state, or local governments.[7] However, if a statute is created by a state legislature or local government, it must not conflict with a federal statute or law. Statutory law includes classifications such as administrative law, criminal law, and civil law, all of which apply in some way to sonographers.

Administrative Law

Because legislative bodies cannot function to both create and enforce all laws, organizations, which have the force of law, are often created to enact regulations.[4] These organizations are referred to as administrative agencies. Thus, a subsection of statutory law, **administrative law**, addresses statutes that are enacted regarding the power of agencies, such as the Internal Revenue Service or the **Occupational Safety and Health Administration (OSHA)**, to regulate and enforce laws.[7] Administrative law impacts sonographers because many of these agencies ensure licensure and practice regulations, while others, like federal government programs such as **Medicaid** and **Medicare**, dictate federal and state healthcare reimbursement and also relate to standards of patient care.[6]

The **Patient Protection and Affordable Care Act of 2010**, often referred to as "Obamacare," is a federal law that is regulated and enforced by numerous administrative agencies. Before the bill became law, many scholars, both medical and legal, felt that the previous healthcare system in the United States had become ineffectual in some regards. In fact, while the United States paid more per capita in healthcare than any other country in the world, it only ranked 37th in the world for quality of care.[2] Also, approximately 45 million individuals were reported to be uninsured in 2013.[2] Obamacare seeks to lower medical costs while at the same time providing options for the uninsured to receive healthcare insurance. Additionally, within Obamacare, preventative treatment testing is a main focus. Medical imaging, which includes sonography, will most likely be directly impacted as portions of law are gradually implemented over the next few years.

Criminal Law

Two main classifications of law that a sonographer should be aware of are **criminal law** and **civil law**. Criminal law involves crimes against the state or society as a whole.[7] Criminal acts include **felonies** and **misdemeanors**. Felonies are crimes that are either punishable by death or by imprisonment in a state or federal institution for more than one year. Felonies include murder, rape, robbery, larceny, arson, burglary, tax evasion, and practicing medicine without a license. Misdemeanors are crimes that are punishable by fines or imprisonment (other than in a prison) for less than one year.[7] Misdemeanors include traffic violations, disturbing the peace, and minor theft.

Criminal cases are brought to suit by the government against a person or group of people who are charged with a crime. The case is composed of a defendant and plaintiff. There are three phases to a lawsuit: pleading phase, discovery phase, and the trial. In the pleading phase, the complaint is lodged against the defendant, and the defense gives an answer. The discovery phase involves the attorneys seeking the facts through investigation and the questioning of the interested parties. The trial is the presentation of the proceeding information to a judge and jury for a decision.[6] If the defendant is found guilty, then the defendant may have to pay a fine, serve prison time, or both.

You may have already undergone a criminal background check prior to entering your educational program. It is important for you to know that criminal background checks are conducted by clinical facilities and are used by your educational institution as part of your clinical training. Depending upon the infraction, the presence of a misdemeanor or felony may inhibit your opportunity for employment in a patient care setting. Also, some felonies may prohibit you from attempting to gain national certification. It would be wise to inform your educational institution and/or employer should an infraction occur while you are in school so that you are cognizant of any possible repercussions that such behavior may have upon your future occupational goals.

Civil Law

Civil law involves crime against an individual, including such crimes as slander, libel, trespassing, and contract violation.[7] Civil law includes a category of law referred to as tort law. A **tort** is a wrong committed against a person or property, which may result in physical injury, damage to personal property, or deprivation of someone's personal liberty or freedom.[7] A tort can be the result of negligence or intentional misconduct. Therefore, torts are divided into either **intentional torts** or **unintentional torts** (Figs. 7-1 and 7-2). Tables 7-1 and 7-2 provide some examples of intentional and unintentional torts.

Sound Off

A tort is a wrong committed against a person or property, which may result in physical injury, damage to personal property, or deprivation of someone's personal liberty or freedom.

Intentional Torts

Though you may suspect that a sonographer would never intentionally harm a patient, civil lawsuits may be filed if a patient feels that you intentionally did something that resulted in his or her injury. Intentional torts result in actions that are done in order to cause harm to another person. These may include **assault, battery, false imprisonment, defamation of character, embezzlement, invasion of privacy, fraud**, and **infliction of emotional distress**.

An assault is a deliberate act in which one person threatens to harm another person, and the victim feels that the attacker has the ability to actually carry out the threat.[6] For example, an assault may be alleged if a sonographer threatens to perform a sonogram on a competent patient against the patient's will. All that is required for an assault is for the patient to fear that he or she will be hurt. On the other hand, battery is the unlawful touching of a person without his or her consent, even if the act is performed

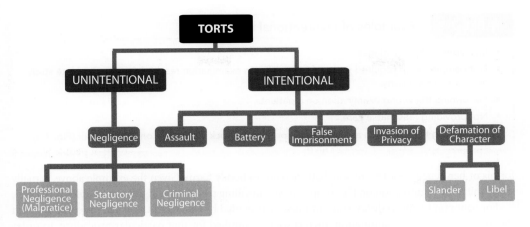

Figure 7-1. Healthcare professionals must appreciate tort law.

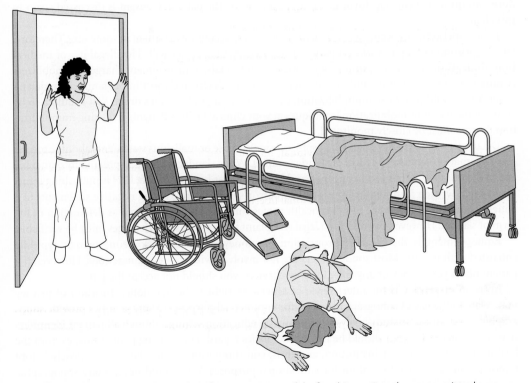

Figure 7-2. The sonographer who was responsible for this patient has committed an unintentional tort and would be considered negligent for failing to lock the wheels on the wheelchair, an action that could have prevented the patient from falling.

TABLE 7-1	Examples of intentional torts
• Immobilization of a patient against his or her will and without a physician's order.	
• Falsely stating that a patient has a disease that he or she does not have.	
• Causing extreme emotional distress resulting in illness.	

TABLE 7-2	Examples of unintentional torts

- Improperly labeling images.
- Not completing all required protocol images for an examination resulting in an incomplete study and missed pathology.
- Performing the wrong examination on a patient.
- Not providing reasonable care.
- Not putting the rails upon a patient's bed or failing to lock the wheels on a wheelchair (Fig. 7-2).

for his or her benefit. For this reason, battery requires bodily harm. Given the example above, actually performing the examination on the competent yet unwilling patient would be both assault and battery.

For sonographic procedures, consent must be provided by the patient. If a patient complies with the instructions of the examination, then consent is implied for that particular procedure. In order to confirm that the patient complies with the procedure, the sonographer should thoroughly explain the examination and ask the patient if he or she understands and approves. For most invasive procedures, **an informed consent form** must be completed by the patient. Consent is discussed again in this chapter.

False imprisonment occurs when a medical professional confines a patient in some way. Therefore, false imprisonment applies when a patient is held against his or her will. The illegal use of medical **immobilization devices** to restrain a patient can result in false imprisonment charges. Immobilizers require the assessment of the individual's need for such a device and most importantly a physician's order. You should never use immobilization devices without a physician's order. You should also be aware of the use of immobilization techniques at your clinical facility. Patients requiring immobilization devices must be closely monitored.

Defamation of character exists when someone makes false or malicious statements about someone else. Defamation can take the form of **slander** or **libel**. While slander is speaking potentially damaging and malicious words about someone that could hinder his or her reputation, libel is publishing information in a written form that is injurious to a person's reputation. Making negative statements to a patient about the competence of other health professionals could be perceived as defamation in the form of slander. However, in order for a legal complaint to be established, damages must be verifiable.

Embezzlement is the illegal appropriation of money or funds by someone who is typically entrusted with its care. Most sonographers are not involved with money transactions. However, if a patient offers you money or anything for your services, you should not accept the gift.

Invasion of privacy is the interference of a person's right to be left alone.[7] Invasion of privacy may relate to the use of sonographic images for commercial purposes. Many facilities provide sonographic images for case study analysis for the use in education settings, though all patient identifiers (e.g., name, age, date, etc.) should be removed. Policies regarding removing patient images from the healthcare setting vary per institution, and thus, you should investigate the policies closely before removing any patient information for educational purposes. You should never share sonographic images that you obtain over the internet or discuss case-specific information with anyone not directly involved in the care of that patient.

Fraud is any attempt to deceive someone. Fraud even involves making false promises to patients regarding their care. To avoid making fraudulent claims, never make promises to patients concerning the outcome of their care like "you will be fine" or "I'm sure your doctor will cure you." On the other hand, the infliction of emotional distress results from intentionally causing emotional or mental suffering. To avoid this, you should provide comfort to your patients without making unreasonable promises.

Unintentional Torts

Unintentional torts are acts that are not intentionally committed but result in an injury to a person. One example of an unintentional tort is **negligence**. Negligence occurs when someone has a duty

TABLE 7-3	Four Ds of negligence
Duty	Exists when a relationship has been established (e.g., sonographer-patient relationship).
Derelict (breach of duty)	The client must prove that the sonographer failed to comply to the standard of care.
Direct cause	The act directly caused the damages or injury to the patient.
Damages (injury)	Applies to the compensation provided for injuries that resulted from the incident.

From Lewis MA, Tamparo CD. *Medical Law Ethics and Bioethics: For Health Professions.* 6th ed. Philadelphia, PA: F.A. Davis Company; 2007.

to provide reasonable care and fails to do so regardless of intentions. Negligence can be established if only a duty exists.[6] In fact, there are four Ds of negligence that must be proven by a patient who charges a healthcare professional with negligence—duty, derelict (breach of duty), direct cause, and damages (injury) (Table 7-3).[4]

Standards, according to the Society of Diagnostic Medical Sonography (SDMS), were previously defined as "statements of the minimum behavioral or performance levels that are acceptable. Something established by authority as a rule for the measure of quantity or quality."[8] A **standard of care** is the care a reasonable and prudent person would provide in a given circumstance. Sonographers have an obligation to perform their professional duties according to the accepted standard of care.

With the goal of establishing standards for the profession, in conjunction with other organizations like the Society of Vascular Ultrasound and American Society of Echocardiography, the SDMS has created Diagnostic Ultrasound Clinical Practice Standards (Table 7-4). The SDMS maintains that certification is considered the standard of practice in ultrasound.[8] Among the list of standards, the SDMS provides for patient information assessment and evaluation, patient education and communication, protocol establishment, and proper documentation.

TABLE 7-4	*Diagnostic Ultrasound Clinical Practice Standards of the Society of Diagnostic Medical Sonography*

Standards are designed to reflect behavior and performance levels expected in clinical practice for the diagnostic medical sonographer. These clinical standards set forth the principles that are common to all of the specialties within the larger category of the diagnostic sonography profession. Individual specialties or clinical areas may extend or refine, but not limit, these general principles according to their specific practice requirements.

Section 1
STANDARD—Patient Information Assessment and Evaluation:

1.1 Information regarding the patient's past and present health status is essential in providing appropriate diagnostic information. Therefore, pertinent data related to the diagnostic sonographic procedure should be collected and evaluated to determine its relevance to the examination. The diagnostic medical sonographer:

    1.1.1 Verifies patient identification and that the requested examination correlates with the patient's clinical history and presentation. In the event that the requested examination does not correlate, either the supervising physician or the referring physician will be notified.

    1.1.2 In compliance with privacy and confidentiality standards, interviews the patient or their representative, and/or reviews the medical record to gather relevant information regarding the patient's medical history and current presenting indications for the study.

    1.1.3 Evaluates any contraindications, insufficient patient preparation, and the patient's inability or unwillingness to tolerate the examination and associated procedures.

(continues)

TABLE 7-4 *Diagnostic Ultrasound Clinical Practice Standards of the Society of Diagnostic Medical Sonography* (Continued)

STANDARD—Patient Education and Communication:

1.2 Effective communication and education are necessary to establish a positive relationship with the patient or the patient's representative, and to elicit patient cooperation and understanding of expectations. The diagnostic medical sonographer:

    1.2.1 Communicates with the patient in a manner appropriate to the patient's ability to understand. Presents explanations and instructions in a manner that can be easily understood by the patient and other healthcare providers.

    1.2.2 Explains the examination and associated procedures to the patient and responds to patient questions and concerns.

    1.2.3 Refers specific diagnostic, treatment, or prognosis questions to the appropriate physician or healthcare professional.

STANDARD—Analysis and Determination of Protocol for the Diagnostic Examination:

1.3 The most appropriate protocol seeks to optimize patient safety and comfort, diagnostic quality, and efficient use of resources, while achieving the diagnostic objective of the examination. The diagnostic medical sonographer:

    1.3.1 Integrates medical history, previous studies, and current symptoms in determining the appropriate diagnostic protocol and tailoring the examination to the needs of the patient.

    1.3.2 Performs the examination under appropriate supervision, as defined by the procedure.

    1.3.3 Uses professional judgment to adapt the protocol and consults appropriate medical personnel, when necessary, to optimize examination results.

    1.3.4 Confers with the supervising physician, when appropriate, to determine if intravenous contrast is necessary to enhance image quality and obtain additional diagnostic information.

    1.3.5 With appropriate education and training, uses proper technique for intravenous line insertion and administers intravenous contrast according to facility protocol.

STANDARD—Implementation of the Protocol:

1.4 Quality patient care is provided through the safe and accurate implementation of a deliberate protocol. The diagnostic medical sonographer:

    1.4.1 Implements a protocol that falls within established procedures.

    1.4.2 Elicits the cooperation of the patient to carry out the protocol.

    1.4.3 Adapts the protocol according to the patient's disease process or condition.

    1.4.4 Adapts the protocol, as required, according to the physical circumstances under which the examination must be performed (e.g., operating room, sonography laboratory, patient's bedside, emergency room, etc.).

    1.4.5 Monitors the patient's physical and mental status.

    1.4.6 Adapts the protocol according to changes in the patient's clinical status during the examination.

    1.4.7 Administers first aid or provides life support in emergency situations.

    1.4.8 Performs basic patient care tasks, as needed.

    1.4.9 Recognizes sonographic characteristics of normal and abnormal tissues, structures, and blood flow; adapts protocol as appropriate to further assess findings; adjusts scanning technique to optimize image quality and diagnostic information.

    1.4.10 Analyzes sonographic findings throughout the course of the examination so that a comprehensive examination is completed and sufficient data is provided to the supervising physician to direct patient management and render a final interpretation.

    1.4.11 Performs measurements and calculations according to facility protocol.

(continues)

TABLE 7-4	*Diagnostic Ultrasound Clinical Practice Standards of the Society of Diagnostic Medical Sonography* (Continued)

STANDARD—Evaluation of the Diagnostic Examination Results:

1.5 Careful evaluation of examination results in the context of the protocol is important to determine whether the goals have been met. The diagnostic medical sonographer:

    1.5.1 Establishes that the examination, as performed, complies with applicable protocols and guidelines.

    1.5.2 Identifies and documents any limitations to the examination.

    1.5.3 Initiates additional scanning techniques or procedures (e.g., administering contrast agents) when indicated.

    1.5.4 Notifies supervising physician when immediate medical attention is necessary, based on examination findings and patient condition.

STANDARD—Documentation:

1.6 Clear and precise documentation is necessary for continuity of care, accuracy of care, and quality assurance. The diagnostic medical sonographer:

    1.6.1 Provides timely, accurate, concise, and complete documentation.

    1.6.2 Provides an oral or written summary of findings to the supervising physician.

Section 2

STANDARD—Implement Quality Improvement Programs:

2.1 Participation in quality improvement programs is imperative. The diagnostic medical sonographer:

    2.1.1 Maintains a safe environment for patients and staff.

    2.1.2 Performs quality improvement procedures to determine that equipment operates at optimal levels and to promote patient safety.

    2.1.3 Participates in quality improvement programs that evaluate technical quality of images, completeness of examinations, and adherence to protocols.

    2.1.4 Compares facility quality improvement standards to external metrics, such as accreditation criteria, evidence based literature, or accepted guidelines.

STANDARD—Quality of Care:

2.2 All patients expect and deserve optimal care. The diagnostic medical sonographer.

    2.2.1 Works in partnership with other healthcare professionals.

    2.2.2 Reports adverse events.

Section 3

STANDARD—Self-Assessment:

3.1 Self-assessment is an essential component in professional growth and development. Self-assessment involves evaluation of personal performance, knowledge, and skills:

    3.1.1 Recognizes strengths and uses them to benefit patients, coworkers, and the profession.

    3.1.2 Recognizes weaknesses and limitations and performs procedures only after receiving appropriate education and supervised clinical experience in any deficient areas.

STANDARD—Education:

3.2 Advancements in medical science and technology occur very rapidly, requiring an on-going commitment to professional education. The diagnostic medical sonographer:

    3.2.1 Obtains and maintains appropriate professional certification/credential in areas of clinical practice.

    3.2.2 Recognizes and takes advantage of opportunities for educational and professional growth.

STANDARD—Collaboration:

3.3 Quality patient care is provided when all members of the healthcare team communicate and collaborate efficiently. The diagnostic medical sonographer:

    3.3.1 Promotes a positive and collaborative atmosphere with members of the healthcare team.

    3.3.2 Communicates effectively with members of the healthcare team regarding the welfare of the patient.

    3.3.3 Shares knowledge and expertise with colleagues, patients, students, and members of the healthcare team.

(continues)

TABLE 7-4	*Diagnostic Ultrasound Clinical Practice Standards of the Society of Diagnostic Medical Sonography* (Continued)

Section 4

STANDARD—Ethics:

4.1 All decisions made and actions taken on behalf of the patient adhere to ethical standards. The diagnostic medical sonographer.

    4.1.1 Adheres to accepted professional ethical standards.

    4.1.2 Is accountable for professional judgments and decisions.

    4.1.3 Provides patient care with equal respect for all.

    4.1.4 Respects and promotes patient rights, provides patient care with respect for patient dignity and needs, and acts as a patient advocate.

    4.1.5 Does not perform sonographic procedures without a medical indication, except in educational activities.

    4.1.6 Adheres to this scope of practice and other related professional documents.

From SDMS Diagnostic Ultrasound Clinical Practice Standards. Retrieved from http://www.sdms.org/positions/clinical-practice.asp

Malpractice is essentially professional negligence.[1] In medicine, this is referred to as medical malpractice. The amount of claims and claims resulting in payment vary per specialty in medicine (Fig. 7-3). The Latin phrase ***res ipsa loquitur*** is a doctrine of negligence, which means "the thing speaks for itself." Basically, this rule of law relates to obvious negligence. These observable situations include such instances as when a physician might leave a medical instrument inside of a patient during surgery, if a patient were to be burned during surgery, or if a patient were injured to another part of his or her body not involved with the necessary field of treatment.[4]

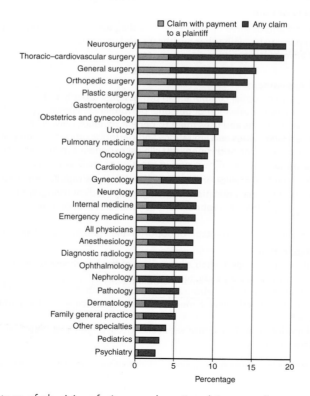

Figure 7-3. Percentage of physicians facing a malpractice claim annually, categorized by specialty.

SONOGRAPHER SCOPE OF PRACTICE

In sonographic clinical practice, medical malpractice may be claimed for several violations, including if a sonographer performed the wrong examination on a patient, or if a sonographer completed a substandard examination resulting in misdiagnosis. To avoid legal concerns, sonographers must perform within the profession's **scope of practice**. A scope of practice defines the role of a professional in the practice of his or her occupation. For the sonographer, the "Scope of Practice for Diagnostic Ultrasound Professionals" published by the SDMS defines the role of the sonographer as a member of the healthcare team (Table 7-5). Included in the scope is the sonographer's obligation to (1) perform patient assessments, (2) acquire and analyze data obtained using ultrasound and related diagnostic technologies, (3) provide a summary of findings to the physician to aid in patient diagnosis and management, and (4) use independent judgment and systematic problem-solving methods to produce high-quality diagnostic information and optimize patient care.[9]

A sonographer should never act as a **diagnostician**. A diagnostician is a physician who provides a patient with a diagnosis. You may encounter sonographers in clinical practice who offer insight into the diagnosis of disease for patients. Sonographers who provide diagnostic information to

TABLE 7-5	*The Society for Diagnostic Medical Sonography Scope of Practice for the Diagnostic Ultrasound Professional*

Preamble:
The purpose of this document is to define the Scope of Practice for Diagnostic Ultrasound Professionals and to specify their roles as members of the healthcare team, acting in the best interest of the patient. This scope of practice is a "living" document that will evolve as the technology expands.

Definition of the Profession:
The Diagnostic Ultrasound Profession is a multi-specialty field comprised of Diagnostic Medical Sonography (with subspecialties in abdominal, neurologic, obstetrical/gynecologic, and ophthalmic ultrasound), Diagnostic Cardiac Sonography (with subspecialties in adult and pediatric echocardiography), Vascular Technology, and other emerging fields. These diverse specialties are distinguished by their use of diagnostic medical ultrasound as a primary technology in their daily work. Certification[a] is considered the standard of practice in ultrasound. Individuals who are not yet certified should reference the Scope as a professional model and strive to become certified.

Scope of Practice of the Profession:
The Diagnostic Ultrasound Professional is an individual qualified by professional credentialing[b] and academic and clinical experience to provide diagnostic patient care services using ultrasound and related diagnostic procedures. The scope of practice of the Diagnostic Ultrasound Professional includes those procedures, acts, and processes permitted by law, for which the individual has received education and clinical experience and in which he/she has demonstrated competency.

Diagnostic Ultrasound Professionals:
- Perform patient assessments
- Acquire and analyze data obtained using ultrasound and related diagnostic technologies
- Provide a summary of findings to the physician to aid in patient diagnosis and management
- Use independent judgment and systematic problem-solving methods to produce high-quality diagnostic information and optimize patient care.

[a]*An example of credentials: RDMS (registered diagnostic medical sonographer), RDCS (registered diagnostic cardiac sonographer), RVT (registered vascular technologist); awarded by the American Registry for Diagnostic Medical Sonography, a certifying body with NCCA Category "A" membership.*
[b]*Credentials should be awarded by an agency certified by the National Commission for Certifying Agencies (NCCA).*
From SDMS *Scope of Practice for the Diagnostic Ultrasound Professional.* Retrieved from http://www.sdms.org/positions/scope.asp

patients may be held liable as this is beyond the legal scope of practice for our occupation. Patients are often unaware that sonographers are trained to produce diagnostic images and that those images are to be read by a qualified interpreting physician who establishes a diagnosis. Therefore, patients may often inquire about the images being taken during the examination and subsequently ask the sonographer for a diagnosis. The only instance in which a diagnosis may be offered to a patient by a sonographer is on the occasion when an interpreting physician specifically requests that you do so under his or her direct supervision. For example, a concerned mother may be exceedingly apprehensive about the welfare of her fetus. Once the examination is completed and the images evaluated, the interpreting physician may request that you inform the patient that the sonogram was normal. But even in this situation, it is best for the interpreting physician to provide the patient with such information.

Sound Off

Sonographers who provide diagnostic information to patients may be held liable, as this is beyond the legal scope of practice for our occupation.

Some sonographic procedures may require the use of a chaperone, especially for male sonographers who must evaluate female patients. In this case, a female chaperone should be delegated to witness the examination. Some examinations that may require a chaperone include endovaginal sonograms, translabial examinations, and breast sonograms. Some department policies may require that *all* sonographers, even females, have a chaperone for such procedures. Indeed, some departments require that female sonographers have a chaperone for testicular sonograms as well. When a chaperone is warranted, it would be wise to document, perhaps on the sonographer's report, who served as the chaperone during the examination.

Medical negligence is also based on the concept of the master-servant doctrine or ***respondeat superior***, which means "let the master answer." This concept centers upon the legal liability that the employer and employee share in a negligence claim. While the sonographer is an employee of the institution in which a claim is made, the sonographer may also be personally held liable for negligence by his or her employer and thus face legal consequences that are brought about by the employer. Table 7-6 provides some helpful measures that may be taken to prevent medical malpractice suits.

Regarding the scope of practice for a sonographer, licensing organizations enforce professional practice standards and thus have the right to revoke certification in some instances. Some sonographers choose to purchase individual **professional liability insurance** to guard against malpractice claims when employer coverage is ambiguous and to protect against personal loss. It is your responsibility to fully understand the scope of coverage of these plans. When considering professional liability insurance, the SDMS claims that one should ask the questions found in Table 7-7.

GOOD SAMARITAN LAWS

All 50 states currently have **Good Samaritan laws**, though the content of those laws may vary drastically. Good Samaritan laws include protection for people who provide emergency care to a stranger from civil or criminal liability as long as (1) the care is given in good faith, (2) the provider acts within his or her scope of practice, (3) the provider uses due care under the circumstances, and (4) the provider does not bill for the service.[7] In some states, you may be required to be a Good Samaritan or risk legal consequences. In others, some laws may protect those who refuse to administer emergency care in fear of legal repercussions. Nonetheless, the chance of a lawsuit resulting from these situations is slim.[4] These laws do not typically pertain to hospital or clinical settings, where your job involves the

TABLE 7-6	Tips for preventing medical malpractice

- Treat each person equally.
- Explain procedures precisely, and obtain the patient's permission.
- Communicate effectively with your patient throughout the procedure.
- Be familiar with your healthcare facility's protocols, policies, and procedures.
- Always practice within the sonographer's scope of practice.
- Never independently perform procedures that you have not been trained to perform. Ask for help.
- Never offer medical advice to patients.
- Never provide diagnostic information to a patient.
- Keep accurate medical records and documents.
- Comply with all state and federal regulations, including HIPAA.
- Keep your work environment safe for patients, and perform quality assurance.
- Practice universal precautions.
- Maintain patient confidentiality.
- Secure informed consent.
- Obtain a chaperone when needed.
- Never leave an incoherent or unconscious patient unattended.
- Learn what legal protection your employer provides.
- Practice ALARA (as low as reasonably achievable). ALARA relates to patient exposure to medical ultrasound. We always want to keep exposure as low as reasonably achievable.
- Properly label images, and identify any alterations that are made to the standard protocol.
- Maintain continuing medical education, and be informed about the changing medical environment.
- Recognize the signs and symptoms of an emergency.

From Dutton AG, Linn-Watson, TA & Torres, LS. (2013). *Torres' Patient Care in Imaging Technology, 8th ed.* Philadelphia: Lippincott, Williams, & Wilkins.

TABLE 7-7	Questions to ask when considering purchasing professional liability insurance

- Has your employer provided you with written verification (such as a certificate of insurance) that you are being covered?
- Does your employer's coverage refer to you by name in the policy?
- Does your employer's policy have a separate limit of liability for you so that coverage cannot be used up by others covered by the same policy?
- Will your employer provide legal counsel representing your interests about who is a fault, even when it is in conflict with your employer's allegations?
- Will your employer advise you of settlement offers made to those suing you before they are made?
- Will your employer reimburse you for loss of income because you are required to attend a trial or participate in pre-trial meetings?
- Will your employer reimburse you for costs of legal representation for licensure and/or administrative review?
- If you moonlight on a contract basis, does your employer's policy cover you?

From SDMS Professional Liability Insurance. Retrieved from http://www.sdms.org/membership/liability.asp.[11]

immediate administration of lifesaving care. You should be aware of the specific Good Samarian laws in the state in which you hope to be employed.

PATIENT RIGHTS

Medical law includes **patient rights**, or the legal rights of the patient, the protection of individual rights, and the rights of the healthcare employee.[1] In the past, legislation has attempted to protect the patient's right to maintain personal control over his or her healthcare. The American Hospital Association (AHA) initially adopted the Patient's Bill of Rights in 1973. The document was revised in 1992, and then, in 2003, the document was replaced with a plain language document referred to as *The Patient Care Partnership: Understanding Expectations, Rights and Responsibilities* (PCP).[12] Table 7-8 provides a brief summary of the PCP. Within the document, patients are ensured considerate and respectful care, the right to privacy, and the right to refuse an examination or treatment.[12]

An underlying theme of the PCP is that of **consent**. Consent is the voluntary agreement or permission that a patient gives a medical professional to allow that professional to touch, examine, and/or perform treatment or a procedure on him or her.[1] There are two general types of consent: **informed consent** and **implied consent**. Informed consent is the act of providing a patient with a proposed procedure or course of treatment, explaining the risks and benefits and ultimately gaining permission to perform the procedure or treatment. Informed consent is obtained by having the patient sign an informed consent document after the procedure or treatment is explained thoroughly. The physician performing the procedure or treatment is solely responsible for the explanation of that procedure and treatment.[1] However, sonographers must understand the procedure, be able to simply explain it to a patient, and are often a witness to the patient's signature of the document. Examples of procedures that require informed consent are thoracentesis, paracentesis, amniocentesis, and any organ biopsies. Implied consent occurs when a patient demonstrates the acceptance of a procedure simply by his or her nonverbal actions. However, the examination must be thoroughly explained to the patient and permission granted. It may be best practice to obtain a written consent form for any examination that could be considered invasive or non-customary in order to retain written documentation.[13]

Patients can refuse an examination for any reason at any time. Sonographers should never perform an examination that a patient refuses or an examination that a patient does not fully comprehend. For those patients who refuse the exam, the sonographer should refer the patient to his or her physician for further guidance. Remember, if the sonographer continues with the procedure that a patient has refused, the sonographer can be held liable for assault and battery. Also, there may be situations in which a sonographer is not proficient in speaking the patient's language, thus leading to the performance of an examination that the patient may not adequately understand. In this situation, the sonographer should obtain an interpreter so that the patient is fully informed about the examination. Effective patient communication techniques are discussed further in Chapter 9.

TABLE 7-8	Summary of the AHA *Patient Care Partnership*

All patients should expect:
- High-quality hospital care.
- A clean and safe environment.
- Involvement in his or her care, which includes discussing medical conditions and treatment options.
- Protection of his or her privacy.
- Help when leaving the hospital.
- Help with billing claims.

From American Hospital Association. *The Patient Care Partnership: Understanding Expectations, Rights and Responsibilities;* 2003. Retrieved March 19, 2015 from http://www.aha.org/advocacy-issues/communicatingpts/pt-care-partnership.shtml

Sound Off

Consent is the voluntary agreement or permission that a patient gives a medical professional to allow that professional to touch, examine, and/or perform treatment or a procedure on him or her.

HIPAA and Patient Confidentiality

One of the largest reforms to American healthcare came in 1996 with the passing of the Health Insurance Portability and Accountability Act of 1996 (HIPAA). The impact of HIPAA is far-reaching. Table 7-9 provides some of the provisions of HIPAA. Essentially, HIPAA requires all of the following: standardization of electronic medical records, administrative data, and financial data; the establishment of unique health identifiers; and security standards to protect **patient confidentiality** (Fig. 7-4). Patient confidentiality relates both to the protection or security of health-related information and maintaining patient privacy.[5] The progression of healthcare toward electronic medical records was inevitable. HIPAA provides guidelines for the protection of and repercussions for the unlawful disclosure of all protected health information in any form. The Health Information Technology for Economic and Clinical Health (HITECH) Act of 2009 further promotes the protection of and use of health information technology. HITECH relates to the enforcement regulations and penalties associated with HIPAA.

Avoiding breaches in patient confidentiality is a crucial part of healthcare. In fact, patients have a right to expect quality care and confidentiality.[1] In order to maintain confidentiality, it is best to consider all patient information regarding the care of the patient as confidential. With modern electronic medical records and digital imaging, access to confidential information has become a great concern for patients. In the clinical setting, those who have access to such information should only be individuals who are providing direct care to the patient. Monitors displaying patient information should also not be easily decipherable to other patients.

HIPAA also reinforces the **statutory duty to report**, which is the obligation of health professionals, including sonographers, to follow state public health laws to report medical conditions or incidents such as venereal disease; contagious diseases such as tuberculosis; wounds inflicted by violence; poisoning; industrial accidents; abortions; drug abuse; and the abuse of children, the elderly, or those with disabilities.[1] In the case of a rape of an adult, state statues vary as to the obligation of the healthcare worker to report, especially in situations when the patient does not want to officially file a police report. It would be wise to be aware of the state statutes concerning the statutory duty to report where you are employed.

TABLE 7-9	Several notable provisions of the Health Insurance Portability and Accountability Act of 1996

- Protection of confidential medical information that identifies patients from unauthorized disclosure or use.
- Curtail the rising cost of medical fraud and abuse.
- Reduction of paperwork.
- Reduction of privacy violations.
- Improving the accuracy and reliability of shared data between healthcare institutions.
- Reduction of healthcare billing fraud.
- Helps workers maintain healthcare coverage between jobs.
- Provides for significant criminal and civil penalties for non-compliance.
- Patients must provide written permission or consent to provide or disclose any of their protected health information for any healthcare reason.

From Judson K, Hicks S. *Glencoe Law and Ethics for Medical Careers.* 3rd ed. New York, NY: McGraw Hill; 2002.

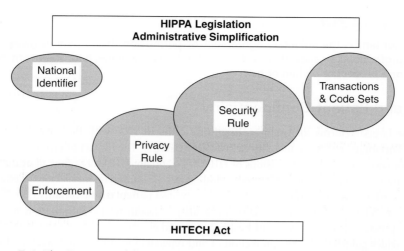

Figure 7-4. The Privacy and Security Rules are part and parcel of the Administrative Simplification Subtitle, which is a part of HIPAA.

Patient Rights Related to End-of-Life Issues

The **Patient Self-Determination Act of 1990**, along with subsequent legislation, sought to establish guidelines concerning the end-of-life desires of patients confronted with serious illnesses. For the patient who does not desire for his or her life to be maintained by mechanical means, **advance directives** can be established. Advance directives are legal documents that are created by a competent person to provide written information concerning his or her desires for treatment if for some reason the patient is unable to make decisions on his or her own.[10] Advance directives provide patients with more choices and options and give them the power of decision long before they lose the ability to make those decisions.[14] There are typically three legal documents that can contain information regarding advanced healthcare directives: a **living will**, a **durable power of attorney for healthcare**, or **healthcare advance directive**.

A living will simply expresses the patient's wishes concerning his or her future medical care. A durable power of attorney for healthcare, also referred to as a healthcare proxy, appoints an agent to act on behalf of the patient to make decisions about that patient's care should the patient lose the ability make his or her own decisions. The combination of the two, the healthcare advance directive, specifies the following: the person who is chosen to make care decisions for the patient, the kind of medical treatment wanted and not desired by the patient, how comfortable the patient wants to be, how the patient wants to be treated, and what the patient wants his or her loved ones to know.[10]

A **do not resuscitate** (DNR) order may also be part of a patient's advance healthcare directive. A DNR is a written physician's order instructing healthcare workers to not perform lifesaving cardiopulmonary resuscitation (CPR). The sonographer must have a written medical order to follow this request.[10] DNR orders may be found attached to a patient's inpatient chart. In the presence of no DNR order, the standard of care indicates that healthcare professionals must attempt to resuscitate if a patient stops breathing or undergoes cardiac arrest.[10] There may also be orders identified as "full code." In this situation, a "full code" often results in a "code blue" being called. A "full code" typically means that all lifesaving techniques must be employed in order to resuscitate a patient following cardiac or respiratory arrest. Students should be aware of code descriptions for each clinical rotation, as these may vary slightly among institutions. Therefore, an important component of clinical orientation is to understand each code and the protocols for enacting each code for every clinical facility that you visit during school. A "code blue" is an emergency situation that typically means that a full CPR is warranted.[10]

SONOGRAPHER DOCUMENTATION

One of the standards found in the SDMS *Clinical Practice Standards for Sonographers* is documentation (see Table 7-4). Sonographers should be aware that the images they obtain are legal documents that become a permanent part of the patient's medical history. Much legal information can be gathered from images regarding imaging technique, image quality, anatomy demonstrated or omitted, and the length of the examination. All of this information can be used to construct a legal argument. It would be wise to evaluate your images with this in mind and always document when and why the examination is not optimal. One of the standards (1.6.3) notes that sonographers should document "any exceptions from the established protocols and procedure." Sonographers should only provide the information requested by the facility or interpreting physician on the sonographer's report. It is ultimately your responsibility to understand how sonographer reports are incorporated into the patient's medical history at your eventual place of employment.

Sonographers are typically not required to log information in a patient's chart. However, you may be asked to complete an incident report or to report patient safety concerns. Incident report requirements vary among institutions. Many incident reports involve the reporting of irregular occurrences that involve patients, employees, or visitors of the institution including falls, deaths, drug or contrast reactions, radiopharmaceutical errors, injuries caused by faulty equipment, or threats of legal actions.[6] Correct documentation and reporting requires that those involved pay close attention to the time of the incident, document the individuals involved (including witnesses), and note the remediation that takes place following the incident.

SUMMARY

This chapter provided an overview of the legal environment in which a sonographer must practice. But laws change, and so the sonographer must be a professional who is attentive to changes and proficient at providing patient care effectively but within the legal scope of practice. Since we live in a litigious society, it is of utmost importance to practice sonography within our means and expertise. We should never cease to continually strive for excellence in patient care. By doing so, we will always promote the safety and well-being of each patient while simultaneously being mindful concerning the standards of practice and ever-evolving role of the sonographer in healthcare. Patients have an implicit right to a sonographer who is fully informed and who practices within the established standards of the profession. If you ever encounter questions that concern the legal aspects of your profession, or if you are asked to perform tasks with which you are uncomfortable, never hesitate to ask for help.

REFERENCES

1. Fremgen BF. *Medical Law and Ethics*. 3rd ed. Upper Saddle River, NJ: Pearson Prentice Hall; 2009.
2. Semelka RC, Elias J. *Current Clinical Imaging: Healthcare Reform in Radiology*. Somerset, NJ: John Wiley & Sons; 2013. ProQuest ebrary. Web. September 2, 2014.
3. Huntsman JM. *Winners Never Cheat: Everyday Values We Learned as Children (But May Have Forgotten)*. Upper Saddle River, NJ: Pearson Education; 2005.
4. Lewis MA, Tamparo CD. *Medical Law Ethics and Bioethics: For Health Professions*. 6th ed. Philadelphia, PA: F.A. Davis Company; 2007.
5. Adler AM, Carlton RR. *Introduction to Radiologic Sciences and Patient Care*. 4th ed. St. Louis, MO: Saunders Elsevier; 2007.
6. Towsley-Cook DM, Young TA. *Ethical and Legal Issues for Imaging Professionals*. 2nd ed. St. Louis, MO: Mosby; 2007.
7. Judson K, Hicks S. *Glencoe Law and Ethics for Medical Careers*. 3rd ed. New York, NY: McGraw Hill; 2002.

8. SDMS Diagnostic Ultrasound Clinical Practice Standards. Retrieved from http://www.sdms.org/positions/clinical-practice.asp

9. SDMS *Scope of Practice for the Diagnostic Ultrasound Professional*. Retrieved from http://www.sdms.org/positions/scope.asp

10. Dutton AG, Linn-Watson, TA & Torres, LS. (2013). *Torres' Patient Care in Imaging Technology. 8th ed*. Philadelphia, PA. Lippincott, Williams, & Wilkins.

11. SDMS Professional Liability Insurance. Retrieved from http://www.sdms.org/membership/liability.asp

12. American Hospital Association. *The Patient Care Partnership: Understanding Expectations, Rights and Responsibilities*; 2003. Retrieved March 19, 2015 from http://www.aha.org/advocacy-issues/communicatingpts/pt-care-partnership.shtml

13. Jasper MC. *Oceana's Law for the Layperson: Healthcare Directives*. New York, NY: Oceana Publications/Oxford University Press; 2007.

14. Loewy EH. *Textbook of Healthcare Ethics*. Hingham, MA: Kluwer Academic Publishers; 1996. ProQuest ebrary. Web. July 16, 2014.

Thinking Critically

1. "Baby's Cardiac Arrest/Brain Damage Lawsuit Settles for $2 Million." Access at http://www.lubinandmeyer.com/cases/newborn-malpractice.html. Read the case history, and answer the following questions:
   - What are the AIUM guidelines for evaluating the fetal heart?
   - What can a sonographer do to avoid this situation?

2. "Woman Sues over Transvaginal Ultrasound." Access at http://www.huffingtonpost.com/2013/09/11/transvaginal-ultrasoundlawsuit_n_3907422.html. Read the limited case article, and answer the following questions:
   - What can a sonographer do to avoid this situation?
   - Should sonography protocols include informed consents for transvaginal sonograms? Explain your answer.

3. Visit SonoWorld.com at http://sonoworld.com/Client/Centers/Legal.aspx. Read the articles provided in the "Legal Issue Center." Discuss your opinions about the article with your fellow classmates.

Chapter 7
Review Questions

1. Which of the following is the legal doctrine of negligence that means "the thing speaks for itself?"
   a. *Respondeat superior*
   b. *Res ipsa loquitur*
   c. *Stare decision*
   d. *Rostitia decision superior*

2. What is the type of statutory law that is enacted regarding the power of agencies to regulate and enforce laws?
   a. Administrative law
   b. Criminal law
   c. Civil law
   d. Common law

3. **Which of the following is an example of an intentional tort?**
   a. Negligence
   b. Malpractice
   c. Assault
   d. Breach of duty

4. **Speaking potentially damaging and malicious words about a coworker would be considered**
   a. negligence.
   b. assault.
   c. libel.
   d. slander.

5. **When a sonographer has a duty to provide reasonable care but fails to do so, this may result in a charge of**
   a. assault.
   b. battery.
   c. negligence.
   d. misdemeanor.

6. **Which of the following is not an intentional tort?**
   a. Embezzlement
   b. Malpractice
   c. Assault
   d. False imprisonment

7. **Which of the following is not one of the four Ds of negligence?**
   a. Deterrence
   b. Duty
   c. Direct cause
   d. Damages

8. **Which of the following would be an example of an unintentional tort?**
   a. Immobilization of a patient against his or her will
   b. Hitting a patient who hit you first
   c. Falsely stating that a patient will soon recover from his or her illness
   d. Performing the wrong examination on a patient

9. **Which of the following is not a diagnostic ultrasound clinical practice standard as described by the SDMS?**
   a. Assesses and monitors the patient's physical and mental status during the examination
   b. Assesses the patient's ability to tolerate procedure
   c. Provides patient care with bias toward none and equal respect for all
   d. Provides minimal diagnosis of imaging for patients and family

10. **Which of the following is not within the sonographer's scope of practice?**
    a. Perform minimally invasive procedures
    b. Acquire and analyze data obtained using ultrasound and related diagnostic technologies
    c. Provide a summary of findings to the physician to aid in patient diagnosis and management
    d. Perform patient assessments

11. Which of the following is defined as statements of the minimum behavioral or performance levels that are acceptable?
    a. Ethics
    b. Laws
    c. Standards
    d. Torts

12. Which of the following is the oldest form of law?
    a. Statutory law
    b. Tort law
    c. Common law
    d. Civil law

13. A sonographer should not include which of the following on a sonographer's report?
    a. At least two differential diagnoses
    b. Comments on any alteration to the standard protocol
    c. Sonographic description of abnormalities identified
    d. Patient data

14. What exists once the sonographer-patient relationship has been established?
    a. Tort
    b. Duty
    c. Diagnosis
    d. Consent

15. Which of the following is not a practice that can help prevent medical malpractice?
    a. Keep accurate medical records and documents
    b. Never offer medical advice to patients
    c. Explain procedures precisely, and obtain the patient's permission
    d. Purchase medical malpractice insurance

16. Which of the following is not included in the Patient's Bill of Rights?
    a. The right to speedy care
    b. The right to respectful care
    c. The right to refuse care
    d. The right to plan care

17. What is a voluntary agreement or permission that a patient gives a medical professional to allow that professional to touch, examine, and/or perform treatment or a procedure on them?
    a. Professional liability contract
    b. Patient's right
    c. Consent
    d. Respondeat superior

18. Which of the following is a crime punishable by death or by imprisonment?
    a. Civil crime
    b. Felony
    c. Misdemeanor
    d. Disparage

19. **Laws are best described as**
    a. mandatory rules of society.
    b. optional rules of society.
    c. rights to be protected.
    d. standards of conduct we should follow.

20. **Which of the following would typically not warrant the signing of an informed consent document?**
    a. Abdominal sonogram
    b. Breast biopsy
    c. Drainage of a Baker cyst
    d. Paracentesis

Basic Principles and Knobology

CHAPTER OBJECTIVES

■ Provide a brief overview of directional terminology and patient positioning.

■ Explain the function of ultrasound modes.

■ Offer a rationalization for the use of common universal controls found on most ultrasound machines.

KEY TERMS

Acoustic gel – substance used to permit the transmission of sound into the human body; also referred to as the coupling gel or ultrasound gel

Acoustic power – control that relates to the amount of energy the transducer is emitting into the patient

Acoustic windows (sonographic window) – optimal locations on the body for placement of the ultrasound transducer to demonstrate both normal anatomy and pathology; the best image acquired by manipulating and placing the ultrasound transducer in the most favorable position; some organs can provide a better acoustic window for improved viewing of adjacent anatomy

Amplitude mode (A-mode) – ultrasound display in which the depth of the returning echo was represented on the x-axis, while the strength (amplitude) of the reflector was represented along the y-axis

Annotation keys – letters of the keyboard that allow for the labeling of images; similar to the display on a computer keyboard

B-color – colorizes the grayscale of the image

Body marker – tool used for labeling different anatomic structures or for identifying where the transducer is placed on a body part

Brightness mode (B-mode) – ultrasound display in which a dot with varying degrees of brightness is used on the screen; the stronger the returning echo, the brighter the dot; also referred to as grayscale sonography

Caret – the transmit zone indicator

Cine loop – a collection of image frames stored temporarily in the system's memory before the image is frozen

Color Doppler imaging – Doppler shift information presented as a color or hue superimposed over a grayscale image

Continuous-wave Doppler – a Doppler device that utilizes two elements—one element that continuously sends ultrasound waves into the body and another element to continuously listen for the returning signal

Coronal plane – plane that divides the body or body part into anterior and posterior portions

Depth – varies the deepness of the echoes that are displayed on the monitor; also referred to as depth range

Doppler technology – relates to the effect of differing frequencies with motion

Dual image – allows the display to be split into two separate images

Electronic calipers – used to measure structures

Ellipse – allows for the measurement of round structures

Freeze – allows for all display data to be started or stopped

HD zoom – allows for the magnification of the image with an adjustment made for resolution; may also be referred to as RES or write zoom

Image store – allows for images to be stored within the hard drive of the machine

Knobology – the study of knobs and how they function

Longitudinal plane – plane that divides the body or body part into right and left portions

Midline – imaginary line that separates the body into equal right and left portions; may also be referred to as the midsagittal plane of the body

Midsagittal plane – plane that divides the body into equal right and left portions; may also be referred to as the midline

Motion mode (M-mode) – demonstrates the motion of structures along a single scan line

Overall gain – adjusts the brightness or the degree of echo amplification of the entire image; may also be referred to as 2D gain

Pedoff probe – a continuous-wave non-imaging transducer

Power Doppler – amplitude mode of Doppler where it is not the shift itself that provides the signal but rather the strength (amplitude) of the shift

Pulsed-wave Doppler – Doppler technique that uses pulses of sound to obtain Doppler signals from a user-specified depth

Realtime imaging – ultrasound imaging technique that allows continual imaging of the body as if one were watching a movie

Reference point – the orientation mark on the transducer; also referred to as the notch or index

Sagittal plane – see longitudinal plane

Sample volume – the area from which information is obtained using pulsed-wave Doppler; also referred to as the sample gate

Scanning plane – term used to describe the transducer's orientation relative to the body or a structure

Slide pots – time gain compensation knobs that allow for the alteration of brightness at a specific depth on the image

Time gain compensation – control that alters the brightness of an image at a specific depth; may also be referred to as depth gain compensation or depth compensation gain

Transducer – instrument used to obtain an image of the human body using ultrasound; also referred to as the ultrasound probe

Transducer orientation – the act of maintaining the correct placement of the transducer on or within the body in order to provide the accurate demonstration of anatomy

Transmit zone – enhances the resolution of an area in the image by electronic focusing; also referred to as the focus

Transverse plane – plane that divides the body or body part into superior and inferior portions

Zoom – allows for the magnification of the image by often increasing the pixel size

INTRODUCTION

This brief chapter provides you with a concise overview of common controls found on most ultrasound machines. Though the locations and titles of these controls may vary, almost all ultrasound machines share the common controls listed in this chapter. This chapter also provides information pertaining to common directional terminology, patient positioning, and transducer care.

DIRECTIONAL TERMINOLOGY AND PATIENT POSITIONING

A person in the anatomic position is standing erect, feet together, with arms by the sides, and the palms and face directed forward, facing the observer. When a sonographer refers to directional terms or anatomy, it is assumed that the patient is in anatomic position. Directional terms can be found in Table 8-1 and Figure 8-1.

Sound Off

Sonographers must have a thorough understanding of normal relational anatomy.

Though many types of sonograms are performed with the patient initially in the supine position—lying on his or her back—there are other positions that the patient may be required to assume during the examination, depending upon the anatomy that must be visualized (Table 8-2 and Fig. 8-2).

TABLE 8-1	Directional terms
Directional Term	**Explanation**
Anterior	Toward the front of the body or body part; in front of another body part
Caudal	See inferior
Contralateral	On the opposite side of the body
Cranial	See superior
Deep	Away from the surface of the body or structure
Distal	Farther from the attachment point or origin of an extremity to the trunk of the body
Dorsal	See posterior
Inferior	Toward the feet or away from the head; a structure lower than another part of the body; the lower part of an organ or structure
Ipsilateral	On the same side of the body
Lateral	Away from the midline of the body or pertaining to the side; situated at or on the side
Medial	Toward the middle of the body or an organ
Posterior	Toward the back or behind another structure
Proximal	Toward the origin or attachment of a structure to the trunk
Superficial	Closer to the surface of the body or structure
Superior (Cephalic)	Toward the head or higher in the body
Ventral	See anterior

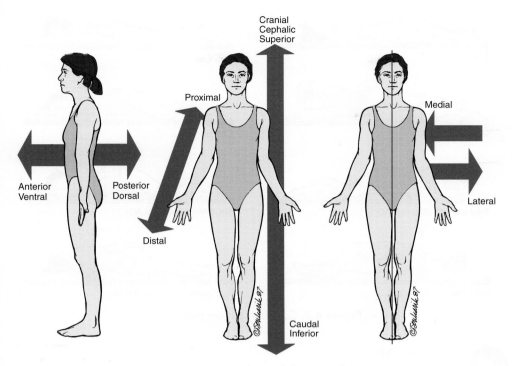

Figure 8-1. Commonly used directional terms.

TABLE 8-2	Patient positions
Patient Position	**Explanation**
Supine	Lying on the back
Prone	Lying face down
Right lateral decubitus (RLD)	Lying on the right side
Left lateral decubitus (LLD)	Lying on the left side
Right posterior oblique (RPO)	Lying semisupine, rolled up on the right side slightly, and elevating the left side
Left posterior oblique (LPO)	Lying semisupine, rolled up on the left side slightly, and elevating the right side
Left anterior oblique (LAO)	Lying semiprone, rolled up on the left side slightly, and elevating the right side
Right anterior oblique (RAO)	Lying semiprone, rolled up on the right side slightly, and elevating the left side
Fowler position	Various inclined positions in which the head of the bed is raised (varies from low to high); the head of the bed is typically raised 18–20 in above the heart with the knees elevated
Trendelenburg	Person in the supine position with the feet raised higher than the level of the head at an angle of 15–30 degrees
Upright	Sitting or standing

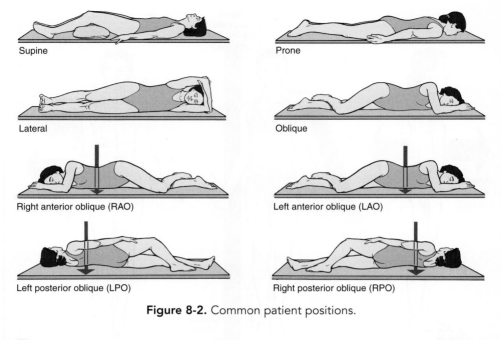

Figure 8-2. Common patient positions.

 ## Sound Off

Throughout sonographic examinations, the patient may have to be placed in many different positions.

TRANSDUCERS

Sonographers use a versatile device referred to as a **transducer** to obtain an image of the human body using ultrasound. The transducer, also referred to as a probe, is capable of converting energy from one form to another. The transducer operates using the pulse-echo principle, as described in Chapter 1 (Fig. 8-3). Essentially, the crystal inside of the transducer produces the ultrasound wave once pulsed with electricity. The wave is sent into the body and then returns to the transducer again. The strength of that echo is displayed on the system's monitor. Transducers come in many shapes and sizes, all of which are created for explicit reasons and utilized for varying sonographic examinations (Fig. 8-4). Subsequently, the shape of the image display varies as well (Figs. 8-5 through 8-7).

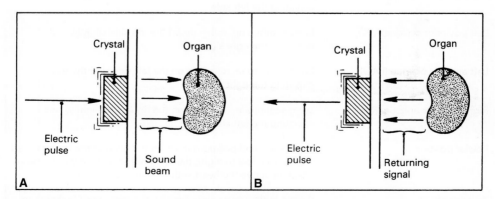

Figure 8-3. Pulse-echo technique. **A.** The transducer pulses ultrasound waves into the body. **B.** The sonographic image is produced when the signal returns to the transducer, causing vibrations. The ultrasound machine interprets the strength of the signal and displays the signal on the monitor accordingly.

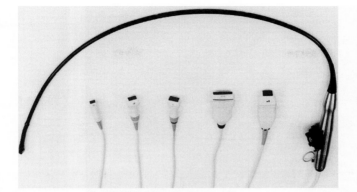

Figure 8-4. Examples of ultrasound transducers utilized for echocardiography. The long transducer (*far right*) is used for transesophageal imaging.

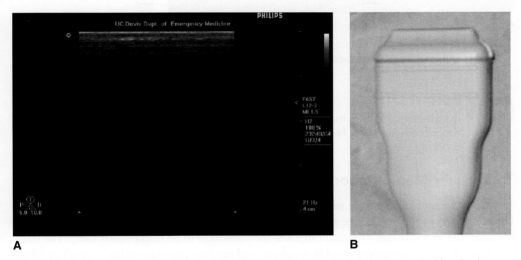

A

B

Figure 8-5. Linear sequenced array transducer. **A.** The image display provided by the linear sequenced array transducer. **B.** An example of a linear sequenced array transducer.

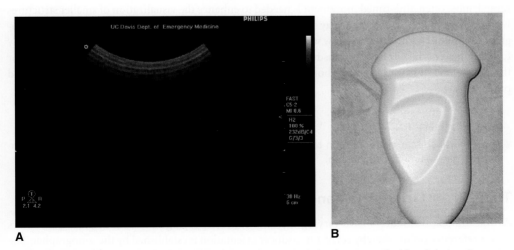

A

B

Figure 8-6. Curvilinear array transducer. **A.** The image display provided by the curvilinear array transducer. **B.** An example of a curvilinear array transducer.

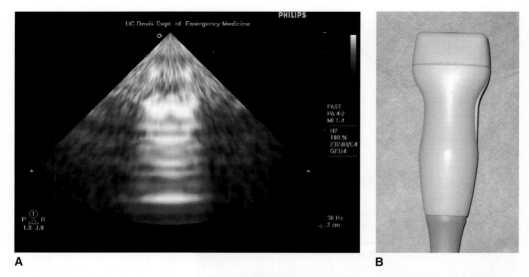

A   **B**

Figure 8-7. Linear phased array transducer. **A.** The image display provided by the linear phased array transducer. **B.** An example of a linear phased array transducer.

Sound Off

Transducers come in many different shapes and sizes according to their purposes. You should become familiar with the most commonly used transducers for your specialty.

Transducer Manipulation

Transducer manipulation on the patient's body requires the use of **acoustic gel**, also referred to as ultrasound gel or coupling gel. The gel acts as a means whereby the ultrasound waves can pass through the body. Gel also provides a lubricant to allow the transducer to be manipulated easily. The transducer, which is most commonly wired to the ultrasound machine (though wireless technology exists), can be slid, angled, heel-toed, and rocked over the patient's body to obtain the required images.

While some drastic movement of the transducer to examine large organs like the liver is warranted, most often, fine-tuned movement is needed to enhance the visualization of smaller structures within the body. The transducer may need to be manipulated to obtain optimal acoustic or sonographic window. An acoustic window was described in Chapter 1 as the optimal location on the body for placement of the ultrasound transducer to demonstrate both normal anatomy and pathology. For the novice, the best way to learn about how to manipulate the transducer is to pick one up and practice.

Sound Off

Transducer manipulation takes practice. Utilize your time wisely, and practice scanning as much as you can.

Transducer Orientation and Scanning Planes

As you can tell, transducers have varying uses and come in varying sizes. However, all transducers have a **reference point** whereby correct transducer orientation is established by the sonographer. The reference point may be referred to as the index or the notch and may be represented by a groove, light, or manufacturer symbol on one part of the transducer (Fig. 8-8). Keeping the index or notch in the

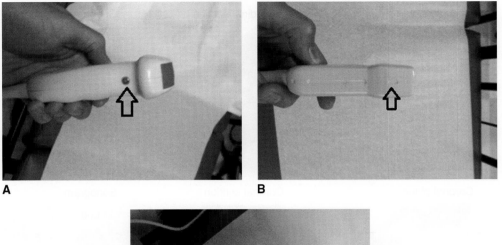

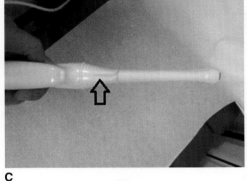

Figure 8-8. The transducer notch or index (*arrows*) provide a point of reference. Notice, each of these transducers (A, B, & C) have a different index.

proper position—**transducer orientation**—is exceedingly important for obtaining correct anatomic orientation. Sonography incorporates imaging of the body in various scanning planes. A **scanning plane** is the term used to describe the transducer's orientation relative to the body or a structure. The following section provides a brief overview of scanning planes used in medical and vascular sonography and transthoracic echocardiography.

 Sound Off

In order to demonstrate the patient's anatomy correctly on the image, you should always know where your reference point, or notch, is located.

Medical and Vascular Sonography Scanning Planes

In general abdominal, small part, and vascular sonography, the three most common scanning planes are the **sagittal plane**, **transverse plane**, and **coronal plane** (Fig. 8-9). A **midsagittal plane**, which may also be referred to as the **midline**, divides the body into equal left and right halves. Thus, any other sagittal plane or parasagittal plane divides the body or structure into unequal right and left portions. Sonographers may also refer to a sagittal plane as a **longitudinal plane**. The transverse plane divides the body or structure into superior and inferior portions, while the coronal plane divides the body or structure into anterior and posterior portions (Fig. 8-10).

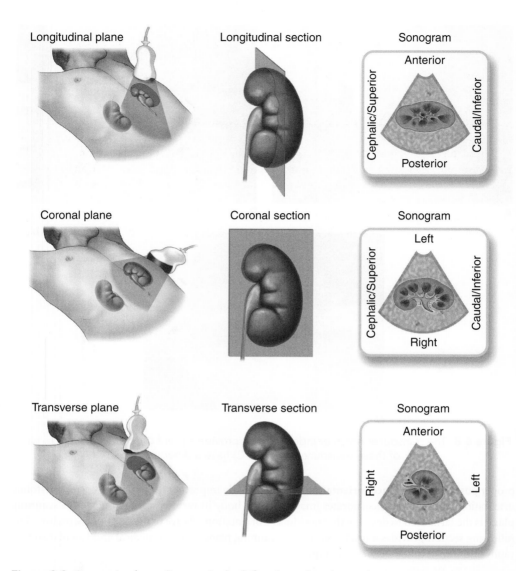

Figure 8-9. Anatomic planes (images in the **left** columns) and transducer orientation (images on the **right**) that are often used in abdominal, small part, gynecologic, obstetrics, and vascular sonographic imaging.

Transthoracic Echocardiography Scanning Planes

For transthoracic echocardiography, the sonographer adjusts the transducer to the heart in order to achieve a variety of views, including suprasternal, parasternal, apical, and subcostal (Figs. 8-11 through 8-14). An echocardiographer may perform the sonographic examination by using his or her left or right hand to manipulate the transducer. Transducer orientation in echocardiography can be challenging because the **acoustic windows** can be exceedingly small between the rib spaces and patient body habitus may inhibit optimal visualization of structures.

Care and Cleaning of Transducers

Ultrasound transducers are expensive. Care must be maintained so that the transducer is consistently in optimal working condition. Do not drop transducers or roll the machine over the cords, as damage may occur. If you identify a crack in the transducer housing, you should report the damage to your immediate supervisor or clinical preceptor.

Transducers should never be autoclaved, as this process will most likely permanently damage the fragile crystals within the transducer, rendering it dysfunctional. Transducers that are employed for topical purposes, such as abdominal, vascular, and transthoracic echocardiography, should be cleaned with a manufacturer-recommended disinfectant solution or disinfectant wipes before and after each examination. The transducer cords should also be cleaned in the same manner.

Ultrasound transducers that are employed for intracavitary purposes, such as endovaginal or transesophageal echocardiography, may be disinfected with some form of glutaraldehyde-based

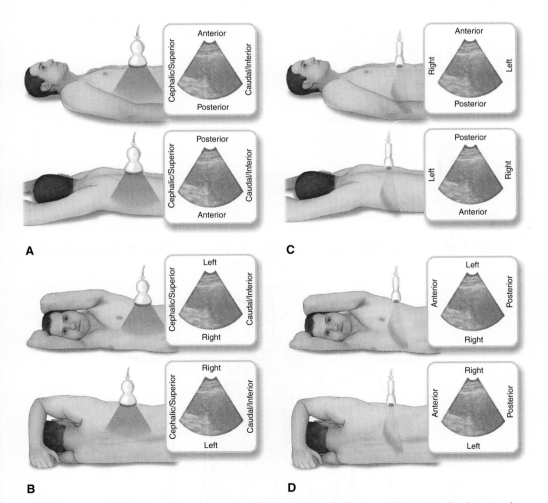

Figure 8-10. Image presentations. **A.** Longitudinal sagittal plane. **B.** Longitudinal coronal plane scanning on the lateral right or left surface. **C.** Transverse plane, anterior or posterior surface. **D.** Transverse plane, right or left lateral surface.

(continues)

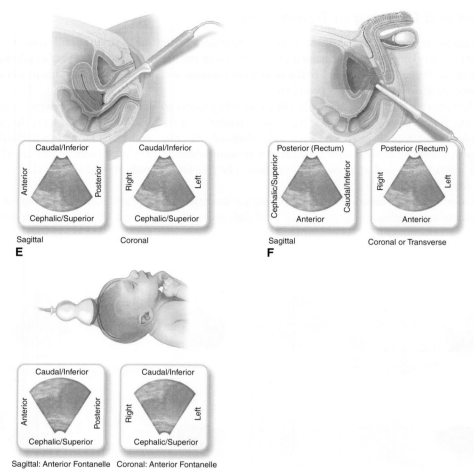

Figure 8-10. (*Continued*) **E.** Endovaginal planes. **F.** Anorectal planes. **G.** Neonatal brain imaging planes.

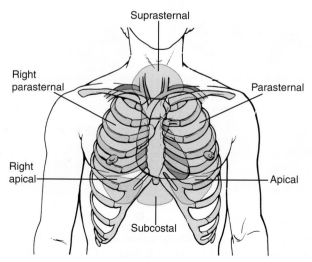

Figure 8-11. This diagram demonstrates the various transducer locations used in echocardiography.

Parasternal Long Axis View

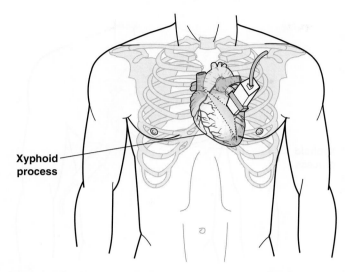

Xyphoid
process

Figure 8-12. Transducer placement for a parasternal long-axis cardiac view.

solution. These transducers are soaked in the solution for the manufacturer's recommended amount of time. Close monitoring and documentation of transducer disinfection is warranted. You should find out how transducers are cleaned and disinfected in each clinical facility that you visit. This topic is further discussed in Chapter 12.

Sound Off
If you identify a crack in the transducer housing, you should report the damage to your immediate supervisor or clinical preceptor.

Subxyphoid View

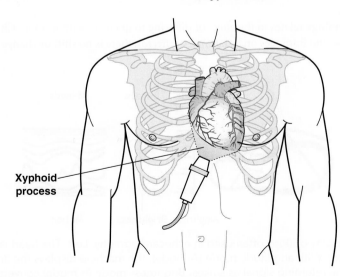

Xyphoid
process

Figure 8-13. Transducer placement for a subxiphoid (subcostal) cardiac view.

Apical Four Chamber View

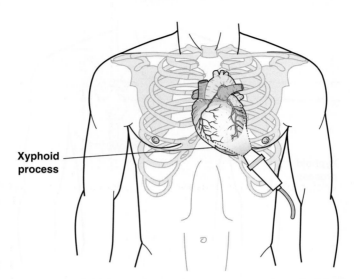

Xyphoid process

Figure 8-14. Transducer placement for the apical four-chamber cardiac view.

B-MODE AND BASIC DOPPLER OVERVIEW

Brightness mode, or B-mode imaging, displays the returning echoes as dots of varying brightness on the ultrasound monitor. With B-mode, the brightness of the dot relates to the strength of the echo that has returned from the body. Modern ultrasound equipment utilizes realtime to obtain images. **Realtime imaging** refers to the ability of the machine to gather information and display it on the screen almost instantaneously. In other words, the information is provided for us so rapidly that it appears to be provided for us on the screen with no delay, as if watching a movie. Combining both B-mode and realtime results in what we use today to obtain our images—the realtime B-scan technique. Echocardiography may utilize A-mode, or **amplitude mode**, as well. A-mode does not produce an image but rather displays the amplitude or strength of the returning echoes as spikes on a scale (Fig. 8-15).[1]

    Doppler technology relates to the effect of differing frequencies with motion. Christian Doppler noted that when sound impinges on a stationary reflector, there is no shift or change in the reflected

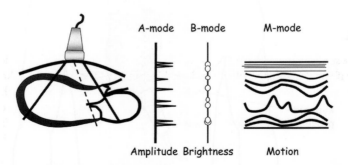

Figure 8-15. Display options often used in echocardiography. *Left*: The heart is imaged with a transducer. With amplitude mode (A-mode), the machine displays the amplitude or strength of the returning signal as spikes. Brightness mode (B-mode) converts those signal spikes to dots of varying brightness. Motion mode (M-mode) plots B-mode on a timeline.

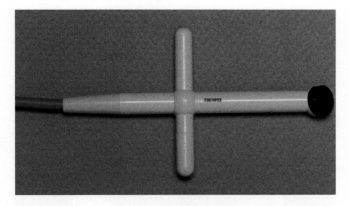

Figure 8-16. A Pedoff probe or continuous-wave (CW) Doppler transducer. A CW transducer contains two elements: one for transmitting and one for receiving.

frequency back to the transducer. However, he also noted that there was a frequency shift if the reflector was moving. If we hook up a speaker, the shift in frequency becomes audible as well. Typically, the structures we analyze with Doppler that are moving are the red blood cells within various blood vessels and organs.[1] The different types of Doppler technology can evaluate the direction of the flow and how fast the blood is flowing (velocity) within the vessel.

Doppler sonography may be described as **continuous-wave** (CW) **Doppler**, **pulsed-wave** (PW) **Doppler**, **color Doppler imaging** (CDI), and **power Doppler**. Continuous-wave transducers employ two crystals, one that sends the sound out and one that listens to the returning echo. For this reason, CW transducers are always on and do not create an image. CW is often utilized in echocardiography with the use of a **Pedoff probe** (Fig. 8-16). Any blood vessel that lies within the path of the ultrasound wave will be measure and displayed in the signal.[1]

Unlike CW, pulsed-wave (PW) Doppler provides an image of anatomy and allows the sonographer to select the depth at which the Doppler measurement will be taken.[1] In other words, a sample or range gate placed in the vessel allows for specific sampling. PW also allows the user to take an accurate measurement of the velocity of the blood within the selected vessel in order to evaluate blood flow for signs of disease (Fig. 8-17). CDI is a color representation of the Doppler shift.[1] The scale for CDI shows direction of flow as a color or a range of colors. Power Doppler, which may also be referred to as Doppler energy or power angio, focuses only on the strength of the Doppler shift. Power Doppler is much more sensitive than standard color Doppler and is better at revealing slower blood flow.[1]

ESSENTIAL UNIVERSAL KNOBOLOGY

Knobology is the study of knobs or the functionality of controls. The title for this section can be somewhat misleading if you think that all ultrasound machines incorporate some sort of knob for controls. This is, of course, not the case. Many of the controls listed below may actually be touch-screen buttons found on a touch-screen monitor. Keep in mind that because all ultrasound machines differ, these controls may also be referred to by other titles as well. It is your obligation to become familiar with the controls and abilities of the ultrasound machines that you are using in the clinical setting.

Sound Off
Every ultrasound machine is different. Spend some time learning the locations and uses of each machine's knobs.

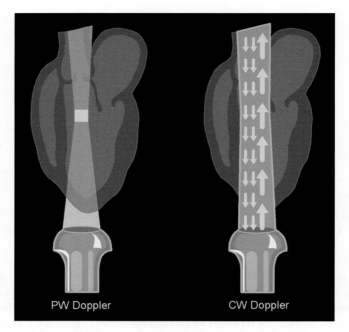

Figure 8-17. Fundamental difference between PW Doppler (*left*) and CW Doppler (*right*). CW Doppler utilizes only one crystal for sending ultrasound and another crystal for listening. For this reason, CW transducers are always listening for the returning signal. In contrast, PW Doppler intermittently transmits sound. Between transmissions, the transducer pauses briefly to listen for the returning signal. This allows the ultrasound system the ability to select a single area of interest to interrogate.

Acoustic Power

The **acoustic power** relates to the amount of energy the transducer is emitting into the patient.[2] Manufacturer power settings are usually set at the minimum for each application setting. Since acoustic power relates to the exposure of the patient to ultrasound, sonographers should be mindful of the settings. Remember, always practice ALARA (as low as reasonably acceptable) when performing a sonogram.

Annotation Keys

The **annotation keys** for an ultrasound machine are arranged similarly to a keyboard for a computer. There should be controls for capitalizing letters, special symbols, and numbers. Special symbols include arrows that are often used to indicate and label anatomy or pathology on a sonographic image.

B-Color

The **B-color** control colorizes the grayscale of the image.[2] Sonographers can select from a number of colors under this setting, including sepia, magenta, and blue. Some sonographers may choose to use B-color to enhance the borders of structures.

Body Markers

Body markers are used for labeling different anatomic structures or for identifying where the transducer is placed on a body part. For example, a body marker may be used in breast imaging to identify the location of a breast lesion. The body marker control may also be used to relate fetal positioning.

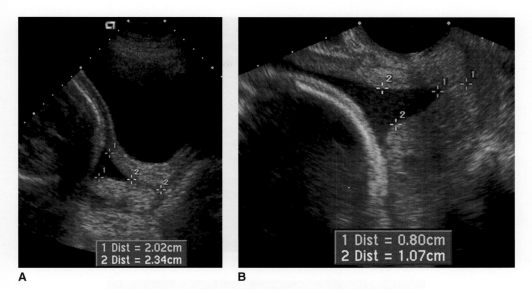

A   B

Figure 8-18. Calipers. Two sets of electronic calipers (cross-shaped, numbered measuring instruments) are noted in both **(A)** and **(B)**, identifying two dimension of the cervix.

Calipers

Sonographers use **electronic calipers** to measure structures during a sonographic examination (Fig. 8-18). Calipers can also be used to measure the depth of structures within the body as well. The selection and input of calipers varies per machine, and the control may be labeled as "distance" or "measure."

Cine (Cine Loop)

Cine loop is a collection of image frames stored temporarily in the system's memory before the image is frozen.[2] Essentially, cine loop allows us to rewind the scan after we use the freeze button. The amount of frames stored varies with each machine. Cine loop is exceedingly useful for moving structures and when a patient cannot hold his or her breath during the examination.

Sound Off

Cine loops are like mini movies of anatomy. This control provides the sonographer with the ability to rewind and view previous imaged anatomy once the image is frozen.

Color (Doppler)

This control activates the CD display. Some delay may be present while the machine accesses the control. Occasionally, rotating this control allows the gain of the color Doppler signal to be increased or decreased as well. Once activated, additional controls will allow for adjustment and optimization of color Doppler.

Continuous-Wave Doppler

The CW control setting actives CW Doppler.

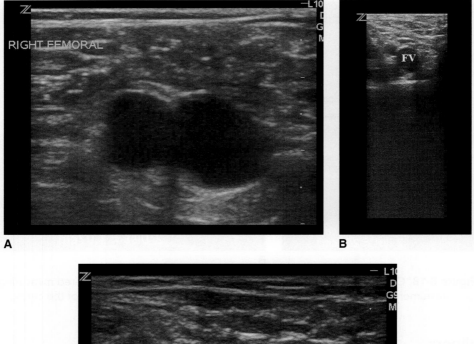

A

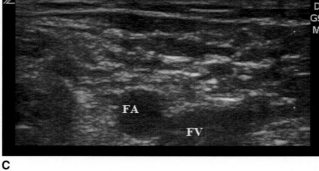

C

B

Figure 8-19. Ultrasound field of depth. **A.** Appropriate depth. **B.** Inappropriate setting of too much depth. Much of the screen is wasted. **C.** Inappropriate setting of not enough depth or imaging that is too shallow. In this case, the femoral artery (FA) and femoral vein (FV) are not centered on the image and are said to be "clipped off."

Depth

The **depth**, or depth range, varies the deepness of the echoes that are displayed on the monitor.[2] Decreasing the depth control results in the display of only superficial structures, while increasing the depth control allows for the visualization of structures farther away from the transducer, or deeper in the body (Fig. 8-19).

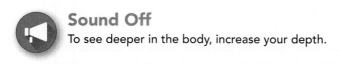

Sound Off
To see deeper in the body, increase your depth.

Dual Image

Dual image allows the display to be split into two separate images. Dual image can be used to compare normal and abnormal anatomy (Fig. 8-20). Realtime scanning may be performed on one side of the display, while the other is frozen. A toggle often allows switching between the frozen and active images.

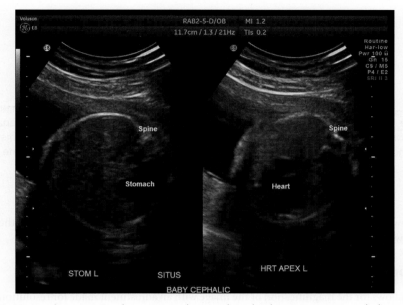

Figure 8-20. Dual image. Dual image can be used to display two images side by side. Seen here, the fetal heart and stomach can be proven to be located in their proper locations using a dual image.

Ellipse

Ellipse allows for the measurement of round structures. This measurement is often employed in obstetric sonography to measure the fetal abdominal circumference (AC) (Fig. 8-21).

Field of View (Extended Field of View)

The field-of-view control gives choices to the sonographer to make maximal use of the screen's potential resolution and yet display all of the relevant area.[2] Extended field of view allows for varying the amount of anatomy to be visualized with a single transducer. Some manufacturers may refer to the image as landscape or seascape (Fig. 8-22).

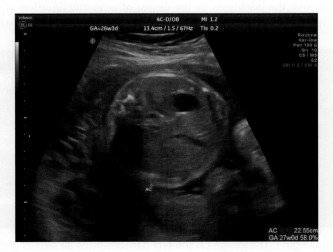

Figure 8-21. Ellipse. Fetal AC is often measured using the ellipse tool. Seen here, the tool provides an outline of the fetal abdomen to obtain an accurate measurement used to date the gestation.

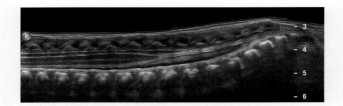

Figure 8-22. Extended field-of-view image. The extended field-of-view image enables the sonographer to display the entire length of various organs or structures. This image demonstrates the use of extended field of view for the newborn or infant spine while searching for evidence of closed spina bifida.

Freeze

Freeze allows for all display data to be started or stopped. Pictures can be stored after the image is frozen. However, some machines do not require that the image be frozen to store.

HD Zoom

HD zoom allows for the magnification of the image with an adjustment made for resolution, offering true magnification.[2] This control may be referred to as RES or write zoom.

Image Store/Print

The **image store** button allows for images to be stored within the hard drive of the machine.

MultiHertz

The MultiHertz control allows the user to choose between different sending frequencies of the transducer. In general, increasing the frequency improves resolution while sacrificing penetration. Decreasing the frequency improves penetration while sacrificing resolution. Therefore, superficial structures are typically better imaged with higher frequencies, while deeper structures are better imaged with lower frequencies.

Overall Gain

The **overall gain** adjusts the brightness or the degree of echo amplification of the entire image (Fig. 8-23).[2] The overall gain is typically measured in decibels. This control may be labeled "2D gain."

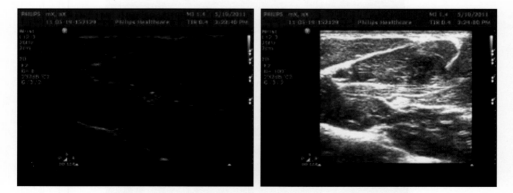

Figure 8-23. Overall gain. The image on the **left** demonstrates an overall gain that has been turned down or adjusted too low, resulting in an image that is too dark to display anatomy correctly. The image on the **right** results from an overall gain that has been adjusted too high, resulting in an image that is too bright.

Sound Off
Increasing the overall gain makes the overall image brighter.

Time Gain Compensation

Time gain compensation (TGC) may also be referred to as depth gain compensation or depth compensation gain. The TGC is often controlled by adjusting **slide pots**, which alter the brightness of an image at a specific depth (Figs. 8-24 and 8-25).[2] TGC compensates for the loss or attenuation of the sound beam as it passes through the body.

Sound Off
TGC allows gain adjustment for a specific area on the image.

Tissue Equalization

Tissue equalization or premium view processing allows for system-controlled image optimization specific to the patients for B-mode and spectral Doppler, which is often independent of the sonographer's adjustments. Manufacturers may use different terms for this technology.

Trace

The trace control allows for a structure to be traced and the distance measured (Fig. 8-26).

Trackball

The trackball allows for the control of cursor for text, cine looping, and various other trackball features similar to the manner in which a mouse functions for a computer. The selection keys (enter/select) are often located adjacent to the trackball.

Transducer Select

Transducer select permits the activation of different transducers. This control may also appear as a diagram or drawing of the transducers.

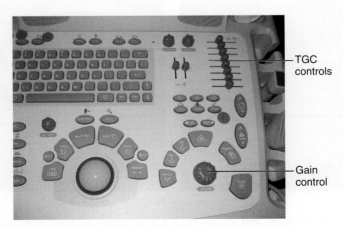

Figure 8-24. Overall gain verses time gain compensation. Difference between overall gain and TGC. Note the gain knob in the lower right. The TGC slide pots are in the upper right of the keyboard and used to adjust segments of the image.

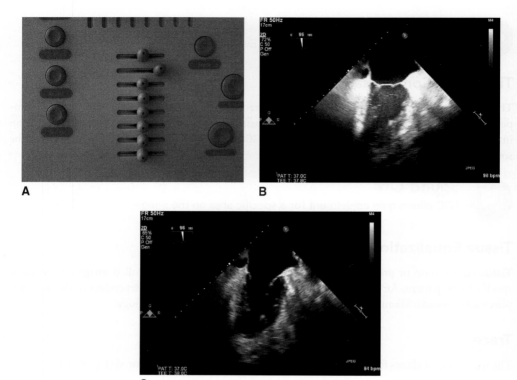

A   **B**

C

Figure 8-25. Time gain compensation. **A.** The TGC is determined by a series of sliding controls referred to as slide pots. The upper controls affect the near field, or the area closest to the transducer face, while the lower controls affect the far field, or the area farthest away from the transducer. **B.** High settings of the second control affect part of the middle of the image. **C.** Improvements to the TGC result in a more uniform brightness and thus better image quality.

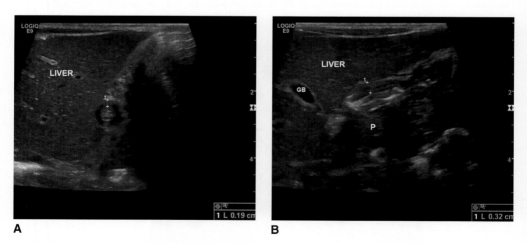

A   **B**

Figure 8-26. Trace. **(A, B, and C)** are images of a thickened pylorus muscle (between calipers). The trace measurement **(D)** is used here to obtain an accurate length of the pyloric channel (between X symbols), resulting in the diagnosis of pyloric stenosis.

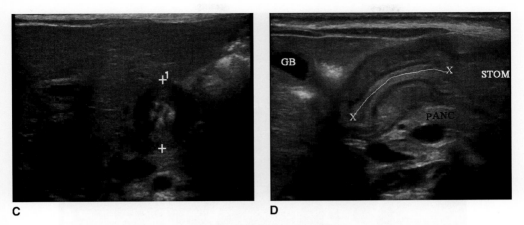

C   D

Figure 8-26. (*Continued*)

M-Mode

The M-mode (or **motion mode**) control setting activates motion mode. M-mode demonstrates the motion of structures along a single scan line (Fig. 8-27). M-mode is used in obstetrics to demonstrate the movement of the fetal heart and in echocardiography to evaluate the motions of various structures within the heart, like the heart valves.

Pulsed-Wave Doppler

The PW control activates and often controls the gain of the PW Doppler (Fig. 8-28). Once activated, additional controls can be altered to adjust the sample gate or **sample volume** and the angle of insonation.

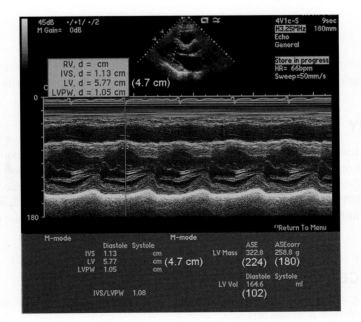

Figure 8-27. M-mode tracing (seen in the middle of this image) is often used in echocardiography to analyze the movement of various heart structures.

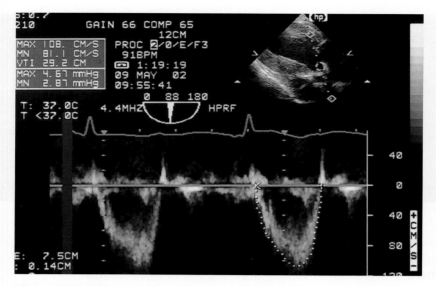

Figure 8-28. PW spectral Doppler velocities used during echocardiography.

Transmit Zone or Focus

The **transmit zone**, or focus, enhances the resolution of an area in the image by electronic focusing. The focus is adjusted by moving the indicator, which may be referred to as the **caret**. Most machines offer multi-focusing as well.

Sound Off

Your transmit zone, or focus, should be adjusted throughout the examination to optimize your image..

Zoom

The **zoom** function allows for the magnification of the image by often increasing the pixel size, thus degrading image resolution. However, the function of the zoom control may vary with manufacturer.

SUMMARY

Sonographers have an obligation to understand the various functions of the ultrasound equipment that they must operate in the clinical setting. In fact, in some clinical settings, several ultrasound manufacturers' equipment may be utilized. This can be a challenge for the novice sonographer and the student. However, you should strive to become familiar with all ultrasound equipment while you are learning. The best way to learn more about the ultrasound machines that you use in clinical is to practice.

REFERENCES

1. Penny SM, et al. *Examination Review for Ultrasound: Sonographic Principles & Instrumentation (SPI)*. Philadelphia, PA: Lippincott Williams & Wilkins; 2011.
2. Sanders RC, Winters T. *Clinical Sonography: A Practical Guide*. 4th ed. Philadelphia, PA: Lippincott Williams & Wilkins; 2006.

Thinking Critically

1. What patient positions have you observed in the clinical setting? Ask your instructor or sonographer why patients are placed in these positions.
2. Briefly describe the pulse-echo principle in your own words.
3. Examine how transducers are cared for in your clinical facility. How are endocavity transducers cleaned? How is the cleaning of endocavity transducers documented? How are all other transducers cleaned between examinations?
4. At your clinical facility, examine each ultrasound machine and become familiar with the controls, including the following tasks also:
   • How to power on the machine.
   • How to select and change transducers.
   • How to freeze and store images.
   • How to adjust the overall gain and TGC.
   • How to access and use color Doppler, PW Doppler, M-mode, and CW Doppler.

Chapter 8
Review Questions

1. **What imaging mode displays the returning echoes as dots of varying brightness?**
   a. A-mode
   b. B-mode
   c. C-mode
   d. M-mode

2. **Which of the following Doppler techniques does not display an image and uses two crystals—one for sending and one for listening?**
   a. B-mode
   b. Color Doppler
   c. Continuous-wave Doppler
   d. Power Doppler

3. **Which control enhances the resolution of the image in a specific area?**
   a. Transmit zone
   b. Overall gain
   c. Focus
   d. Both A and C

4. **Which control allows for the adjustment of the brightness of the entire image?**
   a. Overall gain
   b. Time gain compensation
   c. Focus
   d. Field of view

5. **Which control allows for the adjustment of the brightness of a specific depth within the image?**
   a. Overall gain
   b. Time gain compensation
   c. Focus
   d. Field of view

6. Which control varies the penetration of the echoes displayed on the monitor?
   a. Overall gain
   b. Acoustic power
   c. Depth
   d. B-color

7. Which control would allow the sonographer to select the depth at which the velocity of the blood is measured within a selected vessel?
   a. Pulsed-wave Doppler
   b. Continuous-wave Doppler
   c. Power Doppler
   d. Power angio

8. What term means toward the feet, away from the head?
   a. Cephalic
   b. Superior
   c. Inferior
   d. Lateral

9. What term means located on the opposite side of the body?
   a. Ipsilateral
   b. Lateral
   c. Medial
   d. Contralateral

10. What term means closer to the attachment of an extremity?
    a. Medial
    b. Lateral
    c. Proximal
    d. Distal

11. Which control relates to the amount of energy the transducer is emitting?
    a. Overall gain
    b. Acoustic power
    c. Time gain compensation
    d. Power Doppler

12. The measurement tools utilized in sonography are termed
    a. carets.
    b. calipers.
    c. coaxials.
    d. crosshairs.

13. Which mode displays the strength of the returning echoes as spikes on a scale?
    a. A-mode
    b. B-mode
    c. C-mode
    d. M-mode

14. What term is defined as away from the middle or the midline of the body?
    a. Distal
    b. Anterior
    c. Superior
    d. Lateral

15. **What position is the patient in when he or she is lying on his or her back?**
    a. Anterior
    b. Supine
    c. Prone
    d. Posterior decubitus

16. **What term is described as toward the front of the body?**
    a. Anterior
    b. Medial
    c. Lateral
    d. Proximal

17. **What position is described as lying face down?**
    a. Left lateral
    b. Supine
    c. Prone
    d. Dorsal

18. **Which of the following is not a term for the reference point found on a transducer?**
    a. Notch
    b. Groove
    c. Index
    d. Spike

19. **Which control allows the sonographer to rewind the image?**
    a. Cine loop
    b. Freeze
    c. Field of view
    d. HD zoom

20. **Which control allows the demonstration of motion of the structures along a single scan line?**
    a. Pulsed-wave Doppler
    b. B-mode
    c. M-mode
    d. Power Doppler

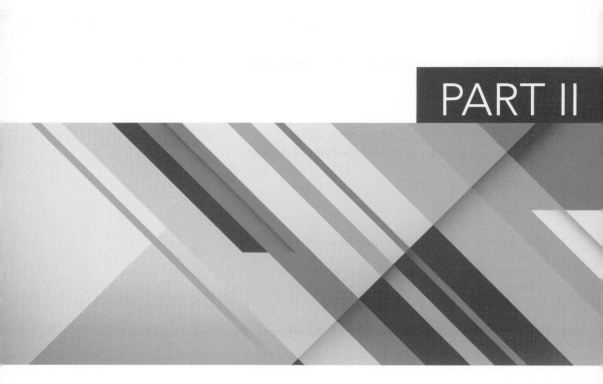

PART II

Introduction to Patient Care

Fundamentals of Communication for Sonographers

CHAPTER OBJECTIVES

- Understand basic human needs and the grieving process.
- Recognize the importance of communication in patient care.
- Appreciate the need to recognize and accept cultural differences.
- Recognize the vital role that effective communication plays before, during, and after each sonographic examination.

KEY TERMS

Active listening – listening that includes maintaining eye contact, nodding, and positioning oneself at the person's level

Affective touch – touch that involves sentiment and thus displays compassion with actions such as holding a patient's hand or placing your hand on the patient's shoulder to display feeling

Bias – our tendency to believe that certain people, ideas, and beliefs are better than others

Body language – involves body movement in communication, such as gestures, facial expressions, and gaze patterns

Communication – the exchange of thoughts, ideas, and information

Cultural awareness – an understanding of one's own culture and the acknowledgment of the cultural differences of others

Cultural competence – an understanding of one's own culture and the ability to accept and interact effectively with people of different cultures

Cultural desire – demonstrates a genuine aspiration by an individual to increase cultural knowledge on a routine basis

Cultural encounter – the face-to-face evidence of cultural competence through interactions

Cultural knowledge – understanding and becoming sympathetic to the attitudes and beliefs of other cultures

Cultural proficiency – the integration of cultural knowledge in practice and the application of that knowledge consistently in patient care

Cultural skill – the ability to assess the patient's needs based on cultural differences

Culture – shared beliefs, values, and behavioral characteristics that provide social structure for a group of people

Effective communication – the creation of meaning in communication in which both the patient and healthcare practitioner exchange information so that the patient can actively participate in his or her care

Ethnicity – a group of people who share a common history or origin

Gestures – body movements or limb movements that express thought or feeling

Grief – a normal human response to loss

Health literacy – the degree to which an individual can obtain, process, and understand his or her health status with regard to making appropriate health decision

Kinesics – see Body language

Noise – anything that negatively affects the communication process

Nontherapeutic verbal techniques – practice that blocks or hinders effective verbal communication

Nonverbal communication – form of communication that includes grooming, clothing, gestures, posture, facial expressions, eye contact, tone, volume of voice, and actions

Prejudice – the formation of an opinion or judgment about someone that is unfounded

Proxemics – physical distance between people when they communicate, including personal space and posture

Race – a related population of people with similar skin color, body structure, hair color and texture, and facial appearance

Stereotyping – forming a belief that is unfair about a group of people with similar characteristics

Task-oriented touch – the physical touch required to perform the sonographic examination

Therapeutic verbal communication – mutually respectful constructive communication that is used to accomplish a particular objective

Touch – nonverbal communication through physical contact

Verbal communication – spoken communication

INTRODUCTION

Communication is critical in healthcare. Sonographers must have the ability to effectively communicate with their patients in order to perform quality patient care. We must first understand the basic human needs of patients and the fact that they may be in the midst of the grieving process; these are fundamental tasks to communication. This chapter provides this underpinning and then succinctly follows that information with a brief overview of communication. Lastly, the framework for performing a sonogram is provided with some detail. As you read the final section on performing a sonogram, it will become clear to you that successful communication plays an imperative role in the daily responsibilities of a sonographer.

PRIMARY HUMAN NEEDS

Abraham Maslow described humans as being governed by a hierarchy of needs. He claimed that we all have basic needs that must be met before one aspires toward more lofty needs.[1] Understanding these needs is an underlying component of both patient care and **communication**. The hierarchy, according to Maslow, is shaped like a triangle or steps (Fig. 9-1). The base of the model comprises physiologic needs. Examples of physiologic needs include water, air, and food. Maslow claimed that once these physiologic needs are met, then one can move up from the base of triangle to fulfill one's safety and security requirements, which is the next level.[1] A step up from security is love and belonging, which includes affiliation, intimacy, and reassurance. Further up are self-esteem,

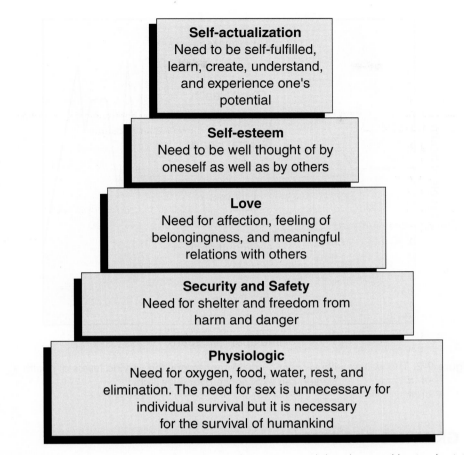

Figure 9-1. Maslow's hierarchy of needs. Maslow suggested that the initial basic physiologic needs must be met before the person can move on to the higher levels.

self-respect, and independence. At the top of the triangle is self-actualization, which includes needs that enrich our lives, such as music, literature, and creative work.

Another theory similar to Maslow's need-based theory is existence, relatedness, and growth (ERG) theory, which was developed by Clayton Aldefer. Aldefer agreed with Maslow in many ways, but unlike Maslow, the ERG theory suggests that individuals can pursue and thus find motivation from needs at more than one level at a time.[2] That is to say, someone can pursue growth in one's career or life while at the same time pursuing self-actualization, either through work or in his or her personal life.

The reason why sonographers should appreciate these and other motivational theories is because we interact with people who are working to meet varying needs throughout the day. Rarely do sonographers meet individuals who are self-actualized. In fact, Maslow believed that there are very few self-actualized.[1] The majority of patients who we meet are most likely in a state of illness. And though not all illnesses are completely debilitating, illness can cause a person to lose a sense of well-being, to question social and economic standing, and to suffer from considerable anxiety.[1] One's health is often paired with illness and depicted as a continuum—the health-wellness continuum. The health-wellness continuum consists of varying degrees of mental and physical health as we travel through our lifespans (Fig. 9-2).

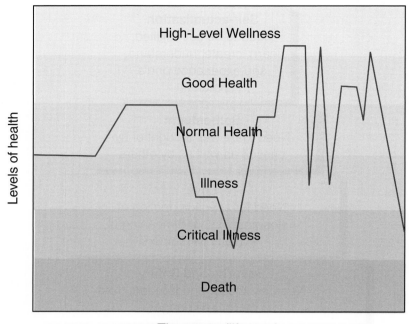

Figure 9-2. The wellness-illness continuum demonstrates the varying levels of health a person can experience over a lifetime.

THE GRIEVING PROCESS

Grief is a normal human response to loss. Dr. Elizabeth Kübler-Ross was among the first to offer insight into the process of dying and grieving.[3] In collaboration with David Kessler, Kübler-Ross described the grieving process in five phases. The first phase of the grieving process is denial. In this stage, patients typically do not accept the truth about their loss or imminent death. The second phase of the grieving process is anger. In this phase, the individual may feel as though he or she is the victim injustice and may appear hateful and blame others, including family members, for his or her problems. The third phase of the grieving process is bargaining. In this phase, the person may feel that if he or she cooperates with tests and physician orders, he or she will be spared from death or loss. The fourth phase is depression, in which the person becomes silent and possibly unresponsive. Finally, in the fifth phase, the person accepts the loss and loses interest in the outside world. Hopefully after grieving, the person eventually faces the reality that life is precious, and he or she can make the most of life.[4]

How someone processes grief can depend upon his or her religion, **culture**, **ethnicity**, and economic standing.[4] In fact, a person can be in several phases of the grieving process at a single time, skip phases, or bounce back and forth among them.[4] Of course, each phase can also vary in length. Sonographers may encounter patients who are undergoing the grieving process, either for themselves, or in some cases such as obstetrics, as a result of fetal or birth complications. For example, a patient may initially deny that her fetus has a fatal disorder and then become angry and depressed before finally accepting the prognosis. Regardless of the grieving phase, sonographers should be supportive of patients and in no way inhibit a patient's right to grieve. Optimistically, the patient will find solace in his or her family and friends during the search for hope.

The following section provides some insight into the importance of communication in our practice as sonographers. Keep in mind that your patient may be in the course of a painfully difficult situation when you encounter him or her. If sonographers can communicate effectively, treat all patients with distinction, and demonstrate positive measures that show the patient that he or she has inherent value, we can supply a counterbalance to unhelpful thoughts that manifest as a result of the grieving process. Remember, a simple smile or providing your patients with someone to talk to may be doing much more to help them than you may ever know.

COMMUNICATION

A major component of sonography and patient care is the proper use of communication. Communication is the exchange of thoughts, ideas, and information.[5] It includes listening, observing, speaking, and writing. To effectively communicate, one must be aware of one's own feelings, values, and attitudes that might cause one to have **bias** or be discriminatory during basic interactions with others. In Chapter 2, we briefly analyzed your personality type. You should return to that brief exercise and assess your own feelings, values, and attitudes toward others, as this could improve the manner in which you communicate.

Five Elements of Communication

There are five major elements that must be present in order for communication to occur: there must be a sender, a message, a receiver, feedback, and context. The sender is the person who creates and relays the message. The message can be in the form of words (verbal), actions (nonverbal), or a combination of both. The receiver is the person who accepts the message from the sender. The response from the receiver is referred to as the feedback.[6] Feedback from the receiver may confirm the receiver's message when the receiver feeds the statement back to the sender.[5] For example, if a patient relays a message to a sonographer, in order to clarify the message, the sonographer may verify that he or she received the correct message by stating the message back to the patient for confirmation. The context is the setting in which the communication occurs, including the mood and the relationship between the sender and the receiver.[5]

Forms of Communication

Effective communication in healthcare is the creation of meaning in communication in which both patient and healthcare practitioners exchange information so that the patient can actively participate in his or her care.[7] Therefore, recognizing the differing needs of patients in regard to communication is critical to effective patient care. Broadly, communication can be described as either verbal or nonverbal. Verbal communication is spoken communication, while **nonverbal communication** includes grooming, clothing, **gestures**, posture, facial expressions, eye contact, tone, volume of voice, and actions.[5] The following sections provide a concise summary of these two different forms of communication and how they can be used by a sonographer.

Nonverbal Communication

The overwhelming majority of communication is nonverbal in format.[5] If you recall from Chapter 2, one exercise related to emotional intelligence provided some analysis into your ability to recognize the variable meaning of facial expressions of others. Nonverbal communication can be used to convey sadness, joy, and anxiety.[8] Nonverbal communication can be divided into **kinesics**, **proxemics**, and **touch**. Kinesics, which may be referred to as **body language**, involves body movement in communication, such as gestures, facial expressions, and gaze patterns.[6] Proxemics entails physical distance between people when they communicate, including personal space and posture. Touch refers to nonverbal communication through physical contact.

In everyday communication, gestures are crucial in relaying the full meaning of words in some situations. For example, the word "stop" combined with an outward projected palm is a strong indicator that the person wants the other to immediately abstain from an action. Gestures, which are body movements or limb movements that express thought or feeling, can provide unspoken communication. For example, if a patient is unable to speak because of recent throat surgery, a simple smile with a head nod can express understanding and acceptance of a process or procedure.

Gestures may also be perceived as negative or positive. Unfortunately, some gestures have different meaning in different cultures, so one must be cautious in the practice of overusing gestures. General good practices include eye-level communication, relaxing your arms and legs, maintaining eye contact approximately 60% to 70% of the time, keeping the head upright, leaning forward to demonstrate interest, and keeping the legs still.[9] Poor body language includes crossing your arms, tapping your fingers, frowning, and looking at your phone or watch while you are interacting with someone.

Proxemics relates to personal space, intimate space, social space, and public space.[9] Most people can tolerate strangers comfortably at a distance of 2 to 3 ft.[9] In order to avoid misinterpretation of intent to violate a patient's personal space during a sonogram, the best approach is to explain beforehand the examination components including what physical tasks are warranted and what touching is involved. This practice will provide a less threatening environment for the patient, gives him or her control, and allows him or her to maintain dignity. Always preserve patient privacy by properly draping or covering the patient throughout the examination as well, and only touch the patient when given permission.

Touch is a primary requirement to perform sonography. Touch can be described in two ways: **task-oriented touch** and **affective touch**. Task-oriented touch is the physical touch required to perform the sonographic examination. This includes assisting patients onto the stretcher or to the bathroom, and the actual performance of the examination. It also includes touching the patient with the transducer as well. Affective touch involves sentiment and thus displays compassion with actions such as holding a patient's hand or placing your hand on the patient's shoulder to display feeling. It can be used for visually impaired patients and in some cases, when a patient displays loneliness, anxiety, insecurity, or fright.[9] Again, cultures display emotions differently, so affective touching may not always be appropriate.

When there is a need to perform a procedure that may be perceived as intimate or sexually invasive, such as a transvaginal or scrotal sonogram, it is best to obtain a chaperone, colleague, or family member to prevent any misinterpretation, especially if the sonographer and patient are of different genders. Continually monitor your patient by confirming that he or she is comfortable and observe facial expressions and gestures for verification as well.

Though it is often an unrecognized facet of communication, the demonstration of respect plays an important role in nonverbal communication, especially during the initial interaction of the sonographer-patient relationship. For example, shaking the patient's hand, opening the door for him or her, and smiling while making eye contact, all demonstrate the sonographer's intrinsic respect for others. Sonography involves much more than performing a sonographic examination; respecting the patient in a manner that is congruent with effective patient care requires us to demonstrate respect consistently through our verbal and nonverbal actions.

Verbal Communication

Verbal communication is spoken communication. Trust between the patient and sonographer will result from the sonographer's ability to initially establish a successful verbal dialogue. For this reason, verbal communication may be separated into therapeutic or nontherapeutic verbal techniques (Tables 9-1 and 9-2). **Therapeutic verbal communication** is mutually respectful constructive communication that is used to accomplish a particular objective.[7,9] Examples of therapeutic verbal communication include direct questioning, open-ended questioning, paraphrasing, clarifying, and silence.

TABLE 9-1	Therapeutic verbal communication techniques	
Therapeutic Verbal Communication Techniques	**Purpose**	**Example**
Closed-ended questions (direct questions)	Often quick "yes" or "no" questions; used to gather specific information	"Where do you hurt?" "Can you hear me?"
Open-ended questioning	Encourages embellishment	"What symptoms are you having?" "How often do you have these symptoms?"
Paraphrasing	Restate what the patient says to demonstrate listening	Patient: "I feel like I need to vomit after I eat." Sonographer: "Eating makes you nauseous, but you do not actually vomit."
Clarifying	Avoids misinterpretation	"Please further explain what you are asking."
Silence	Allows time for thinking and may stimulate more conversation	Silence can be provided while some of the examination is conducted

From Timby BK. *Fundamental Nursing Skills and Concepts.* 10th ed. Philadelphia, PA: Lippincott Williams & Wilkins; 2013.

TABLE 9-2	Nontherapeutic verbal communication techniques
Nontherapeutic Verbal Communication Techniques	**Explanation**
Making false promises	Never make promises you cannot keep or that you do not know will come true. Never tell the patient that everything will be fine, because you do not know that.
Using clichés	Never make statements like "It could be worse" or "It's not over until it's over." Clichés provide baseless hope.
Disagreeing	Disagreeing can intimidate the patient or make him or her feel irrational.
Demanding an explanation	This may put the patient on the defensive.
Changing the subject	Demonstrates that you really do not care what the patient is saying.
Patronizing	Never treat patients condescendingly or like they are children. Treat all patients with respect.
Giving advice	Sonographers should not give medical advice to patients regarding treatment or diagnosis. This discourages independent decision making and is beyond the sonographer's scope of practice.

From Timby BK. *Fundamental Nursing Skills and Concepts.* 10th ed. Philadelphia, PA: Lippincott Williams & Wilkins; 2013.

Silence and the ability to recognize when to be silent are critical in communication. Silence allows the receiver to listen and the patient to verbalize his or her concerns to the sonographer. For that reason, **active listening** is a vital part of the verbal communication process. Active listening includes maintaining eye contact, nodding, and positioning oneself at the person's level. For example, sitting across from a patient instead of standing over him or her when you are communicating would be best to demonstrate active listening.

Nontherapeutic verbal techniques block or hinder effective verbal communication. Examples of nontherapeutic techniques include patronizing a patient, making false promises, and giving advice. Anything that negatively affects the communication process is referred to as **noise**.[6] Though noise can literally mean acoustic noise such as construction occurring outside of a window, it also refers to other distractions, including physical pain that inhibits effective listening, fear or anxiety, language barriers, cultural differences, lack of interest, physical constraints, and hearing or sight impairment.[6]

Additional Potential Barriers to Effective Communication

Differing populations of patients have special needs to be met in order to effectively communicate with them. Tables 9-3 and 9-4 provide some insight into special patient emotional or physical states that could act as potential barriers to effective communication. One of the most common obstacles for

TABLE 9-3	Addressing patient emotions
Patient's Emotional Condition	**Points to Remember**
Irritated	• Identify and acknowledge the patient's anger. • Stay calm, and respond to questions honestly. • Let the patient talk about his or her anger and the reason for the anger. • Apologize if you are the source of the anger. • Obtain a manager if the patient asks for one. • Do not complete the examination if the patient refuses. • For unruly patients, see "combative" section below.
Anxious	• Identify and acknowledge the patient's anxiety. • Be attentive, and recognize what is causing the patient's anxiety. • Make the patient as comfortable as possible. • Be truthful with the patient, and notify the physician of the patient's concerns. • Be supportive, and provide honest answers to questions. • Do not complete the examination if the patient refuses.
Confused	• Speak clearly, and answer questions honestly. • Confirm that the patient understands the examination completely before attempting it. • Do not complete the examination if the patient refuses. • Do not leave the patient alone.
Patient in pain	• A pain scale (often 1 to 10 with 10 being the most severe pain) may be provided by the healthcare facility. • Ask the patient about his or her pain before the exam begins and monitor throughout. If the pain becomes unbearable, stop the examination, and notify the patient's nurse or physician. • Try to make the patient as comfortable as possible. • Do not complete the examination if the patient refuses. • Do not leave the patient alone.

TABLE 9-3	Addressing patient emotions (Continued)	

Patient's Emotional Condition	Points to Remember
Sad or weeping	• Stop performing the sonogram if a patient begins to weep during an examination. • Inquire about weeping, and maintain privacy for a patient who begins to weep. • You may need to allow the patient to use another room or go to the bathroom to collect his or her thoughts. • Provide comfort by holding his or her hand or placing your hand on his or her shoulder if you feel it is appropriate. If not, simply remain quiet until the patient is ready to talk. • Resume the examination with the patient's permission.

Combative	• Be prepared by asking for assistance if the patient is demonstrating combative behavior before the examination.
	• Do not become isolated with a combative patient.
	• Have an emergency exit ready in case you must leave quickly.
	• Adult:
	  • If the examination is underway and the patient becomes combative, stop the examination.
	  • Notify the patient's nurse or physician if the patient is gradually becoming more combative.
	  • If you feel you are in physical danger, protect yourself, leave immediately, and notify security.
	  • If you are trapped, call for help, speak in a calm but firm voice to the patient, let the patient know that you feel uneasy, ask what you can do to remedy the situation, and try to ally yourself with the patient if necessary by claiming that you understand his or her predicament. Once free, notify security immediately.
	• Child:
	  • Stop the examination.
	  • Ask the guardian for assistance.
	  • Notify the patient's nurse or physician if the patient remains combative.
	  • Never leave the patient unattended.

From Dutton AG, et al. *Torres' Patient Care in Imaging Technology.* 8th ed. Philadelphia, PA: Lippincott Williams & Wilkins; 2013.

effective communication in sonography is that of a language barrier. For example, the situation could arise in which the sonographer only speaks English, while the patient only speaks Spanish. There are several means to overcome this challenge. The quickest way to overcome a language barrier and the most effective is to obtain an interpreter. Healthcare interpreters are often employed by healthcare institutions to facilitate appropriate patient care. Also, mobile translation devices that incorporate off-site interpretation using video and audio technology for translation may be utilized in these situations as well. Perhaps the most difficult approach in which a sonographer could counteract the sonographer-patient language barrier is for the sonographer to learn the language of the patient and thereby become proficient as a healthcare interpreter. This would be an outstanding way to develop professionally, and some organizations may provide pay increases for those who become qualified as interpreters.

As demonstrated in the nonverbal communication section, respect demonstrated through effective communication is vital. For example, some patients may appreciate the use of honorific terms, such as Ms., Mr., or Mrs., followed by his or her last name. Also, referring to patients as "honey," "baby," or other colloquial terms may be considered offensive or inappropriate, and doing so does not demonstrate professionalism.

TABLE 9-4	Dealing with patients with different physical conditions

Patient's Physical Condition	Points to Remember
Blind or visually impaired	• Identify yourself to the patient; do not raise your voice. • Ask for his or her assistant to help if the patient is accompanied by someone. • Do not pet or play with a service animal. • Let the patient hold your arm as you guide him or her. • Talk to the patient, and explain where you are going and what procedure you will be performing. • Consistently ask the patient how he or she is doing and if he or she has any questions. • Let the patient know when you are leaving, but never leave him or her unattended.
Child	• In general: • Take time to establish a good rapport with children who can verbally communicate. • Speak to the child at eye level. • Thoroughly explain the procedure in lay terms, including what part of the body is involved. • Avoid the use of medical jargon. • Let the child touch the transducer and the gel. • Show the child the ultrasound machine monitor. • Thoroughly explain the procedure to the guardian. (If the guardian does not speak English, obtain an interpreter.) • Neonates: Explain the procedure to the guardian, keep the child warm, and never leave him or her alone. • Infants and toddlers: Explain the procedure to the guardian, assess the needs and level of independence, maintain privacy and safe surroundings, and never leave the child alone. • Preschoolers: Educate the guardians and patient about the procedure, support independence, maintain privacy, and never leave the child alone. • Adolescents: Educate the guardian (if present) and the patient about the procedure, assess needs, and maintain privacy.
Deaf or hearing-impaired	• Get the patient's attention before speaking to him or her by tapping on his or her shoulder. • Obtain a sign language interpreter for deaf individuals. • Use a small pad of paper and a pen or dry-erase board if needed. • Slow down your speech, and use a deeper voice with more projection for those hard of hearing; avoid chewing gum, and do not yell. • Minimize background noise.
Elderly	• Openly ask the patient about what physical assistance he or she requires, and be prepared to provide it. • Explain the examination to the patient in plain terms. Do not assume that because someone is elderly that he or she does not understand. • Do not treat the patient like a child, but rather treat him or her with compassion and respect. • Do not talk down to him or her (e.g., using terms like "dear" or "sweetie").[9] Depending upon the patient's mental and physical condition, it may be best to not leave him or her alone.

TABLE 9-4	Dealing with patients with different physical conditions (Continued)

Patient's Physical Condition	Points to Remember
Intoxicated	• Explain the examination. • Keep instructions simple, direct, and nonjudgmental. • If the patient becomes combative or refuses the examination, stop immediately, and call for help. • Do not leave the patient alone.
Comatose	• Talk to the patient, and explain the procedure. • Maintain the patient's dignity. • Use compassion and treat the patient with respect as if he or she is aware and alert. • Never leave the patient unmonitored.
Intellectually disabled	• Introduce yourself, and shake the patient's hand. • Do not automatically treat the patient as a child. • Speak to the patient at eye level. • Be patient, flexible, and supportive. • Explain the procedure in plain terms. • Answer any questions honestly. • Provide any physical assistance that is required. • Do not leave the patient alone.
Speech impairment	• If you do not understand the patient, do not pretend to. Ask him or her to clarify or repeat. • Be patient, and take time to communicate. • Try to answer questions with a short answer or nod. • Do not attempt to finish his or her sentences. • If you cannot communicate verbally, ask the patient if he or she would be comfortable writing.

From Dutton AG, et al. *Torres' Patient Care in Imaging Technology.* 8th ed. Philadelphia, PA: Lippincott Williams & Wilkins; 2013; Davis L, Olson D. *Communicating Effectively with People Who Have a Disability.* North Dakota Center for Persons with Disabilities (ND). Retrieved from http://www.labor.state.ny.us/workforcenypartners/forms/communication.pdf; and Elliott-Smith S. Communicating with older patients. *Access* [serial online] 2009;23(9):24. Available from: CINAHL with Full Text, Ipswich, MA. Accessed December 1, 2014.[10,11]

The use of profanity around patients is strongly discouraged, as this will severely reduce the patient's respect for the sonographer and institution and is mostly likely an offense that will be followed quickly by either managerial reprimand or even termination. Profanity, even among coworkers in the workplace, can potentially be overheard by patients and therefore should not be used in the vicinity of a patient care setting. Students should especially abstain from the use of profanity as this demonstrates a lack of professionalism and could potentially harm the reputation of both the student and clinical facility.

Additionally, though we practice sonography in a well-informed society where patients have easy access to medical information online, the overuse of medical jargon can become a barrier to communication, almost sounding like another language to some patients. For this reason, it is best to minimize the use of medical jargon during patient interactions. This does not mean that sonographers should not work to attempt to educate their patients, however (see "Patient Education" discussion).

Finally, incongruence between a patient's verbal and nonverbal communication can occur. For example, a patient may provide permission for a transvaginal sonogram, but when the examination begins, she appears anxious and begins to cry. This incongruent behavior should spark a conversation between the sonographer and the patient. The sonographer should confirm that the patient desires to have the procedure, and if not, the sonographer should immediately stop. Behavior that is not in line with consent must immediately be addressed.

CULTURAL COMPETENCE

We live in a culturally diverse society. It is incumbent upon the sonographer to learn more about the cultural makeup of patients and to ultimately adapt to the uniqueness of the cultures he or she may encounter. The culture of a group of people describes a system of shared beliefs, values, and behavioral characteristics that provide social structure.[1] Culture should not be confused with **race** or ethnicity. The race of someone refers to his or her skin color, body structure, hair color and texture, and facial appearance, while ethnicity is a group of people who share a common history or origin.[4] Sonographers should have a respect for all cultures and thereby be sensitive to the patient's cultural differences. The process of **cultural competence**—also referred to as transcultural awareness—in healthcare relates to an understanding of one's own culture and the ability to accept and interact effectively with people of different cultures in the healthcare setting (Fig. 9-3).[6,12]

According to Josepha Campinha-Bacote, the creator of the Volcano Model that is used to demonstrate the process of cultural competence in healthcare, there are five steps to becoming more culturally competent: (a) **cultural awareness**, (b) **cultural knowledge**, (c) **cultural skill**, (d) **cultural encounter**, and (e) **cultural desire**.[6] The first step toward cultural competence is cultural awareness, which is an understanding of one's own culture and acknowledgment of cultural differences of others. Next, the sonographer should actively increase his or her cultural knowledge by understanding and becoming sympathetic to the attitudes and beliefs of other cultures. With that information in mind, cultural skill, which is the ability to assess the patient's needs based on cultural differences, is the next step. The fourth step is the actual cultural encounter, where the face-to-face evidence of cultural competence is demonstrated. Lastly, as a result of the previous four steps, cultural desire demonstrates a genuine aspiration by the sonographer to increase cultural knowledge on a routine basis.[6,13]

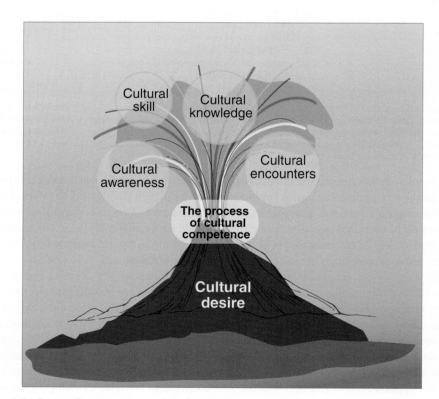

Figure 9-3. Campinha-Bacote's model of cultural competence depicts the process as erupting into a volcano as the sonographer develops skills.[13]

One of the main reasons to progress toward more cultural competence in healthcare is the documented evidence that racial and ethnic minorities, compared to whites, have a higher death rate from cancer, heart disease, and diabetes, regardless of insurance status, income, age, and severity of condition.[14] Bias, **stereotyping**, and **prejudice** contribute to low levels of cultural competence. Bias is our tendency to believe that certain people, ideas, and beliefs are better than others. A stereotype is a belief that is unfair about a group of people with similar characteristics, while prejudice is the formation of an opinion or judgment about someone that is unfounded.[12] Maintaining obstinate baseless convictions about our patients negatively impacts our ability to provide each person with respect and high-quality equitable patient care. The refusal to respect a patient's cultural background can result in legal implications if it can be proven that a sonographer deliberately discriminated (healthcare discrimination) against the patient for any reason in the administration of his or her duties. Cultural disparity can negatively impact sonographer-patient communication, because a patient could be more apprehensive about the examination and subsequently less forthcoming with beneficial clinical history information.[14]

Fortunately, education can overcome cultural disparity. Sonographers who learn about the history, values, and beliefs of the cultural and ethnic groups to which their patients belong can utilize such knowledge to overcome potential communication barriers, resulting in a possible decrease in disparate treatment.[15] The ultimate goal for the sonographer should be to become culturally proficient. **Cultural proficiency** is both the integration of cultural knowledge in practice and the application of that knowledge consistently in patient care.[15] By educating oneself concerning cultural differences, the sonographer ultimately increases his or her ability to effectively communicate with individuals from all over the world.

THE SONOGRAPHIC EXAMINATION: 10 STEPS

Now that an overview of communication has been provided, we can focus on the important role that communication has before, during, and after the sonographic examination. The following section provides some insight into assessing the relevant documents for the examination, interviewing the patient, and several others steps in the process of performing the sonographic examination. In Chapter 2, the following information was condensed into a process called the "Sonographic Reasoning Method" for quick recall in clinical practice. However, the following section expounds upon the process by offering a step-by-step guide to completing a sonographic examination.

Effective communication fundamentally provides the foundation for each sonographic examination we perform. Keep in mind, it is the sonographer's responsibility to maintain communication with the patient throughout the examination. By keeping the communication going, patient anxiety decreases, and this can potentially provide the sonographer with more insight into the patient's current dilemma.

Step 1: Assessment of Relevant Documents

In most hospital settings, the sonographer will be supplied with a requisition for an examination. Table 9-5 provides some of the information provided on the typical imaging requisition document. Every diagnostic sonogram must have a physician's order to be conducted. Though the sonographer may not always have the ability to check the order, one should do so when permitted. For inpatients, the order should be documented in the patient's chart or digital record. Other information can be gathered from the patient's inpatient chart as well, including operative reports and laboratory results. Outpatients may bring in a copy of the physician's order, or an order may be faxed or electronically transferred to the facility.

TABLE 9-5	Components of a requisition
Component	**Explanation**
Examination ordered	Type of sonographic examination.
Gender and age	The gender of the patient, date of birth, and the patient's age will be provided. The race of the patient may be offered as well.
Indication; medical record number	The reason for the examination. It may be described as an ICD-9 or 10 code or provide a primary patient complaint or medical question.
Requisition number	These numbers are vital for identifying the correct patient and the correct examination.
Patient category	Inpatient Outpatient Emergency room patient
Previous studies	Many requisitions list the most recent imaging examinations that the patient has undergone. Examples include CT scan, MRI, and other sonograms. (See the section "Examining Reports and Images.")

Step 2: Examining Reports and Images

Interpreting physicians provide a dictated report for all imaging studies. This report becomes a permanent part of the patient's medical record. Sonographers should analyze all accessible imaging reports, especially those that are most recent and/or pertinent to the anatomy being sonographically inspected. There are several components to the report. The major sections of the report typically include the clinical information or history, examination findings, and the overall impression. Before analyzing the impression, the sonographer should briefly inspect the other parts of the document.

The clinical information or history contained within the imaging report will provide the sonographer with insight into what primary complaints the patient had at the time of the examination. For example, the clinical information may state that the patient complained of right upper quadrant pain and nausea for two days. Clinical history components can be helpful to compare with the patient's current clinical complaints to determine if the complaint is acute or chronic (new or old). Clinical information may contain helpful information regarding recent surgeries and other examinations as well. For example, knowing that a patient's status is post-cholecystectomy can be exceedingly helpful.

The examination findings offer the details of the imaging study. These findings are comprehensive and quite detailed. This section of the document may consist of a paragraph or several pages of examination facts. The location, appearance, and measurements are provided for all pathologic findings, and many normal findings may be mentioned as well. The overall impression, which is a concise summary of the examination, provides the most significant findings. This section is vital for the sonographer to analyze. If questions are raised when you read the overall impression, return to the findings section for greater detail.

Though sonographers are not required to have the ability to decipher images obtained by other imaging modalities, such as CT, MRI, or radiography, a basic appreciation can be helpful. Sonographers do have a thorough understanding of human anatomy and pathology, and for this reason, they can utilize this information to inform them as they view images of human anatomy provided by another imaging modality. For example, CT often offers cross-sectional anatomy of the abdomen, much like a transverse section obtained with sonography. If available, take time to analyze the images found on these studies to advance your diagnostic discernment.

Step 3: Preparing the Examination Room and Protocol Review

The fundamental accessories required for a sonographer to perform his or her job are gel, a stretcher, and an ultrasound machine. Of course, by now you hopefully realize how complex the job of the sonographer is. The sonography room should be designed for ease of performing the specialty in sonography in which you are employed. The ultrasound machine and stretcher should be arranged according to the sonographic examination that will be conducted.

Prior to the examination, you should thoroughly clean the room according to aseptic technique (see Chapter 12). The gel should be warmed to ease the shock of cold gel. All supplies should be readily available, including gloves, positioning sponges, towels, and blankets. Invasive procedures will require additional paperwork and more preparation material, especially those required for sterile examinations. The lighting and the temperature should be both comforting to the patient and sufficient for the sonographer. Being prepared for the examination will decrease the time it takes to perform the examination, while simultaneously portraying professionalism. You should always wash your hands before the examination as well.

Every institution has established protocols for each sonographic examination. Before you fetch the patient for the examination, review the protocol. Students should obtain copies of the protocols and have them available during their clinical rotations. It may be helpful to transfer the protocols to note cards or another easily accessible source. Regardless, you should have them readily available for review. With time, it is optimal to commit each protocol to memory to increase your scanning speed and accuracy. If you have an established protocol, remember that it should be malleable. Always be prepared to make adjustments to your protocol to meet with the standards of each institution that you visit while in school.

Step 4: Introducing Yourself and Patient Confirmation

Going to get a patient from the waiting area and bringing him or her back to the ultrasound room is a basic function of the sonographer. However, it is a significant task, as first impressions are exceedingly important. Sonographers should always demonstrate a professional and friendly demeanor in front of patients. Calling out the patient's last name may be a manner used to identify the patient by some institutions, while others may assign each patient a number that is used for identification. You should smile, make eye contact, and introduce yourself in a gracious way, providing the patient with your first name. Again, referring to adults using honorific terms is professional and demonstrates respect. For children and adolescents, you can use first names. While introductions are made, this time can also be used to make a general assessment of the patient's communication needs. Always use the medical records number, birth date, and any other patient identifiers to confirm that you have the correct patient before performing the examination. Be prepared to provide any physical assistance that the patient may require to help transport him or her to the ultrasound room and assist him or her to the examination stretcher. For patients already lying on a stretcher, introduce yourself in the same manner, and place yourself in a position that is in clear view of the patient.

Step 5: Gathering Clinical History

The sonographer's ability to gather clinical history from the patient can play a critical role in the physician's ultimate mission, which is making the correct diagnosis. Unfortunately, though this step is critical, it can be the most difficult, especially for students. But inexperience with information gathering can be overcome with practice. Also, observation of the sonographer-patient interaction process can provide valuable insight as well.

Once the ambulatory patient is in the sonography room, have him or her sit on the stretcher for the interview process. Appropriate lighting should be provided so that the patient can see your face

TABLE 9-6	Examples of closed-ended and open-ended questions

Closed-Ended Questions	Open-Ended Questions
• Can you hear me? • Have you had a sonogram before? • Does it hurt when I scan here? • Have you had kidney stones?	• How long have you been feeling this pain? • Why did your doctor order a sonogram? • What type of abdominal surgeries have you had? • What medications are you taking?

and so that you can evaluate his or her nonverbal communication as well. Take your place across from the patient in a chair, positioning yourself at eye level to begin the interview. If the patient is recumbent on a stretcher, position yourself in a manner in which the patient can clearly see your face before you begin to ask questions. Your name tag or badge should be readily identifiable to the patient as well.

A sonographer can use closed-ended questions and open-ended questions to obtain clinical history information from a patient (Table 9-6). Closed-ended questions often result in a quick, easy answer like "yes" or "no." They can begin with words like "do" or "who." For example, the sonographer may ask "Do you have a gallbladder?" The patient could then answer "yes" or "no." Closed-ended questions are helpful in filling in the normal gaps that occur during communication and are helpful to begin the patient interview process.

Open-ended questions tend to be much more beneficial for information gathering compared to closed-ended questions. For example, to supplement the previous question about an absent gallbladder, the sonographer could ask the question "Why did you have your gallbladder removed?" Open-ended question frequently begin with "how," "why," or "what." Open-ended questions allow the patient to express him or herself, provide his or her opinion, offer more information for the sonographer, create a better sonographer-patient relationship, and demonstrate time investment and compassion. Lastly, as mentioned earlier, the sonographer should also practice active listening (Table 9-7).

There are two basic forms of information that can be gathered as a result of asking questions during a patient interaction—subjective information and objective information. Subjective information is information that is typically provided through the patient interview process. It is anything that the patient or patient's guardian or family member provides the sonographer related to the patient's history. Objective information is information the sonographer can see, hear, feel, or read or any data reported about the patient. It is factual, concrete data that are proven.

For example, if the patient informs the sonographer that he or she has epigastric pain, back pain, and nausea, this would be an example of subjective information. When the sonographer obtains the laboratory results for the patient and discovers that the patient has an elevated amylase and lipase levels, this is objective information. Furthermore, the sonographer performs a sonogram of the abdomen and discovers evidence of an enlarged, hypoechoic pancreas and peripancreatic fluid; this is additional objective information. For this example, combining the subjective and objective data collected from this examination will most likely result in a diagnosis of acute pancreatitis.

TABLE 9-7	Active listening—remember RASA

R = Receive information without interrupting
A = Appreciate the speaker by demonstrating attentive body language
S = Summarize the other person's key points
A = Ask clarifying questions to check for understanding

From Horevitz E, et al. Examining cultural competence in healthcare: implications for social workers. *Health Soc Work* [serial online] 2013;38(3):135–145. Available from: CINAHL with Full Text, Ipswich, MA. Accessed December 7, 2014.

TABLE 9-8	Educating the patient about sonography
Patient Education	**Explanation**
Examination	Provide the patient with an introduction to the instruments used to obtain images, patient positioning requirements, any breathing techniques, and the approximate time the examination will take.
Medical ultrasound	Provide the patient with information about the safety of medical ultrasound.
Human body	• Provide the patient with an overview of what organs will be analyzed. • Offer insight into the functions of various organs if the patient inquires.
Diagnostic process	• Clarify your role as a sonographer. • Clarify the role of the interpreting physician. • Assure the patient that a report will be provided to his or her ordering physician.

Step 6: Patient Education

Health literacy is the degree to which an individual can obtain, process, and understand his or her health status with regard to making appropriate health decision.[7] Sonographers do have a responsibility to educate their patients about sonography and the medical use of ultrasound. First, this involves a thorough explanation of the examination to the patient or patient's guardian. Patients have a wide range of health literacy, so the overuse of medical jargon should be avoided. However, a basic explanation would provide an overview of how images are obtained, the use of gel, various positions that may be utilized during the examination, and any breathing techniques that may be requested (Table 9-8).

Step 7: Conducting the Sonogram

Conduct the sonogram according to the institution's requirements and in accordance with nationally accepted protocols, such as those recommended by the American Institute of Ultrasound in Medicine. Throughout the examination, maintain open communication with your patient. Once the examination is complete, inform the patient of your next tasks concerning the examination, assist the patient with gel removal, assess your patient's needs, and determine if the patient can be left alone in the room. Before leaving the room, ensure that the lighting is adjusted. It is also best to notify others in the department that the room is occupied.

Step 8: Completing the Sonographer's Report

Sonographer reports vary per institution. Typically, the sonographer report requires that the sonographer provide a basic assessment of the examination. These reports should include sonographic findings, including the locations and sonographic description of pathology, and the measurements of various normal and abnormal structures. However, sonographer reports should not contain a diagnosis, as this is beyond the scope of the sonographer's job duties. Writing sonographer reports is a responsibility at which one can become more efficient through observation and practice.

Step 9: Sonographer Interaction with Interpreting Physician

Sonographers are often required to present cases. In Chapter 2, Table 2-14 provided some "must-know" information needed prior to presenting a case to an interpreting physician. Working collaboratively with interpreting physicians is often an enjoyable part of being a sonographer. Providing input into the development of a diagnosis is a unique assignment for the sonographer and one that is exceedingly exclusive to the sonographer among imaging professionals. Because sonographers work independently and have a thorough understanding of human anatomy, sonographic anatomy, and pathology, they are afforded the opportunity to play a vital role in the diagnostic process. Often, an interpreting physician may ask a sonographer about varying sonographic pathologic processes in the hopes of better appreciating the entire clinical picture. These instances allow for the collaboration of thoughts and can provide a time for the proficiency and knowledge of the sonographer to be demonstrated.

Professional communication skills are exceedingly important. Physicians demand and rightly deserve respect from sonographers. Physicians should be referred to respectfully as with the title of "Dr." preceding his or her last name. Most conflicts between sonographers and physicians occur as a result of poor communication. The sonographer should accept that the ultimate responsibility of the interpreting physician is to provide a diagnosis and that clear communication must be provided. With the patient's well-being in mind, any ambiguity that exists should be eliminated. Always be honest with the physician, and do not be afraid to tell him or her if you do not know the answer to a question. In patient care, it is always better to be honest than to conceal uncertainty.

Step 10: Discharging the Patient

After all of the examination requirements and presenting the case has been performed, the sonographer should provide the patient with discharge instructions. Before allowing the patient to leave, you should determine if the patient is required to stay for any further testing, and assure the patient that a report will be provided to his or her physician. Lastly, if the interpreting physician allows you to provide the patient with any results, do so in a caring and respectful manner. Providing a quick "thank you" to the patient is always a kind gesture as well.

SUMMARY

Preserving good communication is an ongoing, dynamic task for the sonographer. It is one of our most essential requirements. The majority of our patients come to us in a weakened physical or mental state. The ability to communicate with them effectively, regardless of the situation, is critical for proper patient care. This chapter provided some insight into how patients with various limitations should be approached and how effective communication can make a positive difference. The physical or mental limitations of our patients should never dissuade us from communicating with them, for our goal should always be to consistently strive to provide satisfactory patient care to him or her in an equitable manner.

REFERENCES

1. Maslow AH. A theory of human motivation. *Psychol Rev* 1943;5:370–396.
2. Alderfer CP. An empirical test of a new theory of human needs. *Organ Behav Hum Perf* 1969;4(2):142–175.
3. Kübler-Ross E, Kessler D. *On Grief and Grieving*. New York, NY: Scribner; 2005.
4. Dutton AG, et al. *Torres' Patient Care in Imaging Technology*. 8th ed. Philadelphia, PA: Lippincott Williams & Wilkins; 2013.

5. Chitty KK, Black BP. *Professional Nursing: Concepts & Challenges*. 6th ed. Maryland Heights, MO: Saunders; 2011.

6. McCorry LK, Mason J. *Communication Skills for the Healthcare Professional*. Baltimore, MD: Lippincott Williams & Wilkins; 2011.

7. Boykins D. Core Communication Competencies in Patient-Centered Care. *ABNF J* [serial online] 2014;25(2):40–45. Available from: CINAHL with Full Text, Ipswich, MA. Accessed November 19, 2014.

8. LWW. *Fund of Nursing Made Incredibly Easy*. Philadelphia, PA: Lippincott Williams & Wilkins; 2007.

9. Timby BK. *Fundamental Nursing Skills and Concepts*. 10th ed. Philadelphia, PA: Lippincott Williams & Wilkins; 2013.

10. Davis L, Olson D. *Communicating Effectively with People Who Have a Disability*. North Dakota Center for Persons with Disabilities (ND). Retrieved from http://www.labor.state.ny.us/workforcenypartners/forms/communication.pdf

11. Elliott-Smith S. Communicating with older patients. *Access* [serial online] 2009;23(9):24. Available from: CINAHL with Full Text, Ipswich, MA. Accessed December 1, 2014.

12. Makely S. *Professionalism in Healthcare*. 3rd ed. Upper Saddle River, NJ: Pearson Prentice Hall; 2009.

13. Campinha-Bacote J. Coming to know cultural competence: an evolutionary process. *Int J Human Caring* [serial online] 2011;15(3):42–48. Available from: CINAHL with Full Text, Ipswich, MA. Accessed December 7, 2014.

14. Anitori E. Assessing cultural awareness of practicing cardiac sonographers. *JDMS* 2014;30(6):307–313.

15. Horevitz E, et al. Examining cultural competence in healthcare: implications for social workers. *Health Soc Work* [serial online] 2013;38(3):135–145. Available from: CINAHL with Full Text, Ipswich, MA. Accessed December 7, 2014.

Thinking Critically

1. Have one of your classmates pretend to have an illness. Practice the patient interview process by asking closed-ended and open-ended questions.

2. At your clinical facility, review various imaging reports from differing studies. If you discover words within the report that are unfamiliar, look them up or ask the sonographer to explain their meanings.

3. Review a copy of your clinical facility's sonographer report forms. Practice filling out the forms after each examination that you observe.

4. Find out how the sonographers at your clinical facility approach language and other communication barriers. For example, what do they do if the patient speaks a different language than they do? What if a patient is hearing-impaired?

Chapter 9
Review Questions

1. Which of the following would not be recommended when caring for a visually impaired patient?
   a. Let him or her hold your arm as you guide him or her.
   b. Introduce yourself to his or her service animal by petting it gently.
   c. Ask him or her questions without raising your voice.
   d. Consistently keep communications going to reduce anxiety.

2. Which of the following would be an example of nontherapeutic communication?
   a. Making false promises
   b. Using open-ended questions
   c. Using closed-ended questions
   d. Clarifying

3. **Which of the following would not typically be a barrier to communication?**
   a. Excessive use of medical jargon
   b. Language disparity between the sonographer and patient
   c. The use of profanity
   d. Paraphrasing what the patient has stated

4. **Which of the following relates to personal space, public space, and social space?**
   a. Body language
   b. Proxemics
   c. Kinesics
   d. Touch

5. **Which type of touch involves sentiment?**
   a. Effective
   b. Task-oriented
   c. Therapeutic
   d. Affective

6. **Which of the following relates to body language, such as gestures, facial expressions, and gaze patterns?**
   a. Touch
   b. Proxemics
   c. Kinesics
   d. Verbal communication

7. **Which of the following is not one of the five elements of communication?**
   a. Message
   b. Receiver
   c. Hearing
   d. Feedback

8. **What is defined as the ability to assess the patient's needs based on cultural differences?**
   a. Cultural skill
   b. Cultural knowledge
   c. Cultural composition
   d. Nonverbal cultural appraisal

9. **What is defined as anything that negatively affects the communication process?**
   a. Distraction
   b. Affective communication
   c. Noise
   d. Bias

10. **What term refers to a person's skin color, body structure, hair color and texture, and facial appearance?**
    a. Ethnicity
    b. Race
    c. Culture
    d. Stereotype

11. **Which of the following is the second step in the grieving process?**
    a. Loss of interest
    b. Blame
    c. Denial
    d. Anger

12. **What fundamental human needs are located at the base of Maslow's Hierarchy of Needs pyramid?**
    a. Physiologic needs
    b. Safety and security
    c. Self-actualization
    d. Defense and projection

13. **What term is defined as shared beliefs, values, and behavioral characteristics among a group of people?**
    a. Race
    b. Ethnicity
    c. Type
    d. Culture

14. **Active listening includes all of the following except:**
    a. Summarizing the other person's key points
    b. Providing affective touch
    c. Demonstrating attentive body language
    d. Asking clarifying questions to check for understanding

15. **Which of the following would not be a therapeutic verbal communication technique?**
    a. Silence
    b. Paraphrasing
    c. Giving advice
    d. Using closed-ended questions

16. **Which of the following would be an example of an open-ended question?**
    a. Why did you have your uterus and ovaries removed?
    b. Does your arm hurt here?
    c. Have you had anything to eat today?
    d. Have you had an ultrasound before?

17. **What is the understanding of one's own culture and the ability to accept and interact effectively with people of different cultures?**
    a. Cultural skill
    b. Cultural awareness
    c. Cultural competence
    d. Cultural comprehension

18. **Which of the following is typically not included on an imaging requisition?**
    a. Gender and age of the patient
    b. Patient category
    c. Indication
    d. Results of other imaging studies

19. **Which of the following is typically not included on an imaging report?**
    a. Examination findings
    b. Clinical information
    c. Overall impression
    d. Sonographic findings

20. **Which of the following information would not be an appropriate patient education component?**
    a. Diagnosis
    b. Ultrasound
    c. Human body
    d. Sonographic examination

10

Fundamental Patient Care

CHAPTER OBJECTIVES

■ Learn how to apply proper patient care techniques in obtaining vital signs and patient mobilization.

■ Explain the active role a sonographer should play in monitoring vital signs.

■ Identify abnormalities and variances in vital signs by understanding normal ranges for blood pressure, pulse, respiration, and body temperature.

■ Recognize how to assess a patient's mobility and provide adequate patient care.

KEY TERMS

Ambulatory – when referring to a patient, describes someone who is capable of walking about; not bedridden

Antecubital fossa – a triangular region on the anterior aspect of the elbow where the brachial artery is located

Aortic valve – heart valve located between the left ventricle and aorta

Arrhythmia – abnormal rhythm of the pulse; also referred to as dysrhythmia

Atrial septum – the band of tissue that separates the atria of the heart

Atrioventricular node – the electrical relay station between the atria and the ventricles of the heart

Automaticity – the ability of the heart to start, operate, and function independently

Bicuspid valve – the heart valve between the left atrium and left ventricle

Blood pressure – the amount of blood flow ejected from the left ventricle of the heart during systole and the amount of resistance the blood meets due to systemic vascular resistance

Body temperature – the measurement of the degree of tissue heat deep within the body

Bradycardia – a slower than normal heart rate

Bradypnea – a slower than normal breathing rate

Cardiac cycle – one sequence of contraction (systole) and relaxation (diastole) of the heart

Cardiac myocytes – muscle cells of the heart

Cardioverter defibrillator – a device placed in the chest or abdomen that attempts to correct abnormal heart rhythms

Depolarization – process by which the cardiac muscle cells change their charge from a negative to positive intracellular state

Diastole – the filling phase of the cardiac cycle

Dyspnea – difficult or labored breathing

Dysrhythmia – abnormal rhythm of the pulse; also referred to as arrhythmia

Einthoven triangle – the three-lead arrangement for electrocardiography that often accompanies an echocardiogram

Electrocardiogram – a graphic record of the electrical current as it progresses through the heart

Endocardium – the innermost layer of the heart wall

Epicardium – the outmost layer of the heart wall

Essential hypertension – high blood pressure with no known cause; also referred to as primary hypertension

Foley catheter – a urinary catheter that drains urine using a tube and is held in place by a balloon that is inflated inside of the urinary bladder

Homeostasis – the body's ability or tendency to maintain internal equilibrium by adjusting its physiologic processes

Hyperthermia – elevation in body temperature; also referred to as pyrexia or fever

Idiopathic – no known cause

Infiltration – the displacement and accumulation of fluid from an intravenous needle into the surrounding tissue

Infusion pump – an electronic device that regulates intravenous therapy using pressure to infuse solutions into the body

Inpatient – patient who has been admitted to a hospital and typically stays overnight

Interventricular septum – the band of tissue that separates the ventricles of the heart

Intravenous infusion – the administration of fluids into a vein

Leads – electrocardiographic electrodes

Left atrium – the chamber of the heart that receives oxygen-rich blood from the lungs and then pumps it into the right ventricle

Left ventricle – the chamber of the heart that receives blood from the left atrium and pumps it into the aorta to be disseminated throughout the body

Motion mode – mode used to display motion of the reflectors

Myocardium – the muscular portion of the heart wall

Normal sinus rhythm – the cardiac cycle of the heart functioning normally

Nosocomial infections – hospital-acquired infections

Oscilloscope – the screen on which electrocardiograms are displayed

Outpatients – patients who travel to the hospital for a procedure and leave the same day; many are ambulatory (able to walk unassisted), though some may need transport assistance

Pacemaker – an electronic device placed in the chest to regulate abnormal heart rhythms

Paracentesis – a procedure that uses a needle to drain fluid from the abdominal cavity for diagnostic or therapeutic purposes

Phlebitis – inflammation of a vein

Portable sonograms – sonographic procedures performed away from the sonography department

Pulmonary embolus – a blood clot that has become lodged in an artery supplying blood to the heart

Pulmonic valve – heart valve located between the right ventricle and pulmonary artery

Pulse – the result of blood that is pushed through the arterial system of the body by the beating heart

Pyrexia – elevation in body temperature; also referred to as hyperthermia or fever

Repolarization – process by which cardiac muscle cells return to a more negatively charged intracellular state; the resting state of the cardiac muscle cells

Respiration – the exchange of oxygen and carbon dioxide in the lungs

Right atrium – chamber of the heart that receives deoxygenated blood from the body

Right ventricle – chamber of the heart that receives blood from the right atrium and moves it into the pulmonary circulation for reoxygenation

Secondary hypertension – high blood pressure with an underlying known cause

Sinoatrial node – the heart's natural pacemaker

Sphygmomanometer – instrument used to obtain a blood pressure measurement

Systole – the contraction phase of the cardiac cycle

Tachycardia – a rapid heart rate

Tachypnea – rapid breathing

Thoracentesis – a procedure that uses a needle to drain fluid from the thoracic cavity for diagnostic or therapeutic purposes

Thrombus – blood clot

Tragus – the small pointed eminence on the anterior aspect of the external ear

Tricuspid valve – the heart valve located between the left atrium and left ventricle

Venipuncture – the surgical puncture of a vein to provide access to obtain a blood sample or for intravenous therapy

Vital signs – fundamental physiologic functions of the body that can be utilized to monitor homeostasis, including body temperature, pulse, blood pressure, and respiration

Volumetric controller – a device used to mechanically compresses intravenous tubing at a certain frequency to infuse the IV solution at a specified rate

INTRODUCTION

This chapter will provide a review of basic patient care and assessments performed in the sonography department. It will then go on to explain how to obtain vital signs, including some causes of abnormal vital signs. A discussion of patient assistance methods will offer instruction related to transporting and transferring patients, as well as caring for patients who may have special medical needs in the sonography department. For the echocardiography student, this chapter will also review fundamental heart anatomy and electrocardiography.

PATIENT ASSESSMENT

The sonographer's obligation in monitoring **vital signs** is fundamental, and these simple tasks are central to providing high-quality patient care. Several primary mechanisms must be kept in balance in order for our bodies to function properly (Table 10-1). **Homeostasis** is the body's ability and tendency to maintain internal equilibrium by adjusting its physiologic processes. Before an invasive procedure, such as a **thoracentesis, paracentesis**, or ultrasound-guided biopsy, sonographers may be asked to obtain baseline vital signs. Also referred to as cardinal signs, these include **body temperature, pulse, blood pressure**, and **respiration**. Sonographers may also be asked to monitor these vital signs throughout a procedure.

TABLE 10-1	Vital signs
Primary Mechanisms for Homeostasis	**Definition**
Body temperature	The measurement of the degree of tissue heat deep within the body
Pulse	The result of blood that is pushed through the arterial system of the body by the beating heart
Respiration	The exchange of oxygen and carbon dioxide in the lungs
Blood pressure	The amount of blood flow ejected from the left ventricle of the heart during systole and the amount of resistance the blood meets due to systemic vascular resistance

TABLE 10-2	Body temperatures ranges by age
Age Group	**Temperature Ranges**
3 mo–3 y	99.0°F (37.2°C)–99.7(37.7°C)
5–13 y	97.8°F (36.7°C)–98.6°F (37°C)
Adult	97.8°F (36.7°C)–99°F (37.4°C)

Dutton AG, Linn-Watson TA, Torres LS. *Torres' Patient Care in Imaging Technology.* 8th ed. Philadelphia, PA: Lippincott Williams & Wilkins; 2013.[1]

Sound Off

Sonographers are often asked to obtain vital signs or monitor vital signs during procedures. It is imperative to have the skills necessary to correctly perform and document vital signs.

Body Temperature

Body temperature is the measurement of the degree of tissue heat deep within the body. Though body temperature can vary, the body is constantly striving to maintain a stable temperature in order for all of the tissues of the body to function properly. This balance is achieved through thermoregulation. The hypothalamus, located within the brain, is vital in regulating heat loss and is often referred to as the thermostat of the body. The normal average body temperature is 98.6°F (37°C), though it may vary slightly among different age groups (Table 10-2).

It is important to note that average body temperatures also vary depending on the location where the temperature is measured (Table 10-3). Body temperature can be taken orally (O), rectally (R), in the axilla (Ax), via the tympanic membrane (T), or via the temporal artery (TA). Sonographers should be cognizant of the patient's physical condition and emotional state and take these into account before choosing the best site for measuring body temperature.

The most common site for a temperature to be taken is within the mouth, or orally. To obtain the oral temperature, a digital thermometer is placed within the mouth under the tongue. The thermometer may be disposable or one that can be used repeatedly. The sonographer, if asked to obtain a body temperature, must always be aware of infection control and should therefore wear gloves at all times. The instrument should be thoroughly cleaned with alcohol before and after each use.

TABLE 10-3	Average body temperatures by measurement sites
Body Temperature Site	**Average Temperature**
Oral	98.6°F (37°C)
Rectal	98.6°F (37°C)
Tympanic membrane	99.6°F (38°C)
Axilla	97.6°F (36.4°C)–98.0°F (36.7°C)
Temporal artery	99.6°F (38°C)

Dutton AG, Linn-Watson TA, Torres LS. *Torres' Patient Care in Imaging Technology.* 8th ed. Philadelphia, PA: Lippincott Williams & Wilkins; 2013.[1]

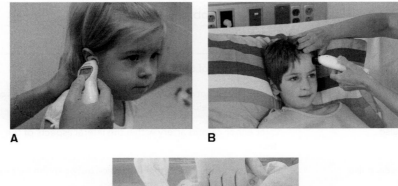

A

B

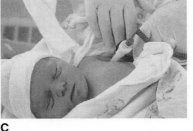

C

Figure 10-1. Examples of uncommon sites for obtaining the temperature such as the tympanic membrane **(A)**, temporal artery **(B)**, and the axilla **(C)**.

Often, thermometer covers are supplied by the medical facility. However, the instrument should still be routinely cleaned with alcohol even if a cover is used. A digital reading will appear on the thermometer, and correct documentation of the site and temperature should be performed.

There are several atypical locations where a temperature may need to be obtained (Fig. 10-1). The tympanic membrane thermometer, or aural thermometer, is a small, handheld device that is inserted into the ear. These thermometers also have covers and should be routinely cleaned. The rectal thermometer could be a mercury glass thermometer, though digital versions are available as well. The temporal artery temperature requires a temporal thermometer to be placed over the temporal artery. This thermometer interprets infrared heat waves emitted by the temporal artery to obtain a temperature.

An elevation in body temperature is commonly known as a fever, though it may also be referred to in the clinical setting as **hyperthermia** or **pyrexia**. The febrile patient, one who has a fever, may be suffering from inflammation or infection. Symptoms of fever include an increased pulse, increased respiration, aches, skin that is hot to the touch, chills, and possibly even loss of appetite.

Sound Off

The febrile patient, one who has a fever, may be suffering from inflammation or infection.

Pulse (Appendix 3, Procedure 10-1)

The heart, the pump of the cardiovascular system, provides the body with oxygen-rich blood. As the left ventricle of the heart contracts, blood is forced out of the heart and into the arteries. Therefore, the pulse is the result of blood that is pushed through the arterial system of the body by the beating heart. In the adult, the heart contracts 60 to 100 times per minute.[2]

The pumping action of the heart can be felt, or palpated, by the sonographer in several locations (Table 10-4; Fig. 10-2). These arteries are all superficially located and therefore easily accessible. Though vascular sonographers and cardiac sonographers may evaluate other sites, the primary

TABLE 10-4	Location of arteries for obtaining pulse rates
Pulse Site	**Position**
Apical pulse	Over the apex of the heart (using a stethoscope)
Brachial pulse	In the groove between the biceps and triceps muscles of either arm above the elbow at the **antecubital fossa**
Carotid pulse	Over either carotid artery within the lateral aspects of the neck
Dorsalis pedis pulse (Fig. 10-4)	At the top of the feet within the space between the extensor tendons of the great and second toes
Femoral pulse	Over the femoral artery within either groin
Popliteal pulse	At the posterior surface of the knee
Posterior tibial pulse	On the medial side of either ankle
Radial pulse	Over the artery located at the base of the thumb within the wrists
Temporal pulse	Anterior to the ear, slightly superior to the **tragus**

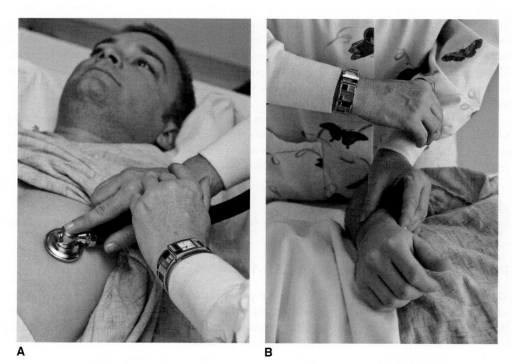

A   B

Figure 10-2. Pictures of various pulse locations. **A.** Apical. **B.** Radial.

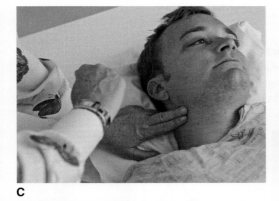

C

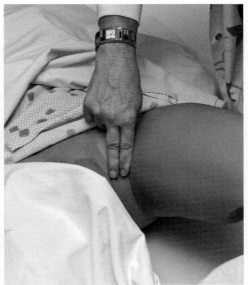

D

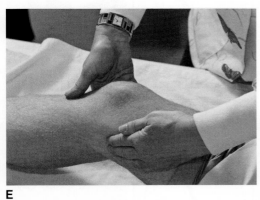

E

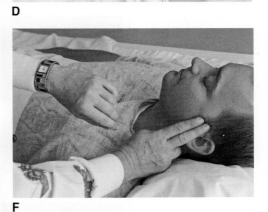

F

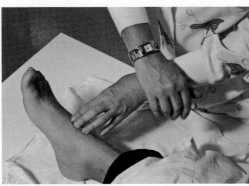

G

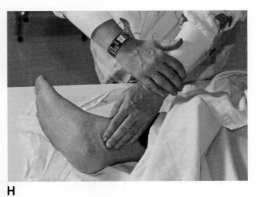

H

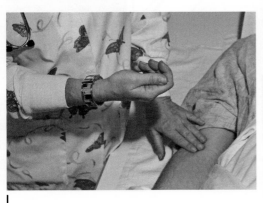

I

Figure 10-2. (*Continued*) **C.** Carotid. **D.** Femoral. **E.** Popliteal. **F.** Temporal. **G.** Dorsalis pedis.
H. Posterior tibial. **I.** Brachial.

location to obtain a pulse in an adult patient is the radial artery located at the base of the thumb in the wrist. To obtain a pulse, the sonographer uses the index finger and middle finger over the location of the artery that has been chosen (Fig. 10-3). Sonographers and other healthcare professionals should never use their own thumbs to assess the pulse, as the thumb has its own pulse. Care should also be

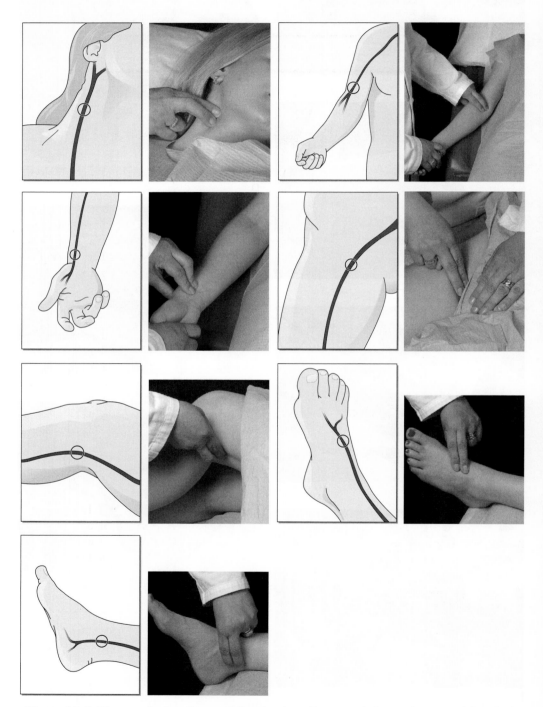

Figure 10-3. Diagram for locating peripheral pulses. From *top left* to *right*: carotid, brachial, radial, femoral, popliteal, dorsalis pedis, posterior tibial.

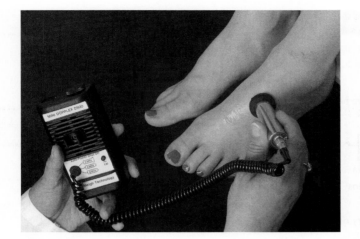

Figure 10-4. A handheld Doppler device can be used to evaluate the dorsalis pedis pulse.

taken not to compress the artery too firmly, as excessive compression could reduce the strength of the pulse and therefore lead to a miscalculation. The pulse rate, often referred to as the heart rate, reflects how rapidly the heart contracts. The pulse rate is calculated in beats per minute (bpm). Therefore, it is best practice to count total number of beats for an entire minute. The average bpm will vary for adults, children, infants, and the fetus (Table 10-5). The fetal pulse, or heart rate, cannot be obtained through routine means. Instead, documentation is performed using a Doppler device or **motion mode** (M-mode) technology during an obstetric sonographic examination. M-mode displays a visual representation of the moving fetal heart.

Sonographers should not only evaluate the bpm, but they should also appraise the rhythm of the pulse and its strength. The pulse should be both normal in rhythm and strong. An abnormal rhythm of the pulse is referred to as **arrhythmia** or **dysrhythmia**. A rapid heart rate is referred to as **tachycardia**, and a slower than normal heart rate is referred to as **bradycardia**. Tachycardia in an adult is considered to be 100 to 150 bpm, while bradycardia is below 60 bpm.[2] Several conditions could result in an abnormal heart rate (Tables 10-6 and 10-7). In certain situations, it is best to continually monitor the patient's heart rate. This monitoring can be achieved with the use of several different devices (Table 10-8).

Blood Pressure (Appendix 3, Procedure 10-2)

Sonographers may have to monitor a patient's blood pressure (BP), and often a baseline BP is obtained before an invasive procedure. BP is the measurement of the pressure of blood in an artery as it is forced against the arterial walls. It is measured in millimeters of mercury (mm Hg) and is essentially the amount of blood flow ejected from the left ventricle of the heart and the amount of

TABLE 10-5	Pulse rates by age
Age Group	**Pulse Rate**
Adults	Ranges between 60 and 100 bpm
Child	Ranges between 70 and 120 bpm

Adler AM, Carlton RR. *Introduction to Radiologic Sciences and Patient Care.* 4th ed. St. Louis, MO: Saunders Elsevier; 2007.[3]

TABLE 10-6	Possible causes of tachycardia

- Anemia
- Anger
- Anxiety
- Congestive heart failure
- Exercise
- Fear
- Fever
- Hypoxemia
- Medications
- Pain
- Respiratory disorders
- Shock

Adler AM, Carlton RR. *Introduction to Radiologic Sciences and Patient Care.* 4th ed. St. Louis, MO: Saunders Elsevier; 2007.[3]

TABLE 10-7	Possible causes of bradycardia

- Depression
- Hypothermia
- Medications
- Physically fit athletes
- Resting
- Severe pain

Timby BK. *Fundamental Nursing Skills and Concepts.* 10th ed. Philadelphia, PA: Lippincott Williams & Wilkins; 2013;[2] Adler AM, Carlton RR. *Introduction to Radiologic Sciences and Patient Care.* 4th ed. St. Louis, MO: Saunders Elsevier; 2007.[3]

TABLE 10-8	Pulse monitoring devices

Device	Description
Electrocardiogram	Electrodes are placed on the patient's chest to observe the heart rate. Electrical activity of the heart is displayed on a monitor.
Arterial line	A catheter inserted into an artery is used to monitor the heart rate and BP. Feedback from a pressure transducer within the artery displays the heart rate on a monitor.
Pulse oximeter (Fig. 10-5)	A device, which uses light, is placed on the patient's finger, foot, toe, ear lobe, nose, temple, or forehead to assess the hemoglobin oxygen saturation in the arterial blood and the patient's pulse rate to be displayed on a monitor.

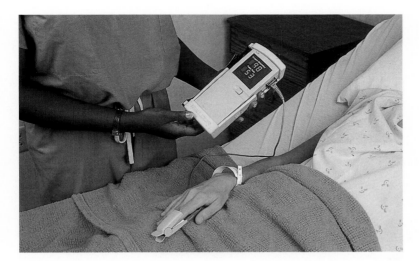

Figure 10-5. A pulse oximeter is often used to monitor the oxygen content of the blood and to collect other data.

resistance that blood meets during systemic vascular resistance. **Systole** is the highest amount of pressure or the highest point reached during the contraction of the left ventricle, while **diastole** is the lowest point that the pressure drops during relaxation of the left ventricle. The most accurate BP is taken when the patient is either sitting or lying down. The most important factor is the position of the arm that is used for obtaining the BP, which must be at the level of the heart.

A person's BP depends upon many factors; you should know these factors, as a dramatic change in BP can indicate severe and possibly life-threatening problems (Table 10-9). To obtain a BP, the sonographer will typically have to use a stethoscope and a **sphygmomanometer**, though occasionally

TABLE 10-9	Factors that can affect BP
Factor	**Result**
Activity	Exercise raises BP temporarily, while rest lowers BP.
Age	• Infants have higher BP compared to adults. • Young people tend to have lower BP. • Older patients tend to have higher BP.
Body position	• BP should be taken with the patient sitting or lying down. • BP may be lower in standing patients.
Gender	Men tend to have higher BP than do women.
Medication	Some medications lower BP, while others raise BP.
Postprandial (after eating)	BP should not be taken after drinking coffee or caffeinated beverages or after a large meal.
Stress or pain	BP increases when the sympathetic nervous system releases epinephrine in response to stress or pain.
Time of day	BP tends to be lower in the morning after rest and higher at night.

Timby BK. *Fundamental Nursing Skills and Concepts.* 10th ed. Philadelphia, PA: Lippincott Williams & Wilkins; 2013.[2]

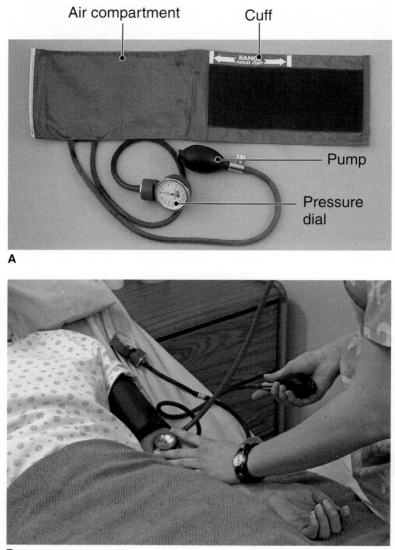

Figure 10-6. Obtaining BP. BP is obtained using a sphygmomanometer **(A)**, commonly referred to as a BP cuff. The cuff is placed around the patient's arm, it is inflated, and the pressure is evaluated using a stethoscope **(B)**.

electronic BP devices may be available (Fig. 10-6). Appendix 3 provides a step-by-step process for measuring BP. Table 10-10 also provides normal ranges for BP.

 Sound Off

The most accurate BP is taken when the patient is either sitting or lying down.

Hypertension may be described as **essential hypertension** or **secondary hypertension**. Essential hypertension is high BP that has no known cause, or is said to be **idiopathic**, while secondary hypertension has a known cause. Hypertension can be a disorder that gradually affects a patient. It is important for patients to have routine BP analysis if hypertension has been discovered as a family trait.

TABLE 10-10	Average BP by age
Age Group	**Normal Ranges of BP**
Adults	Systolic = 100–140 mm Hg Diastolic = 60–90 mm Hg Normal = <120/80
Adolescents	Systolic = 85–130 mm Hg Diastolic = 45–85 mm Hg

Dutton AG, Linn-Watson TA, Torres LS. *Torres' Patient Care in Imaging Technology*. 8th ed. Philadelphia, PA: Lippincott Williams & Wilkins; 2013;[1] Molle EA, Kronenberger J, West-Stack C. *Lippincott Williams and Wilkins' Clinical Medical Assisting*. 2nd ed. Philadelphia, PA: Lippincott Williams & Wilkins; 2005.[4]

Though hypertension is a multifaceted disorder, it has been associated with high cholesterol levels and the subsequent development of arteriosclerotic disease. Secondary hypertension can be caused by many conditions, including renal disorders, trauma, and some drugs. Hypotension is typically not as concerning. However, patients who have a sudden onset of hypotension could have some underlying disease, such as a ruptured abdominal aortic aneurysm, that is a true medical emergency. Patients with acute hypotension may complain of dizziness, confusion, or blurred vision. Other causes of hypotension include trauma and heat exhaustion.

Respiration (Appendix 3, Procedure 10-3)

Though a seemingly straightforward task, the recognition of an abnormal respiratory rate can be lifesaving. Respiration consists of an inspiratory phase and an expiratory phase. The diaphragm, the structure that separates the chest cavity from the abdominal cavity, is the major muscle of ventilation. During the inspiratory phase, the patient takes in oxygen through the mouth, filling the lungs, and moving the diaphragm inferiorly. With expiration, the diaphragm moves superiorly, pushing the carbon dioxide out of the lungs and out of the mouth. Though we cannot observe the movement of the diaphragm, we can examine the process of ventilation by visually monitoring the motion of the chest. With inspiration, the chest rises; with expiration, the chest falls. Each respiration is counted for a full minute, and the average respiration rate depends upon the person's age group (Table 10-11). A patient should not be aware that his or her respiratory rate is being evaluated, because he or she may alter the breathing upon recognition that it is being assessed.

Sound Off

A patient should not be aware that his or her respiratory rate is being evaluated, because he or she may alter the breathing upon recognition that it is being assessed.

TABLE 10-11	Average respiration rate by age
Age Group	**Average Respiratory Rate**
Adults	12–20 breaths per minute
Children (<10)	20–30 breaths per minute
Infants	30–60 breaths per minute

Adler AM, Carlton RR. *Introduction to Radiologic Sciences and Patient Care*. 4th ed. St. Louis, MO: Saunders Elsevier; 2007.[3]

TABLE 10-12	Possible causes of tachypnea

- Anxiety
- Central nervous system abnormalities
- Decreased oxygen levels in the blood
- Exercise
- Fever
- Heart failure
- Infection
- Pain
- Trauma

Adler AM, Carlton RR. *Introduction to Radiologic Sciences and Patient Care.* 4th ed. St. Louis, MO: Saunders Elsevier; 2007.[3]

Tachypnea is an abnormally high rate of respirations, while **bradypnea** is an abnormally low rate of respirations (Tables 10-12 and 10-13). Abnormalities of respiration can be recognized not only by evaluating the number of breaths but also by assessing the quality of the respirations. **Dyspnea**, or difficulty breathing, can be caused by a number of abnormalities, including congestive heart failure, asthma, and choking. Therefore, while evaluating respiration, the sonographer should determine the depth and pattern of the respirations. The depth of the respirations is evaluated based on whether the breaths are shallow, normal, or deep. The pattern of respirations would yield whether the respirations are regular or sporadic.

PATIENT ASSISTANCE

Whereas nurses may spend an entire 12-hour shift responsible for the care of only a few patients, sonographers and other imaging professionals often encounter many patients each day. For this reason, sonographers should appreciate the different concerns of these unique patient groups. There are three main patient groups: **outpatients**, **inpatients**, and emergency room patients. In the hospital setting, sonographers often encounter all three of these groups, all of which have varying **ambulatory** needs, such as requiring a stretcher or wheelchair transfer. However, in the office setting, most patients are able to transport themselves with minimal assistance.

It is the obligation of the sonographer to provide adequate patient care to all patients, regardless of their ambulatory needs. Therefore, you must be capable of evaluating your patients for the personal assistance that they require. The following sections will provide basic information regarding special assistance situations that you may encounter in your work as a sonographer.

Evaluating the Patient's Mobility

Probably the best way to determine whether a patient requires special assistance is to simply ask him or her. If the patient has the ability to articulate his or her needs, he or she can explain what assistance is desired in most situations. However, patients may not be capable of communicating their special ambulatory needs. For this reason, Table 10-14 provides some tips for evaluating a patient's mobility.

TABLE 10-13	Possible causes of bradypnea

- Drug overdose
- Hypothermia
- Trauma

Adler AM, Carlton RR. *Introduction to Radiologic Sciences and Patient Care.* 4th ed. St. Louis, MO: Saunders Elsevier; 2007.[3]

TABLE 10-14	Evaluating the patient's mobility

- Look for the ability to walk. Note if the patient can walk normally without any assistance.
- Look for deviations from normal body alignment. The patient may have had recent surgery, trauma, or muscle damage.
- Look for limitations in range of motion. Any stiffness, instability, swelling, inflammation, pain, limitation of movement, or muscle atrophy should be noted.
- Note any respiratory, cardiovascular, metabolic, and musculoskeletal problems that will need to be addressed before, during, or after the sonographic examination.
- Note the patient's ability to comprehend the transfer process and his or her ability to understand the sonographic procedure.
- Ask the patient if he or she is capable in assisting with the move.

Dutton AG, Linn-Watson TA, Torres LS. *Torres' Patient Care in Imaging Technology*. 8th ed. Philadelphia, PA: Lippincott Williams & Wilkins; 2013.[1]

For inpatients and emergency room patients, you should ask the patient's nurse about any special assistance that the patient may require. For outpatients, you should ask the caregiver, which may be a family member, about those concerns. The following sections will provide some information concerning transporting and transferring patients. Keep in mind that you should never hesitate to ask for the help of your colleagues in assisting patients. Patient safety requires that you plan ahead and be prepared for any emergencies.

Transferring and Transporting Patients (Appendix 3, Procedures 10-4, 10-5, 10-6, and 10-7)

Though sonographers do not typically move patients from gurneys or stretchers, you should be aware of how patients are transferred from stretchers and wheelchairs to another location. Procedures 10-4 through 10-7 found in Appendix 3 provide transfer methods from gurneys and wheelchairs. Also, sonographers may be involved in transporting patients to the sonography department. Therefore, you must not only be capable of recognizing the ambulatory needs of your patients but also be capable of carefully transferring patients in a manner that prevents any potential harm to them. Remember, you are responsible for the patient's well-being while he or she is in your care. Table 10-15 provides some steps to take if you are asked to transport a patient from another department to the sonography department.

 Sound Off

You are responsible for the patient's well-being while he or she is in your care.

TABLE 10-15	Steps to take when transporting patients

1. Inform the patient's nurse that you will be transporting the patient.
2. Inquire about any special transport needs. Evaluate the patient's ability to ambulate. Always ask for help if you need it during any part of the transport.
3. If the chart is accessible, obtain the chart. In some inpatient situations, the chart must accompany the patient. You may also be required to locate the order in the chart.
4. Establish the correct identity of the patient by evaluating his or her wristband or hospital-provided patient identification.
5. Transport the patient to the sonography department.
6. Relate any unique patient needs to those responsible for his or her care if you must leave the patient with another healthcare team member.

Circumstances Requiring Unique Assistance

Care for Patients with Intravenous Infusion

Inpatients and emergency room patients often require the use of intravenous (IV) infusion. Since sonographers do not typically perform **venipuncture** or make adjustments to the flow parameters of an IV, this section will focus on how to care for a patient with an **intravenous infusion**. A patient may require a simple IV infusion controlled by gravity in which an IV bag is hung from an IV pole and IV tubing attaches the IV bag to the patient. An alternate manner of dispensing an IV solution incorporates an electronic IV **infusion pump** that regulates IV infusion (Fig. 10-7).

For those patients with IV solution hung from an IV pole, the IV bag must be continually located higher than the infusion site, typically 18 to 24 inches above the site of the infusion.[2] If this arrangement is not maintained, the patient may have retrograde filling of blood into the tubing. IV bags should never be placed on the patient's lap or bed while transporting. If you notice that there is blood within the tubing, immediately raise the IV bag.[2]

Electronic infusion can be maintained by two methods. An infusion pump, a device that utilizes pressure to infuse solutions into the body, is one method that may be employed. This manner of infusion creates sufficient pressure to push fluid into the vein. Another method uses a **volumetric controller**, which mechanically compresses the tubing at a certain frequency to infuse the IV solution at a specified rate. Both of these methods are programmed by the patient's nurse as prescribed by a physician. Sonographers should not adjust the flow rate of an IV device. These devices also require electricity and should be plugged into a wall outlet when accessible.

 Sound Off

IV bags should never be placed on the patient's lap or bed while transporting.

Audible alarm signals may alert the sonographer during a sonographic procedure that something is wrong with IV administration, such as air within the tubing or an obstruction to flow. Often, the IV tubing becomes kinked or twisted as the patient moves. Having the patient straighten his or her arm out may remedy this problem. Should the alarm continue to sound, it is best to notify the patient's nurse. You should never adjust flow parameters.

Care must also be taken to prevent the dislodging of the IV catheter from the patient's IV site. If a patient complains of pain, discomfort, burning, or swelling in the IV site, the patient may be having

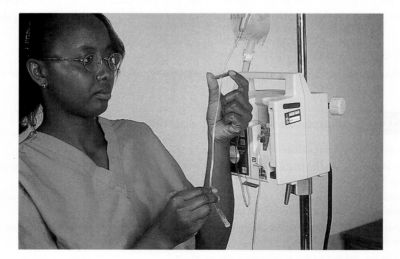

Figure 10-7. IV infusion pump. The pump is programmed by a nurse to administer medications as prescribed by a physician.

transfusion complications, such as an allergic reaction, IV **infiltration**, **phlebitis**, or other complications. Infiltration is the escape of IV fluid into the tissue. With infiltration, the area around the site will appear swollen. Phlebitis is inflammation of the vein causing the area around the site to swell with other complications including redness, warmth, and discomfort along the vein.[2] In any of these observable situations, you should inform the patient's nurse as soon as possible. Though less common, conditions such as **thrombus** formation and **pulmonary embolus** can result from the use of IV infusion.[2] For this reason, you should closely monitor patients who require IV infusion.

Care for Patients with Urinary Catheters

Sonographers do not typically have to insert urinary catheters, but we do perform sonograms on patients who require such devices. There are several types of urinary catheters (Fig. 10-8). A closed drainage system is a device used to collect urine from a catheter. One of the most readily used forms of

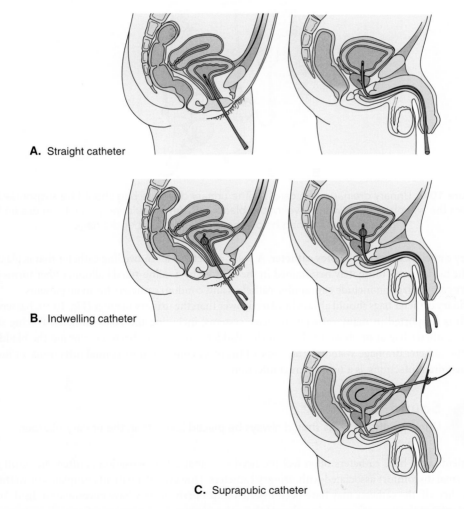

A. Straight catheter

B. Indwelling catheter

C. Suprapubic catheter

Figure 10-8. Bladder catheterization techniques. **A.** To obtain a urine sample, a straight catheter is used. It is inserted through the urethra and into the bladder. Once the urine is drained, the catheter is removed. **B.** An indwelling catheter, also known as a Foley catheter or a retention catheter, will remain in the body to continuously drain urine into a bag. It has a balloon on the end of the catheter to keep it in place within the bladder. **C.** A suprapubic catheter is inserted directly into the bladder through a surgical incision made above the pubic bone.

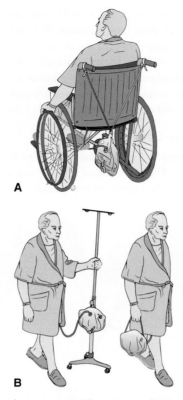

A

B

Figure 10-9. Urinary drainage bag care. **A.** The urinary drainage bag should be suspended from the wheelchair below the level of the bladder. **B.** An ambulating patient can use an IV pole to keep the bag below the bladder for proper drainage.

urinary catheterization is the **Foley catheter**. A Foley catheter is an indwelling catheter that is placed into the bladder and ultimately maintained in the bladder by a saline-filled balloon. Other forms of urinary catheterization include suprapubic catheters and condom catheters for male patients.

Urinary catheter bags should always be placed lower than the urinary bladder (Fig. 10-9). Bacterial growth is supported in many catheter drainage systems, including the Foley catheter. Placing the urinary catheter bag at or above the level of the bladder can result in bacteria entering the bladder from the catheter drainage system. In fact, one of the most common **nosocomial infections**, or hospital-acquired infections, is a urinary tract infection.

Sound Off

Urinary catheter bags should always be placed lower than the urinary bladder.

Patients who have catheters often feel the need to urinate. This sensation is often the result of the normal discomfort associated with urinary catheters. However, if a patient complains of wetting him or herself, the catheter may have been inserted improperly or may have become dislodged. You should inform the patient's nurse in either of these situations.

For emergency room or inpatient gynecologic and early obstetric sonogram, some institutions may require the filling of the urinary bladder in order to enhance the visualization of female pelvic organs or the early gestation. Sonographers may be required to clamp off the Foley catheter tubing to retro-fill the urinary bladder with saline. However, other institutions may perform a limited transabdominal sonogram, quickly followed by an endovaginal sonogram. It is your obligation to

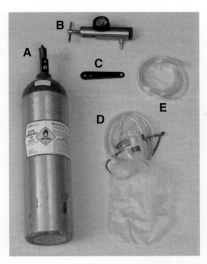

Figure 10-10. Portable oxygen therapy delivery system components. **A.** Oxygen tank. **B.** Pressure regulator and flowmeter assembly. **C.** Oxygen tank wrench. **D.** Nonrebreather mask. **E.** Nasal cannula.

understand your institution's policy and procedure regarding the necessity for a full urinary bladder in these special situations. Should your institution require retro-filling of the urinary bladder, proper aseptic techniques must be utilized to prevent infections.

Care for Patients on Oxygen Therapy

Patients with compromised pulmonary function often require the use of oxygen therapy while in the sonography department (Fig. 10-10). Oxygen is considered a medication and therefore must be prescribed by a physician before being administered to a patient. Oxygen is measured in liters per minute (LPM), and administration levels can range between 1 and 15 LPM or higher, depending upon the delivery method.[2]

Patients who are transported to the sonography department may be receiving oxygen therapy via an oxygen tank and nasal cannula, nasal catheter, or face mask. A nasal cannula is the most common manner in which oxygen is delivered to a patient. It is a plastic device with two hollow prongs that deliver oxygen directly into the patient's nostrils. The cannula is held in place by looping the tubing over the patient's ears.

The nasal catheter and face mask are less common oxygen administration methods. The nasal catheter is placed through one of the patient's nostrils and into the pharynx. Oxygen administration via this method can have hazards, such as over-distention of the stomach with air and drying out of mucous membranes in the throat. Patients who require this method can become disoriented and may be prone to pulling the tubing out. The sonographer must be mindful and take care not to dislodge the tubing and to monitor the patient closely during a sonographic examination. The face mask delivery method is a mask that is secured over the head with an elastic strap. This method is typically used for only a limited amount of time. The mask may also have an attached humidifier that contains a small amount of water.

Once the patient has reached the sonography department and has been placed in the sonography room, it is best to unhook the patient from the oxygen tank and use the wall outlet oxygen unit instead. Both the oxygen tank and the wall unit will have some source of LPM device, most likely a flow meter, that indicates the amount of oxygen that should be maintained during the examination (Fig. 10-11). Before unhooking the oxygen administration from either the wall or the tank, evaluate how many LPM have been prescribed.

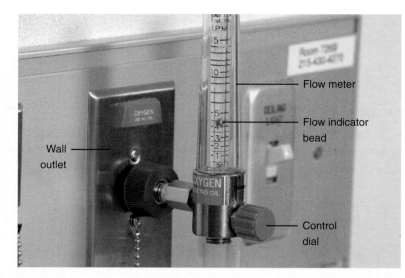

Figure 10-11. A flowmeter. Within the hospital setting, flowmeters like this one are readily available in patient rooms and occasionally within sonography examination rooms. Oxygen delivery requirements should be met using wall units like this one when the patient is not being transported.

Care should be taken when working with oxygen because of its combustibility potential. Oxygen tanks should be treated with caution, as they are under pressure and could potentially explode. Also, take care to prevent sparks or flames from occurring where oxygen is being administered.

Sound Off

Before unhooking the oxygen administration from either the wall or the tank, evaluate how many LPM have been prescribed.

Assisting Patients with Bedpans or Urinals

Though considered beyond the routine duties of a sonographer, in the course of your work, you may be asked to assist patients with bedpans or urinals (Fig. 10-12). In the hospital setting, clean bedpans and urinals are provided in most imaging departments. Tables 10-16 and 10-17 provide steps that will help you assist a patient in need of a bedpan or urinal. Always wear gloves and enlist the aid of another team member if needed.

Portable Sonography

Sonographers are often required to visit other departments within the hospital to perform **portable sonograms** (Table 10-18). The ultrasound machines must be thoroughly cleaned before transportation, especially if you are traveling to areas such as the intensive care nursery, where infection control is of utmost importance. Transducers should also be cleaned before leaving the sonography department, and cleaning supplies should accompany the machine on portable ventures. Some hospital policies or procedures may require that the sonographer access the patient's chart to check for written orders. Always be cognizant of infection control warning signs that are posted outside of patient rooms and follow your institution's protocol before entering the room. You should always inform the patient's nurse that you are about to perform the sonogram and ask for any special patient care instructions.

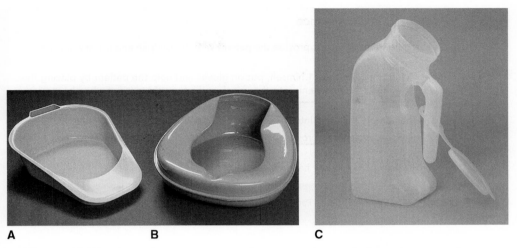

Figure 10-12. Urinary assistance. **A.** Small pans may be used when a larger pan is too cumbersome, as in the case of children. **B.** The standard bedpan is used by patients who are unable to get out of bed. For men, this type of pan is used for defecation. For women, it may be used for voiding and defecating. **C.** A urinal is used by men who cannot get up to void. It can be used while he is lying down or sitting.

Sound Off

The ultrasound machines must be thoroughly cleaned before transportation, especially if you are traveling to areas such as the intensive care nursery, where infection control is of utmost importance.

TABLE 10-16	Bedpan assistance

1. Obtain the bedpan and toilet tissue or wipes, and provide assistance if needed.
2. Close the examination room door to maintain patient privacy.
3. Show the bedpan to the patient, and explain the procedure to him or her.
4. Put on clean, disposable gloves.
5. Be sure the patient is covered with a sheet.
6. If the patient is able, have the patient bend his or her knees and lift his or her buttocks off of the stretcher high enough to place the bedpan under the patient. If possible, offer some assistance with your other arm. If the patient cannot raise his or her hips, he or she must roll over for the placement of the bedpan.
7. Instruct the patient to get into a sitting position above the bedpan. Do not leave the patient alone in this position.
8. Place toilet tissue where the patient can reach it.
9. Provide the patient with some privacy and turn around if the patient is stable.
10. When the patient has finished using the bedpan, help the patient off the pan by having the patient lie flat and lift his or her buttocks off of the bedpan.
11. Empty the contents into the toilet, and dispose of the bedpan appropriately.
12. Provide the patient with one wet washcloth to wash his or her hands, and one dry washcloth to dry his or her hands.
13. Remove your gloves, and wash your hands thoroughly.

Dutton AG, Linn-Watson TA, Torres LS. *Torres' Patient Care in Imaging Technology*. 8th ed. Philadelphia, PA: Lippincott Williams & Wilkins; 2013.[1]

TABLE 10-17	Urinal assistance

1. If the patient is able to help himself, provide the patient with the bedpan and privacy until he is done.

2. If the patient cannot perform Step 1 himself, put on gloves and help the patient by placing the urinal between his legs. Place his penis into the urinal, and inform the patient when he may void.

3. Remove the urinal. Empty the urine into the toilet and dispose of the urinal appropriately.

4. If he did not need your assistance, provide him with a wet washcloth to wipe his hands and a dry washcloth to dry his hands.

5. Remove your gloves, and wash your hands thoroughly.

Dutton AG, Linn-Watson TA, Torres LS. *Torres' Patient Care in Imaging Technology*. 8th ed. Philadelphia, PA: Lippincott Williams & Wilkins; 2013.[1]

TABLE 10-18	Portable sonography

1. Verify the request for the sonographic examination.

2. Gather all helpful clinical findings by analyzing previous imaging reports and evaluating the patient's laboratory findings if applicable.

3. Unplug, clean, and prepare the ultrasound machine.

4. Obtain warm gel, towels, and any other supplies needed for the trip.

5. Before entering the room, notify the patient's nurse that you have arrived, and ask if there are any special mobility concerns, infection control requirements, or other needs unique to the patient.

6. If required, check the order in the patient's chart.

7. Before entering the room, evaluate again for infection control warning signs or special personal protective equipment required.

8. Call the patient by his or her preferred name.

9. Introduce yourself to the patient.

10. Verify the patient's identification with at least two patient identifiers.

11. If a family member is present, explain that he or she may need to leave the room (if required).

12. Explain the procedure to the patient and assess the patient's ability to understand and cooperate.

13. Visually inspect the room for placement of the ultrasound machine. Evaluate the location of IVs, oxygen, tubes, lines, catheters, and other medical equipment. Adjust the equipment, being mindful not to unplug it.

14. Position the ultrasound machine adjacent to the patient's bed.

15. Drape the patient appropriately for the sonogram while maintaining patient dignity.

16. Perform the sonogram.

17. Clean the patient off, and unplug the machine.

18. Reposition any moved medical equipment back to its original position.

19. Assess the situation for any patient safety concerns before you leave.

20. Inform the patient's nurse that the examination is complete (if required).

INTRODUCTION TO ELECTROCARDIOGRAPHY FOR ECHOCARDIOGRAPHY STUDENTS

A valuable diagnostic tool that is often used in conjunction with echocardiography is the electrocardiogram (ECG or EKG). An ECG is a graphic record of the electrical current as it progresses through the heart (Fig. 10-13).[4] Echocardiographers may be asked to attach the electrodes, or **leads**, to the patient's anterior chest and upper abdomen. Typically, results of an ECG are displayed on the screen of an **oscilloscope**. An ECG may be performed for many reasons, including an irregular heartbeat, possible damage to heart tissue, or changes in heart muscle thickness demonstrated on an echocardiogram.

In echocardiography, sonographic imaging is performed in realtime, and image clips, or short videos, are stored for image interpretation. This allows the physician to evaluate the heart dynamically. During the echocardiography examination, an ECG is also performed. A display of the ECG

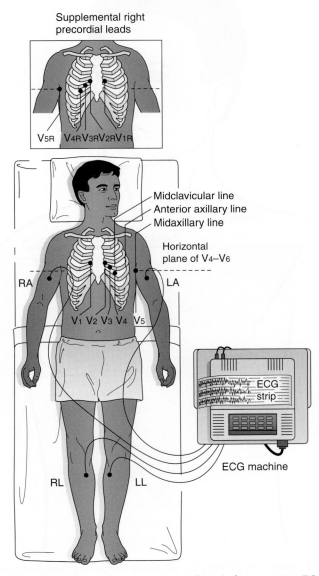

Figure 10-13. Typical arrangement of leads for a routine ECG.

reading is placed on the screen concurrently with the sonographic image. This provides the echocardiographer and physician the ability to correlate timing of the heart motions displayed via sonography with the **cardiac cycle** demonstrated with ECG. For this reason, this section will provide a brief explanation of cardiac cycle and arrhythmias.

Lead Placement

For echocardiography, a three-lead arrangement, **Einthoven triangle**, is utilized (Fig. 10-14). In this arrangement, the heart sits in the middle of the imaginary triangle formed by the placement of the leads. To form Einthoven triangle, one lead is placed on the chest in the region of the right shoulder,

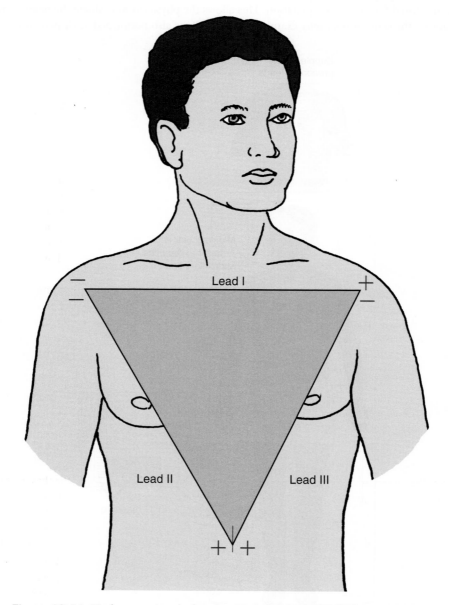

Figure 10-14. Einthoven triangle for electrocardiography lead placement during echocardiography.

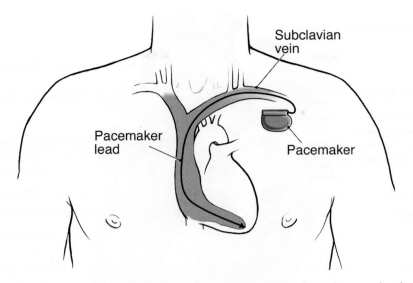

Subclavian
vein

Pacemaker
lead

Pacemaker

Figure 10-15. Cardiac pacemaker. The pulse generator is implanted just under the skin.

one lead is placed in the region of the left shoulder, and a third lead is placed on the left side of the torso in the abdominal region. Care should be taken to prevent placing the leads on an area that is covered with an excessive amount of hair, as the leads may not adhere to the skin surface adequately. Leads should not be placed on top of or in close proximity to a **pacemaker** (Fig. 10-15). Pacemakers are often obvious findings and will likely be recognizable by the noticeable lump they create under the skin in the upper chest. An implantable **cardioverter defibrillator** will appear similarly to a pacemaker. You may need to ask the patient which type of device has been implanted. The cardiac ultrasound machine has ECG cables, which can then be attached to the leads. Be mindful of your facility's protocol regarding care for patients with pacemakers or cardioverter defibrillators.

Protocols for image acquisition based on ECG findings are variable. However, a common protocol provides that two cardiac cycles should be obtained during one clip acquisition. If an optimal running strip cannot be obtained, the machine should be reset to acquire the images by time. In this situation, image acquisition will consist of seconds. Depending on the patient's heart rate and rhythm, a two- or three-second clip may be used. It is better to obtain clips by beats than by time, because the video will play more seamlessly when reviewed by an interpreting physician.

Simplified Heart Anatomy and Circulation

The heart is a double pump with one pump responsible for pumping deoxygenated blood from the body to the lungs to be reoxygenated, and the other pump responsible for pumping oxygenated blood from the lungs to the rest of the body (Fig. 10-16). The heart walls are composed of the **myocardium**, the muscular portion; **endocardium**, the inner layer; and **epicardium**, the thin outer layer. The heart has four chambers: **right atrium**, **left atrium**, **right ventricle**, and **left ventricle**. The apex of the heart points inferiorly while the base is superior. The band of tissue separating the ventricles is referred to as the **interventricular septum** (IVS), while a similar band of tissue separating the atria is referred to as the **atrial septum**. The **tricuspid valve** is located between the right atrium and right ventricle, and the **bicuspid** (mitral) **valve** is located between the left atrium and left ventricle.

Deoxygenated blood returning from the upper body to the heart enters the superior vena cava, and the deoxygenated blood from the lower part of the body returns to the heart via the inferior vena cava. These two structures empty blood directly into the right atrium. From the right atrium, the blood travels through the tricuspid valve and into the right ventricle. The contraction of the right

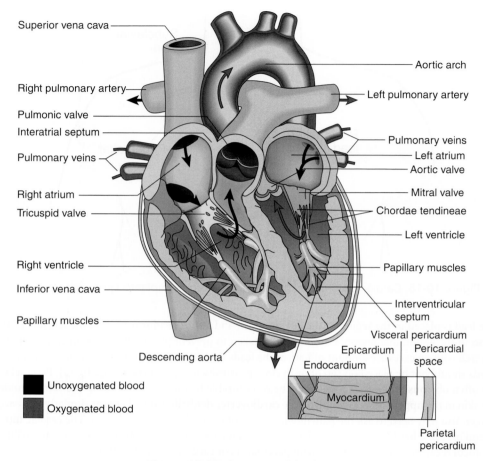

Superior vena cava

Aortic arch

Right pulmonary artery

Left pulmonary artery

Pulmonic valve

Interatrial septum

Pulmonary veins

Pulmonary veins

Left atrium

Aortic valve

Right atrium

Mitral valve

Tricuspid valve

Chordae tendineae

Left ventricle

Right ventricle

Papillary muscles

Inferior vena cava

Interventricular septum

Papillary muscles

Visceral pericardium

Epicardium

Pericardial space

Endocardium

Descending aorta

Unoxygenated blood

Myocardium

Oxygenated blood

Parietal pericardium

Figure 10-16. Anatomy of the heart.

ventricle sends the blood through the **pulmonic** (semilunar) **valve** into the lungs via the pulmonary artery. The pulmonary artery branches send the deoxygenated blood to each lung, where reoxygenation takes place.

Oxygenated blood returns to the heart from the lungs by way of the pulmonary veins and into the left atrium. The blood travels through the left atrium to the left ventricle by means of the bicuspid valve. The contraction of the left ventricle causes the blood to travel through the **aortic valve** and into the aortic arch. From there, the blood can either be sent to the upper body via the branches of the aortic arch or to the lower body via the descending aorta.

The heart is supplied with blood via the paired coronary arteries and their branches. The left coronary artery supplies blood to the walls of the atria and ventricles and to the IVS. The remainder of the blood supply to the heart is via the right coronary artery, which also supplies blood to the vital **sinoatrial** (SA) **node** or sinus node, which is the heart's natural pacemaker, and the **atrioventricular** (AV) **node**, which is the relay station between the atria and ventricles.

The Cardiac Conduction System

Electrical stimulation by the SA node, the pacemaker of the heart, results in the contraction of the heart (Fig. 10-17). One cardiac cycle is said to be one contraction (systole) of the heart, followed by relaxation (diastole). The muscle cells of the heart, **cardiac myocytes**, are stimulated by sodium, calcium, and potassium ions.[1] The myocytes, when at rest, are said to be polarized, and thus have a negative charge. When they become depolarized (**depolarization**), the myocytes become positive. When the SA node

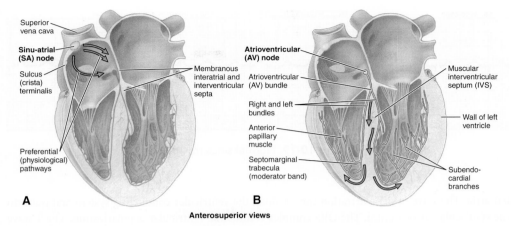

Figure 10-17. Conducting system of heart. **A.** Impulses (*arrows*) originate at the SA node, located at the superior end of the sulcus terminalis, and then travel through the atrial musculature to the AV node. **B.** The impulses (*arrows*) received by the AV node, in the inferior part of the interatrial septum, are then conducted through the AV bundle and all of its branches to the myocardium, the muscular portion of the heart. The AV bundle begins at the AV node and divides into the right and left bundles at the junction of the membranous and muscular parts of the IVS.

initiates an electrical pulse, potassium rushes out of the myocytes, and sodium rushes in.[1] Calcium is released within the myocytes as well and regulates cardiac contraction. Depolarization produces a wave that is passed through the myocardium like an electrical current, ultimately leading to the contraction of the heart chambers. The atria are the first chambers to contract, as the electrical conduction progresses quickly through the heart. **Repolarization** occurs as the cells return to a resting state, and the cardiac cycle restarts.[1] The SA node will fire between 60 and 100 times per minute to initiate the same process.[5]

Normal Sinus Rhythm

Figure 10-18 provides the **automaticity** of the cardiac cycle when the heart is functioning normally in a **normal sinus rhythm**. The P wave records the depolarization and contraction of the right and

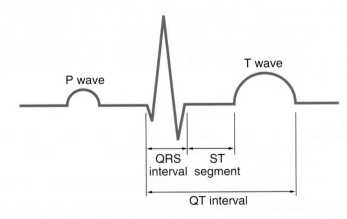

Figure 10-18. Basics of EKG. The P wave records the depolarization and contraction of the right and left atria. The wave of depolarization travels along the ventricular conducting system and out into the ventricular myocardium. The QRS complex records the ventricular depolarization. The T wave represents ventricular repolarization. The other segments are described in the text.

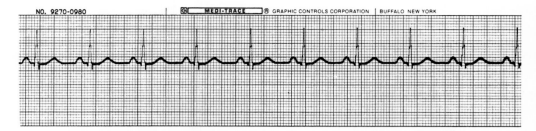

Figure 10-19. Normal sinus rhythm.

left atria. The wave of depolarization travels along the ventricular conducting system and out into the ventricular myocardium. The QRS complex records the ventricular depolarization. The T wave represents ventricular repolarization.

Several other segments can also be analyzed on an ECG. The ST segment follows the QRS complex and represents the time from the end of ventricular depolarization to the start of ventricular polarization.[5] The PR interval measures the time from the start of atrial depolarization to the start of ventricular depolarization. The PR segment measures the time from the end of atrial depolarization to the start of ventricular depolarization. The ST segment records the time from the end of ventricular depolarization to the start of ventricular depolarization. The QT interval measures the time from the start of ventricular depolarization to the end of ventricular repolarization. The QRS interval measures the time of ventricular depolarization.[5] The U wave may be demonstrated as well and may or may not represent a pathologic condition, as its precise physiologic meaning is not completely understood.[5] Normal sinus rhythm can be recognized in Figure 10-19. Examples and explanations of electrocardiographic dysrhythmias are provided in Appendix 4.

SUMMARY

One challenging aspect of patient care in sonography is the temporary relationships we have with our patients. We may encounter dozens of patients with many different physical challenges each day. This chapter provided a brief overview of patient care skills in sonography, including a brief analysis of ECG for echocardiography students. You should be prepared to face the daily patient care challenges that await you by knowing the basics and gradually enhancing your skills through clinical practice. Your patient's life may depend upon your ability to recognize the need to obtain assistance, so never hesitate to ask for help.

REFERENCES

1. Dutton AG, Linn-Watson TA, Torres LS. *Torres' Patient Care in Imaging Technology.* 8th ed. Philadelphia, PA: Lippincott Williams & Wilkins; 2013.
2. Timby BK. *Fundamental Nursing Skills and Concepts.* 10th ed. Philadelphia, PA: Lippincott Williams & Wilkins; 2013.
3. Adler AM, Carlton RR. *Introduction to Radiologic Sciences and Patient Care.* 4th ed. St. Louis, MO: Saunders Elsevier; 2007.
4. Molle EA, Kronenberger J, West-Stack C. *Lippincott Williams and Wilkins' Clinical Medical Assisting.* 2nd ed. Philadelphia, PA: Lippincott Williams & Wilkins; 2005.
5. Thaler MS. *The Only EKG Book You'll Ever Need.* 7th ed. Philadelphia, PA: Lippincott Williams & Wilkins; 2012.

Thinking Critically

1. A 65-year-old male patient presents to the sonography department for an invasive proce-
   dure at 8:00 AM. His history includes diabetes and hypertension.
   - Explain how you would obtain a pulse, BP, respiration, and temperature on this patient.
   - Discuss the importance of placing the patient in the proper position and environment for
     obtaining vital signs.
   - Discuss some factors that could affect the patient's BP that morning.
   - List some valid clinical history questions that should be asked of this patient.
2. You are asked to assist a coworker in transporting a patient to the sonography department.
   The patient is on a stretcher and has an IV and a urinary catheter. What steps would you take
   to safely transport the patient?
3. A male patient asks you to assist him with a urinal. Explain the steps you would take to
   provide that assistance.
4. Practice obtaining the following pulses:
   - Carotid pulse
   - Dorsalis pedis pulse
   - Popliteal pulse
   - Posterior tibial pulse

Chapter 10
Review Questions

1. **Which of the following is the most common site to obtain a pulse in the adult?**
   a. Popliteal fossa
   b. Antecubital fossa
   c. Radial artery
   d. Ulnar artery

2. **Which of the following refers to a rapid heart rate?**
   a. Bradycardia
   b. Tachycardia
   c. Pyrexia
   d. Hypercardia

3. **Which of the following is a common nosocomial infection?**
   a. HIV infection
   b. Urinary tract infection
   c. HBV infection
   d. Meningitis

4. **A urinary catheter should always be located:**
   a. Above the patient's head
   b. Above the patient's chest
   c. Below the patient's bladder
   d. Above the patient's bladder

5. **What is the term for difficulty breathing?**
   a. Dyspnea
   b. Dysthermia
   c. Dytheria
   d. Dysrhythmia

6. **Which of the following would not typically result in increased respirations?**
   a. Heart failure
   b. Anxiety
   c. Hypothermia
   d. Pain

7. **Which of the following is not true of respiration?**
   a. Expiration results in the diaphragm moving superiorly.
   b. Inspiration results in the diaphragm moving inferiorly.
   c. The patient should not be told that you are observing respirations.
   d. Bradycardia is a decrease in the number of respirations.

8. **Which term describes the body's ability to maintain internal equilibrium?**
   a. Physiology
   b. Normal sinus rhythm
   c. Depolarization
   d. Homeostasis

9. **Typical oxygen therapy ranges between**
   a. 4 and 12 LPM.
   b. 5 and 14 LPM.
   c. 1 and 4 LPM.
   d. 1 and 15 LPM.

10. **The normal range for adult respirations is**
    a. 1 to 29 breaths per minute.
    b. 12 to 20 breaths per minute.
    c. 20 to 30 breaths per minute.
    d. 30 to 60 breaths per minute.

11. **The normal blood pressure for an adult is**
    a. 120/80 mm Hg.
    b. 100/45 mm Hg.
    c. 110/39 mm Hg.
    d. 145/120 mm Hg.

12. **Which of the following would not typically lead to a decreased respiratory rate?**
    a. Fever
    b. Drug overuse
    c. Hypothermia
    d. Trauma

13. **Which of the following would be least likely to affect blood pressure?**
    a. Medication
    b. Gender
    c. Age
    d. Drowsiness

14. **Which of the following is not a cause of bradycardia?**
    a. Exercise
    b. Medications
    c. Hypothermia
    d. Depression

15. **What is the typical pulse rate for an adult?**
    a. Between 40 and 50 bpm
    b. Between 60 and 100 bpm
    c. Between 90 and 100 bpm
    d. Between 40 and 90 bpm

16. **Which of the following is not a means of monitoring pulse?**
    a. Arterial line
    b. Sphygmomanometer
    c. Electrocardiogram
    d. Pulse oximeter

17. **Which of the following is the pulse site in the neck?**
    a. Popliteal pulse
    b. Dorsalis pedis pulse
    c. Carotid pulse
    d. Apical pulse

18. **What is the term for an abnormal rhythm of the pulse?**
    a. Arrhythmia
    b. Pyrexia
    c. Dyspnea
    d. Bradycardia

19. **What is the normal average oral body temperature?**
    a. 87.9°F
    b. 99.0°F
    c. 99.6°F
    d. 98.6°F

20. **What is the pulse obtained on the medial side of the ankle?**
    a. Radial pulse
    b. Temporal pulse
    c. Popliteal pulse
    d. Posterior tibial pulse

Medical Emergencies

CHAPTER OBJECTIVES

■ Appreciate the importance of assessing the patient's cognitive and neurologic state prior to performing and during a sonographic procedure.

■ Describe terminology related to medical emergencies.

■ Recognize the signs and symptoms of various medical emergencies.

■ Understand the steps that are appropriate for sonographers to take in cases of medical emergencies.

KEY TERMS

Anaphylactic shock – shock that is the result of an extreme allergic reaction

Arterial stenosis – narrowing of an artery

Ataxia – lack of voluntary muscle coordination

Bronchospasm – spontaneous and abnormal narrowing or constriction of the bronchi (airways)

Capillary permeability – the ability of large molecules or plasma to pass through the capillary lumen, leading to edema in surrounding tissue, which can result from septic shock

Cardiac arrest – the sudden cessation of the heart's pumping function

Cardiac tamponade – pressure placed on the heart by blood or fluid accumulation around the heart that causes heart dysfunction

Cardiogenic shock – the failure of the heart's left ventricle, resulting in the inability of the heart to pump an adequate amount blood to the vital organs

Cerebrovascular accident – a stroke; the result of an obstruction or occlusion of a cerebral artery within the brain, leading to hemorrhage either into the brain parenchyma or around the brain

Constrictive pericarditis – the inflammation of the pericardium of the heart that results in limiting the function of the heart

Cyanosis – the bluish discoloration of the skin caused by the lack of oxygen in the blood

Diabetes mellitus – a metabolic disorder characterized by hyperglycemia that results from either an insufficient production of insulin by the pancreas or an inadequate utilization of insulin by the cells of the body

Diabetic ketoacidosis – an acute complication of diabetes that results from insufficient insulin and subsequent overproduction of glucose by the liver (hyperglycemia)

Diaphoresis – profuse perspiration

Do not resuscitate (DNR) order – a physician's written order instructing healthcare workers not to perform lifesaving cardiopulmonary resuscitation

Dysphasia – difficulty swallowing

Emergency crash cart – an organized, portable cart that contains necessary emergency equipment and medicines

Emergency response team – group of healthcare individuals in the hospital, including doctors and nurses, who are on standby and trained to provide emergency lifesaving treatment

Epilepsy – a disorder characterized by seizures

FAST – American Stroke Association acronym for stroke emergencies; stands for *face drooping, arm weakness, speech difficulty, and time to call 911*

Gestational diabetes – diabetes associated with pregnancy

Grand mal seizure – type of seizure that involves the entire body

Heart attack – the loss of blood supply to a certain part of the heart

Hypercoagulable – characteristic of a blood disorder that increases the risk of developing blood clots

Hyperglycemic hyperosmolar nonketotic syndrome – type 2 diabetes complication characterized by hyperglycemia without the presence of ketones, loss of consciousness, and dehydration

Hyperpnea – increased depth of breathing

Hypoglycemia – low blood sugar

Hypovolemic shock – type of shock resulting from the loss of blood or other body fluids

Neurogenic shock – type of shock often caused by dysfunction of the nervous system, typically following nervous system trauma and resulting in the loss of normal function

Orthostatic hypotension – low blood pressure caused by a rapid change in position from lying down to sitting or standing up

Pallor – paleness of the skin

Peripheral vasodilation – dilation of the veins and arteries within the peripheral circulation

Polydipsia – excessive thirst

Polyphagia – excessive hunger

Polyuria – excessive urination

Pulmonary embolus – a blood clot, or thrombus, located within one of the pulmonary arteries (the arteries that supply blood to the lungs) and often the result of a deep vein thrombosis

Pulmonary hypertension – high blood pressure within the pulmonary blood vessels

Respiratory arrest – the sudden cessation of breathing secondary to lung dysfunction

Seizures – alterations in consciousness that result from misfiring neurons within the cerebral cortex

Semi-Fowler position – patient position in which the patient is supine with the head raised 30 degrees

Septic shock – type of shock that occurs as an immune system reaction to an invasion of bacteria

Shock – the body's response to a pathologic condition such as illness, trauma, or severe physiologic or emotional stress

Sims position – patient position in which the patient lies on one side with the lower arm behind the back and the upper thigh flexed

Supine hypotensive syndrome – drop in maternal blood pressure secondary to the fetus compressing the maternal inferior vena cava

Syncope – fainting

Transient ischemic attack – stroke resulting from transient (temporary) ischemia (loss of blood supply) to the brain

Vasovagal reaction – a common cause of fainting brought on by involuntary stimulation of the vagus nerve and resulting in decreased blood flow to the brain, lightheadedness, nausea, and possibly vomiting

INTRODUCTION

Nearly all sonographers are required to maintain the basic life support (BLS) certification for healthcare providers for cardiopulmonary resuscitation (CPR) certification. In fact, this is most likely a requirement for you in your sonography education program. For this reason, this chapter will not include BLS training. This chapter will focus instead on the basic assessment of a patient's neurologic and cognitive function, as well as information related to shock, seizures, stroke, pulmonary embolism, diabetic emergencies, and signs of cardiac arrest.

THE ROLE OF THE SONOGRAPHER IN EMERGENCY SITUATIONS

Sonographers must be capable of dealing with patients who are in poor physical condition. Even outpatients can present unique challenges secondary to a weakened physical state because of the preparation required for diagnostic imaging. For example, diabetic patients are not typically accustomed to NPO (*nil per os*, or nothing by mouth) requirements. As a result, diabetic patients are at a higher risk for complications if they have to fast in preparation for a diagnostic examination. See the section titled "Diabetic Emergencies" in this chapter.

Emergency situations may result from physiologic reactions that occur rapidly and without warning, including **shock**, **syncope**, **pulmonary embolus**, diabetic emergencies, **cerebrovascular accident** (CVA), **seizures**, and cardiac and respiratory crises. For this reason, a baseline assessment of the patient's neurologic and cognitive function should be performed prior to the sonographic examination. Hopefully, this baseline will allow the sonographer to recognize when alterations in a patient's neurologic or cognitive function occur.

Sound Off

Even outpatients can present unique challenges secondary to weakened physical states because of the preparation required for diagnostic imaging.

Typically, the sonographer's first step in an emergency response within a hospital setting is to notify the **emergency response team**. In most institutions, this is referred to as "calling a code" or "Code Blue." You will most likely be required to perform CPR before the emergency response team arrives. Sonographers must also know the location of the institution's **emergency crash cart**. There may even be different pediatric and adult emergency crash carts, so you should know the difference. Once the emergency response team arrives, sonographers may be asked to assist with chest compressions during CPR or to move out of the way.

Although an outpatient office setting may exercise emergency responses similar to those of a hospital, the institution may instead require that you call 911 in emergency situations. You would still be expected to rapidly administer BLS until the arrival of the emergency medical response team. As a critical part of the healthcare team, sonographers must be capable of recognizing emergency situations, while acting appropriately and quickly. Ultimately, it is your responsibility to know the procedures and protocols for emergency response at your clinical facility and future place of employment.

ASSESSING THE PATIENT'S NEUROLOGIC AND COGNITIVE FUNCTION

Before a sonographic examination, sonographers should perform a basic assessment of the patient's neurologic and cognitive function. This quick step is essential for providing adequate individualized patient care. Complex neurologic assessment is certainly beyond the scope of the sonographer. However, one can use the simplified alert/confused/drowsy/unresponsive (ACDU) scale as described in Table 11-1 to perform a basic assessment of the patient's level of consciousness prior to beginning the sonographic examination. A coma scoring scale, the Glasgow coma scale, is another scale developed for grading consciousness (Table 11-2). Three areas of emphasis are described in the Glasgow Coma Scale: awareness or eye openness, motor response, and verbal response. Though some understanding of these scales may be warranted, typically sonographers do not have to explicitly grade a patient's level of consciousness or neurologic state, but they should be capable of making general observations. If you note any drastic changes in a patient's level of consciousness during the sonographic examination, you should get help immediately and report the change right away to the patient's physician or nurse.

TABLE 11-1	Adapted ACDU scale for sonographers
1. Is the patient *alert*?	Look at the patient. Is she awake and taking in her surroundings? If so, she is alert.
2. Is the patient *confused*?	Listen to the patient. Does he speak clearly? Does he understand instructions? Does he know who he is? Does he know where he is? Does he know what day it is? If so, he is oriented. If not, he is confused.
3. Is the patient *drowsy*?	A patient with some level of consciousness can respond with her voice or by moving her eyes or part of her body. Does the patient fall asleep as soon as voice stimulation stops? If so, the patient is drowsy.
4. Is the patient *unresponsive*?	If the patient makes no response, he is considered unresponsive.

Adam S, Odell M, Welch J. *Rapid Assessment of the Acutely Ill Patient.* Hoboken, NJ: Wiley-Blackwell, 2010. ProQuest ebrary. Web. 30 September 2014.[1]

Sound Off

If you note any drastic changes in a patient's level of consciousness during the sonographic examination, you should get help immediately and report the change right away to the patient's physician or nurse.

TABLE 11-2	Stages of shock	
Stage	**Description**	**Physical Manifestation**
1. Compensatory stage	Blood is shunted away from the lungs, skin, kidneys, and gastrointestinal tract and sent to the brain and heart.	1. Cold, clammy skin 2. Nausea and dizziness 3. Shortness of breath (rapid respirations) 4. Increased anxiety 5. Decreased blood pressure and increased pulse
2. Progressive stage	Reduction in fluid circulations, resulting in acute renal failure, liver failure, gastrointestinal failure, and hematologic failure.	1. Significantly decreased blood pressure and increased pulse 2. Rapid and shallow respirations 3. Tachycardia 4. Chest pain 5. Confusion and lethargy 6. Renal, hepatic, gastrointestinal, and hematologic failure symptoms
3. Irreversible stage	Irreparable damage to organs and systems occurs.	1. Low blood pressure 2. Complete renal and liver failure 3. Lactic acidosis 4. Recovery unlikely

Dutton AG, Linn-Watson TA, Torres LS. *Torres' Patient Care in Imaging Technology.* 8th ed. Philadelphia, PA: Lippincott Williams & Wilkins; 2013.

TYPES OF EMERGENCIES

Shock

Shock is the body's response to a pathologic condition such as illness, trauma, or severe physiologic or emotional stress. The shock continuum is the progression of adverse effects on the normal physiologic processes of the body as a result of shock. This continuum is expressed in stages (Table 11-2). The compensatory stage is characterized by the initial changes in the body's physiology as the body attempts to compensate. Next, during the progressive stage, the body systems begin to fail secondary to inadequate perfusion. The final stage of shock is the irreversible stage, at which time the body suffers irreparable damage. There are several types of shock: **hypovolemic shock**, **cardiogenic shock**, **neurogenic shock**, **septic shock**, and **anaphylactic shock** (Fig. 11-1).

Hypovolemic shock results from the loss of blood or other body fluids. If shock results from the severe loss of blood, as in the case of trauma or internal bleeding, the condition may be termed "hemorrhagic shock." However, hypovolemic shock can also result from severe dehydration caused by diarrhea, vomiting, or profuse sweating.[3] Sonographers could encounter patients from the emergency room who have the potential for experiencing hypovolemic shock. For example, patients who are suffering from a ruptured aneurysms, traumas, or ruptured ectopic pregnancies could have significant internal bleeding and could progress rapidly toward hypovolemic shock while in the sonography examination room. Early clinical signs of hypovolemic shock include excessive thirst, cold or clammy skin, and **cyanosis**—bluish discoloration of the skin starting at the lips and nails.[2]

 Sound Off

Patients who are suffering from ruptured aneurysms, traumas, or ruptured ectopic pregnancies could have significant internal bleeding and could progress rapidly toward hypovolemic shock while in the sonography examination room.

Cardiogenic shock is essentially the failure of the heart's left ventricle, resulting in the inability of the heart to pump an adequate amount blood to the vital organs.[2] Echocardiography patients tend to be hospitalized for myocardial infarctions, dysrhythmias, or other cardiac pathologies, so awareness of the signs of cardiogenic shock must be a main concern for echocardiographers. In

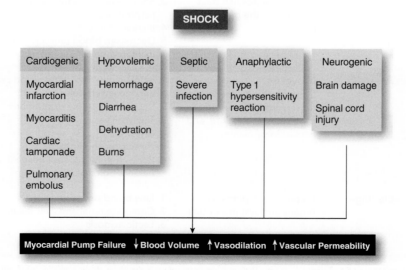

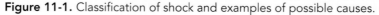

Figure 11-1. Classification of shock and examples of possible causes.

addition to the other aforementioned signs of shock in Table 11-2, clinical symptoms of cardiogenic shock also include chest pain that radiates to the jaw, cyanosis, and a rapid change in consciousness. Obstructive shock is a category of cardiogenic shock that can result from a pulmonary embolus, **cardiac tamponade**, **pulmonary hypertension**, **arterial stenosis**, **constrictive pericarditis**, or tumors within the heart.[2]

While cardiogenic shock results from the heart's inability to perfuse the body, distributive shock results from the inability of the peripheral blood vessels to return blood to the heart. Distributive shock results in pooling of the blood in the peripheral blood vessels, decreased blood pressure, and decreased tissue perfusion. There are three types of distributive shock: neurogenic, septic, and anaphylactic.[2]

Neurogenic shock results in **peripheral vasodilation**. It is often caused by dysfunction of the nervous system, typically following nervous system trauma and resulting in the loss of normal function.[2] However, neurogenic shock can also be caused by severe pain or a lack of glucose.[2] Septic shock results from the immune system's reaction to an invasion of bacteria into the body. To fight the bacteria, the body releases chemicals that increase **capillary permeability** and vasodilatation, which, if not managed, lead to shock.[2]

Anaphylactic shock, also referred to as anaphylaxis, is the result of an extreme allergic reaction. In the imaging department, imaging studies that utilize iodine-containing contrast solutions, such as CT, may cause allergic patients to develop anaphylactic reactions from the iodine. Technologists who perform procedures involving contrast agents must obtain a detailed medical history, including documentation of any food or medicine allergies. The body responds to this hypersensitive reaction by releasing hormones that cause widespread vasodilation with subsequent pooling of blood within the peripheral circulation. The smooth muscle in the respiratory tract also contracts, which can lead to **bronchospasm** and edema of the airways and larynx.[2] Clinical manifestations of anaphylaxis vary from mild to severe. Mild allergic reactions include nasal congestion, itching, sneezing, and anxiety, while moderate reactions can further lead to dyspnea, coughing, and wheezing. Severe anaphylactic reactions include a sudden onset of the mild and moderate symptoms, quickly followed by decreased blood pressure, obstruction of the airway from edema, **dysphasia**, vomiting, seizures, and cardiac arrest.[2]

Sound Off

In the imaging department, imaging studies that utilize iodine-containing contrast solutions, such as CT, may cause allergic patients to develop anaphylactic reactions from the iodine.

Contrast agents are readily utilized in sonography in Europe, and the future of sonography in the United States includes more applications of contrast agents as well. In fact, echocardiography now utilizes contrast agents in the form of microbubbles sold under assorted name brands. Though these contrast agents have long been considered safe, there have been reported adverse reactions in some studies, including premature ventricular contractions.[4,5] There is also a slight chance that anaphylactic reactions can occur. For this reason, sonographers must closely monitor patients undergoing contrast-enhanced sonographic procedures, and protocols should be developed to ensure a quick response to emergency situations. Sonographers should be aware of possible side effects and informed as to how these side effects are treated.

The sonographer's response to any form of shock should be to immediately call for emergency assistance in the hospital setting or call 911. Do not leave the patient. Place the patient in a position that best facilitates breathing, such as the **semi-Fowler position** or sitting (Fig. 11-2).[2] In the hospital setting, you may be required to ask someone to deliver the emergency crash cart to the patient's bedside. Monitor the patient's vital signs, and be prepared to administer CPR and offer the emergency team assistance. Make note of the time and the assistance provided during and after the incident for documentation.

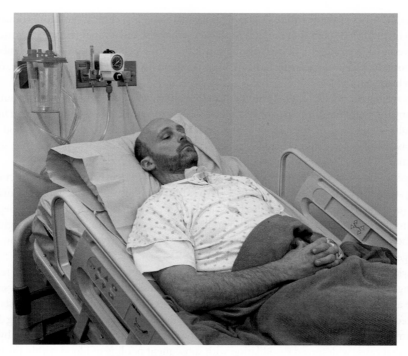

Figure 11-2. Semi-Fowler position.

Sound Off

You should know where the crash carts are in your department. In the hospital setting, you may be required to ask someone to deliver the emergency crash cart to the patient's bedside.

Syncope

Syncope, also referred to as fainting, is the temporary loss of consciousness. Syncope typically results from deficient blood supply reaching the brain. However, syncope can also be caused by heart disease, hunger, poor ventilation, extreme fatigue, and emotional distress or trauma.[2] The clinical manifestation of syncope includes **pallor**, dizziness, nausea, **hyperpnea**, tachycardia, and cold or clammy skin.[2] Several patient populations are more prone to syncope. Older patients may suffer from **orthostatic hypotension**, which occurs when changing position from supine to sitting or standing. These patients can injure themselves, so you should allow your patient to sit up slowly and pause briefly before standing. Always provide elderly patients with standing assistance. Fasting patients may also be prone to fainting, as their bodies may be in a weakened state. Patients taking certain medicines that may cause them to feel dizzy or light-headed also have an increased likelihood of fainting.

Sound Off

You should allow your patient to sit up slowly and pause briefly before standing to prevent orthostatic hypotension.

Obstetric patients, especially those late in gestation, may suffer from dizziness secondary to compression of the maternal inferior vena cava by the fetus, a condition known as **supine hypotensive syndrome** (Fig. 11-3). The patient may become pale, warm, weak, dizzy, or feel out of sorts. In some situations, the patient may temporarily lose consciousness. To prevent fainting in the obstetric

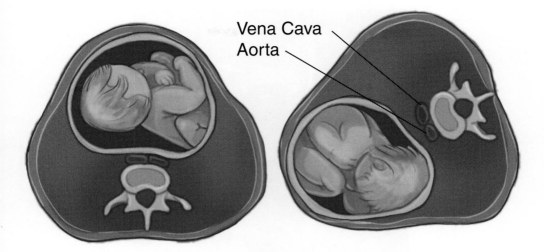

Supine position   Side-lying position

Figure 11-3. Supine hypotensive syndrome. When the pregnant woman lies flat on her back, the weight of the fetus and uterus can compress the aorta and vena cava against the spine. Consequently, the amount of blood returning to the heart is compromised, pressure falls, and supine hypotensive syndrome occurs (*image on the left*). By placing the patient on her side (*image on the right*), the pressure is relieved, and the patient should feel better soon.

patient, the sonographer should place the patient on her side or in a sitting position and provide her with a cool washcloth for her forehead, and the symptoms should resolve.[6] If the patient continues to feel ill, you should call a nurse.

Sound Off
Obstetric patients, especially those late in gestation, may suffer from dizziness secondary to compression of the maternal inferior vena cava by the fetus. This is referred to as supine hypotensive syndrome.

Lastly, patients may experience a **vasovagal reaction**, or vasovagal attack, during a procedure, especially transrectal, carotid studies, and invasive procedures, secondary to the stimulation of the vagus nerve as a result of anxiety.[6] A vasovagal attack is a common cause of fainting. Patients may experience symptoms consistent with syncope, including a decrease in blood pressure and pulse, pallor, nausea and vomiting, dizziness, and cold or clammy skin.[2]

If a patient does faint, the sonographer should call for assistance, place the patient in a supine position, and elevate the patient's legs slightly. If a patient is standing and faints, you should try to get behind the patient, if possible place your knee behind the patient's knee, and slowly let the patient down to the ground (Fig. 11-4). Care should be taken to prevent any injuries that the patient may suffer as he or she falls without injuring yourself. Make note of the time and the assistance provided during and after the incident for documentation.

Seizures

A seizure results from the misfiring of neurons within the cerebral cortex. Seizures typically alter consciousness and may last for several minutes or only seconds. Seizures may occur as the symptoms of many different syndromes. They are also associated with severe stress, trauma, brain tumors and brain tumor removal, and birth trauma.[2] They can be triggered by odors or flashing lights, though many are random.[2] Seizures are a hallmark feature of **epilepsy**.

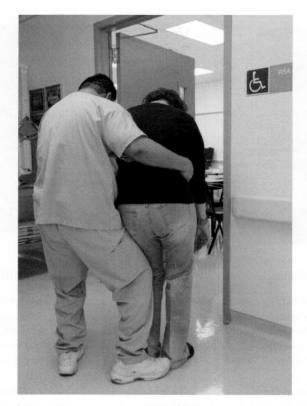

Figure 11-4. For a falling patient, try to get behind him or her, place your knee behind the patient's knee, and safely lower him or her to the floor.

A generalized seizure, also referred to as a **grand mal seizure**, involves the entire body. With this type of seizure, the patient often becomes rigid with his or her eyes wide open. The patient may have jerky body movements and rapid respiration. The patient could utter sharp cries, froth at the mouth, vomit, urinate, and/or defecate.[2] Complex seizures and simple seizures are not as readily detected upon visual examination. Patients may suffer from mild facial grimacing, lip smacking, and confusion with no loss of consciousness. If a seizure occurs in a patient, the sonographer should immediately call for assistance and take steps to prevent any patient injuries (Table 11-3). Make note of the time and the assistance provided during and after the incident for documentation.

TABLE 11-3	Response to a patient having a seizure

1. Call for help.
2. Stay with the patient.
3. Do not attempt to insert anything in the patient's mouth.
4. Protect the patient's head from injury by placing a pillow under it.
5. Do not restrain the patient's limbs, but protect them from injury.
6. Do not move the patient.
7. Provide the patient with privacy.
8. After the seizure, place the patient in the **Sims position** or recovery position to allow any fluid within the mouth to drain.

Dutton AG, Linn-Watson TA, Torres LS. *Torres' Patient Care in Imaging Technology.* 8th ed. Philadelphia: Lippincott Williams & Wilkins; 2013.

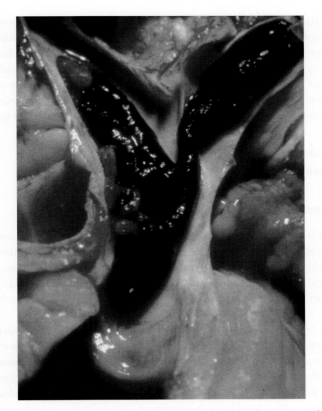

Figure 11-5. Pulmonary embolism. The dark material within this main pulmonary artery is pulmonary embolus.

Pulmonary Embolus

A pulmonary embolus (PE) is a blood clot, or thrombus, located within one of the pulmonary arteries, the arteries that supply blood to the lungs (Fig. 11-5). This thrombus obstructs the flow of the blood to the lungs and can result in a mortality rate of nearly 50%.[2] Some patients are more prone to developing PEs, including those who are older, live a sedentary lifestyle or have had prolonged immobilization, have had recent trauma, are pregnant, or are in a **hypercoagulable** condition.[2]

Risk factors also include estrogen use, recent hip or abdominal surgery, cancer, cardiac disease, and previous deep venous thrombosis. In fact, most pulmonary emboli travel from the deep venous systems within the legs. Clinical symptoms include dyspnea, tachypnea, tachycardia, **diaphoresis**, syncope, cyanosis, hypotension, and even sudden death.[2] If a patient experiences any of these, you should stop your procedure, call for emergency assistance, and have someone obtain the emergency crash cart. Do not leave the patient. Make note of the time and the assistance provided during and after the incident for documentation.

Cerebrovascular Accident (Stroke)

A CVA is commonly referred to as a stroke. It is the result of an obstruction or occlusion of a cerebral artery within the brain, resulting in hemorrhage either into the brain parenchyma or around the brain.[2] Strokes are often spontaneous events that range in severity. A mild stroke may be referred to as **transient ischemic attack** (TIA) or mini-stroke. As the name implies, these strokes are the result of transient (temporary) ischemia (loss of blood supply) to the brain. However, a TIA is of great concern because it can be an early indicator of an imminent, more severe stroke.

Some signs of stroke, according to the American Stroke Association, are described in its **FAST** acronym related to stroke emergencies: *f*ace drooping, *a*rm weakness, *s*peech difficulty, and *t*ime to call 911.[7] Other signs and symptoms of a CVA include possible severe headache, numbness in the extremities or face, confusion, difficulty hearing, dizziness, **ataxia**, and loss of consciousness.[2,7] If clinical symptoms occur during a procedure, the sonographer should immediately end the procedure, summon emergency assistance, and prepare to assist the emergency team. Do not leave the patient. Make note of the time and the assistance provided during and after the incident for documentation.

Sound Off

If a stroke is suspected, think FAST!

Diabetic Emergencies

Diabetes mellitus is a metabolic disorder characterized by hyperglycemia that results from either an insufficient production of insulin by the pancreas or an inadequate utilization of insulin by the cells of the body (Fig. 11-6). Hyperglycemia is an excess of sugar in the blood. Diabetes mellitus can produce clinical symptoms such as **polyuria**, **polydipsia**, and **polyphagia**.[2] This chronic disorder gradually damages small blood vessels and many organs of the body, including the kidneys and liver.

There are three types of diabetes: type 1 diabetes mellitus is usually insulin-dependent and diagnosed before the age of 30; type 2 diabetes mellitus, which is the most common form, has a gradual onset and usually occurs in people older than 40 years; and type 3, or **gestational diabetes**, occurs in pregnant women. Several acute complications can result from diabetes mellitus, including **hypoglycemia**, **diabetic ketoacidosis**, **hyperglycemic hyperosmolar nonketotic syndrome** (HHNS), and coma. Hypoglycemia, or low blood sugar, is a common concern in the imaging department, as many procedures require patients to fast. In order to prevent a diabetic emergency, diabetic patients should be a scheduling priority for early morning examinations that require fasting. Because of inadequate food intake, the diabetic patient can suffer from high levels of insulin and thus be more prone to a rapid onset of complications.

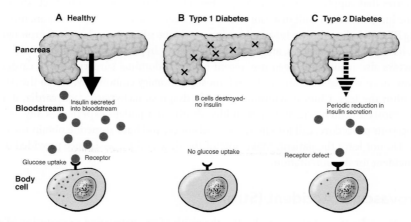

Figure 11-6. Normal insulin function and type 1 and 2 diabetes. **A.** The normal pancreas releases insulin into the bloodstream. Insulin enables the cells of the body the ability to use glucose effectively. **B.** Type 1 diabetics lack insulin production, resulting in no glucose uptake by the cells. **C.** Type 2 diabetics have normal, increased, or decreased insulin production by the pancreas, but the cells of the body have defective receptors, resulting in poor insulin uptake by the cells.

Diabetic ketoacidosis, which is more common for type 1 diabetic patients, is an acute complication of diabetes that results from insufficient insulin and hyperglycemia. Because of the high level of sugar in the blood, one physical feature of diabetic ketoacidosis is sweet-smelling breath. Other clinical symptoms of a diabetic emergency include tachycardia, headache, blurred or double vision, extreme thirst, and possible abdominal pain, nausea, and vomiting. HHNS or coma related to type 2 diabetes is typically the result of severe dehydration and can occur rapidly.[2]

In cases of suspected hypoglycemia, some healthcare employers may advise that the sonographer provide the patient with a sugary snack, such as orange juice or candy, while others strictly prohibit this practice. Nevertheless, it is your obligation to understand your role in these situations. Either way, you should immediately stop the procedure and request assistance. If the patient suddenly faints, it may be difficult to know if the cause is diabetes related, and thus, the previously mentioned emergency response for syncope should be followed. Do not leave the patient. Make note of the time and the assistance provided during and after the incident for documentation.

Sound Off

You should find out your facility's protocol for hypoglycemic patients before you give a patient a sugary snack, orange juice, or candy.

Emergencies Requiring Immediate Cardiopulmonary Resuscitation

Though BLS is beyond the scope of this chapter, sonographers must be alert to the signs and symptoms of **cardiac arrest**, **respiratory arrest**, and airway obstructions. Cardiac arrest should not be confused with a heart attack. While cardiac arrest is the sudden cessation of the heart's pumping function, a **heart attack** is the loss of blood supply to a certain part of the heart. However, a heart attack can lead to a cardiac arrest. Table 11-4 provides a brief explanation of the clinical manifestation of these emergencies and how you should respond. In all of these situations, once emergency assistance

TABLE 11-4	Emergency situations requiring CPR	
CPR Emergency	**Description**	**Clinical Manifestation**
Airway obstruction	Food or foreign object lodged in the throat that can lead to respiratory arrest (see below).	• Universal sign of choking (both hands around the throat) • Labored, noisy breathing • Anxiety • Abdominal or neck muscle breathing • Cyanosis • Diaphoresis
Cardiac arrest	The heart abruptly stops its pumping function with the subsequent loss of breathing and consciousness.	• Loss of consciousness • No pulse • No breathing • Dilated pupils • Possible seizures
Respiratory arrest	Typically resulting from an airway obstruction, such as the tongue or a foreign object that is not removed in a timely manner, it can also be caused by disease, drug overdose, injury, or coma.	• Unresponsiveness • Weak to eventual nonexistent pulse • Chest movement stops • No air detectable from the nose or mouth

Dutton AG, Linn-Watson TA, Torres LS. *Torres' Patient Care in Imaging Technology.* 8th ed. Philadelphia: Lippincott Williams & Wilkins; 2013.

is notified, you should perform BLS. It is your obligation as a medical professional to maintain CPR certification and to be up to date on current standards.

As previously noted in Chapter 7, a **do not resuscitate (DNR) order**, or "no code," may also be part of a patient's advanced healthcare directive. A DNR is a physician's written order instructing healthcare workers not to perform lifesaving CPR. Sonographers must have a written medical order to follow this request. DNR orders may be found attached to a patient's inpatient chart. In the presence of no DNR order, the standard of care indicates that healthcare professionals must attempt to resuscitate if a patient stops breathing or undergoes cardiac arrest.[2] There may also be orders identified as "Full Code." A "Full Code" may be also be referred to as a "Code Blue" in some institutions.[2] A "Code Blue" is an emergency situation that typically means that a full CPR is warranted.[2] However, it is your responsibility to investigate your institution's policies concerning all healthcare directives, especially codes and DNR orders.

Sound Off

It is your responsibility to investigate your institution's policies concerning all healthcare directives, especially codes and DNR orders.

SUMMARY

Because patients are placed in our care, often in a dark and secluded sonography room, we must be capable of recognizing emergency situations. Our ability to recognize these situations and act quickly can save someone's life. For these reasons, you must maintain CPR certification and continually be capable of recalling lifesaving steps that must be taken in emergency situations. Many patients visit the sonography department in a weakened state of health. By performing a basic assessment, you can gauge their initial communication and health needs. Never leave a patient alone who is in need of emergency treatment, and never fail to ask others for help when emergencies arise. This chapter listed several unexpected medical situations that would challenge your abilities as a sonographer to provide adequate patient care at a time when your patients need you most.

REFERENCES

1. Adam S, Odell M, Welch J. *Rapid Assessment of the Acutely Ill Patient.* Hoboken, NJ: Wiley-Blackwell, 2010. ProQuest ebrary. Web. 30 September 2014.
2. Dutton AG, Linn-Watson TA, Torres LS. *Torres' Patient Care in Imaging Technology.* 8th ed. Philadelphia, PA: Lippincott Williams & Wilkins; 2013.
3. Molle EA, Kronenberger J, West-Stack C. *Lippincott Williams and Wilkins' Clinical Medical Assisting.* 2nd ed. Philadelphia, PA: Lippincott Williams & Wilkins; 2005.
4. Ter Haar G. Safety and bio-effects of ultrasound contrast agents. *Med Biol Eng Comput* [serial online] 2009;47(8): 893–900. Available from: Business Source Complete, Ipswich, MA. Accessed October 6, 2014.
5. Armstrong WF, Ryan T. *Feigenbaum's Echocardiography.* 7th ed. Philadelphia, PA: Lippincott Williams & Wilkins; 2010.
6. Sanders RC. *Clinical Sonography: A Practical Guide.* 4th ed. Philadelphia, PA: Lippincott Williams & Wilkins; 2006.
7. American Stroke Association FAST. Retrieved from http://www.strokeassociation.org/STROKEORG/WarningSigns/Stroke-Warning-Signs-and-Symptoms_UCM_308528_SubHomePage.jsp

Thinking Critically

1. Review the current steps of CPR as recommended by the American Heart Association by visiting the following links:
   * http://www.heart.org/HEARTORG/CPRAndECC/CPR_UCM_001118_SubHomePage.jsp
   * http://www.cprcertificationonlinehq.com/aha-cpr-guidelines-latest-jan-2014/

2. Obtain the emergency response number and codes to your clinical facility, write them down, and keep them with you when you are at clinical.

3. How does your clinical facility go about handling DNR orders and other healthcare directive requests? What is the sonographer's role in these situations should an emergency occur?

Chapter 11
Review Questions

1. **What is typically the first step for the sonographer in most emergency situations in the hospital system?**
   a. Perform CPR.
   b. Provide a private place for the patient.
   c. Alert the emergency response team.
   d. Call a code.

2. **Which of the following is also referred to as a mini-stroke?**
   a. Transient ischemic attack
   b. Dysphasia
   c. Heart attack
   d. Vasovagal reaction

3. **What type of shock results from the loss of blood or other body fluids?**
   a. Neurogenic shock
   b. Hypovolemic shock
   c. Anaphylactic shock
   d. Cardiogenic shock

4. **Which type of shock results in peripheral vasodilation due to nervous system dysfunction?**
   a. Neurogenic shock
   b. Hypovolemic shock
   c. Anaphylactic shock
   d. Cardiogenic shock

5. **What term describes bluish discoloration of the skin?**
   a. Pallor
   b. Syncope
   c. Hyperpnea
   d. Cyanosis

6. **What type of occurrence can result from a patient's apprehension about an invasive procedure?**
   a. Supine hypotension syndrome
   b. Bronchospasm
   c. Vasovagal reaction
   d. Cardiac tamponade

7. **What stage of the shock continuum results in lactic acidosis?**
   a. Compensatory
   b. Irreversible
   c. Progressive
   d. Immediate

8. **What medical emergency consists of the heart abruptly stopping its function and the loss of consciousness?**
    a. Heart attack
    b. Respiratory arrest
    c. Cardiac arrest
    d. Airway obstruction

9. **Which of the following would not be considered a typical symptom of diabetes mellitus?**
    a. Polyuria
    b. Polydipsia
    c. Polyphagia
    d. Polymenorrhea

10. **What is a typical cause of pulmonary embolism?**
    a. Seizure
    b. Deep vein thrombosis
    c. Heart attack
    d. Arterial stenosis

11. **You are performing a sonogram on an outpatient with a history of epilepsy. Suddenly, the patient becomes rigid, her eyes stretch wide open, and she begins to jerk. What is the most likely diagnosis?**
    a. Syncope
    b. Respiratory arrest
    c. Pulmonary embolus
    d. Seizure

12. **What term describes an increased depth of breathing?**
    a. Apnea
    b. Dyspnea
    c. Hyperpnea
    d. Diaphoresis

13. **Which of the following describes heart dysfunction as the result of pressure caused by fluid around the heart?**
    a. Cardiac tamponade
    b. Cardiomegaly
    c. Cardiac arrest
    d. Cardiopathy

14. **Low blood pressure caused by a rapid change in position is referred to as**
    a. bronchospasm.
    b. brachycephaly.
    c. orthostatic hypotension.
    d. supine hypotensive syndrome.

15. **What type of shock is associated with an invasion of bacteria and the body's subsequent reaction?**
    a. Anaphylactic shock
    b. Neurogenic shock
    c. Septic shock
    d. Cardiogenic shock

16. **What term is defined as profuse perspiration?**
    a. Diaphoresis
    b. Cyanosis
    c. Pallor
    d. Shock

17. **Which of the following would cause an obstetric patient who is at 32 weeks' gestation to experience syncope symptoms during an obstetric sonogram?**
    a. Orthostatic hypotension
    b. Supine hypotensive syndrome
    c. Transient ischemic attack
    d. Epileptic seizure

18. **Which type of diabetes is diagnosed most often when patients are younger than 30 years old?**
    a. Type 1
    b. Type 2
    c. Type 3
    d. Hyperglycemic hyperosmolar nonketotic syndrome

19. **What should the sonographer do in the case of a patient who has a DNR?**
    a. Perform CPR.
    b. Nothing.
    c. Follow the protocol for DNR orders for your institution.
    d. Administer medication.

20. **What type of shock is associated with an extreme allergic reaction?**
    a. Cardiogenic shock
    b. Neurogenic shock
    c. Septic shock
    d. Anaphylactic shock

12

Infection Control for the Sonographer

CHAPTER OBJECTIVES

- Describe the cycle of infection.
- Understand the means of transmission for several common pathogenic microorganisms.
- Appreciate the need to use standard precautions and personal protective equipment.
- Define the role of the sonographer in the fight against infection.

KEY TERMS

Airborne precautions – precautions taken to prevent the spread of pathogens through the air

Airborne transmission – transmission method of either airborne droplet nuclei or particles small enough to be inhaled that contain infectious agents that remain infective over time and distance

Asymptomatic – showing no symptoms

Bacteria – one-celled microorganisms of varying shapes that contain both DNA and RNA

Bloodborne pathogen – a disease-causing microorganism that is contained within the human blood

Botulism – potentially deadly illness caused by toxins from bacteria that can result in paralysis in muscles

Carrier – a mode of transmission of an infectious disease; examples include hands, a sneeze, or an inanimate object

Centers for Disease Control and Prevention – U.S. agency that tracks and investigates public health trends and concerns

Chlamydia – sexually transmitted disease caused by the bacterium *Chlamydia trachomatis*

Chronic hepatitis – the chronic inflammation of the liver that may be the result of long-standing viral hepatitis

Cirrhosis – condition defined as hepatocyte death, fibrosis, and necrosis of the liver

Clinically silent – no apparent signs or symptoms resulting from a disease or disorder; asymptomatic

Clostridium difficile – a spore-forming bacterium that releases toxins into the bowel

Colonization – the presence of bacteria on a body surface that does not cause disease in the person

Communicable – capable of being transmitted between persons

Contact precautions – measures used to block the spread of pathogens by either direct or indirect contact

Contact transmission – transference of microorganisms from one infected person to another person by direct touch or by indirect transmission from a contaminated intermediate object or person

Contagious – communicable by contact

Disinfection – the process that inactivates virtually all recognized pathogenic microorganisms except for spores on inanimate objects

Droplet precautions – precautions that block the spread of pathogens within moist droplets larger than 5 μm

Droplet transmission – infection transmission by respiratory droplets carrying infectious pathogens directly from the respiratory tract of the infectious individual to susceptible mucosal surfaces of the recipient, generally over short distances

Echinococcus granulosus – a parasitic disease of tapeworms that can infect a human

Endocavity sonogram – a sonogram that involves inserting the transducer into a body orifice such as the mouth, anus, or vagina

Enteric precaution – special precautions taken when there is potential for someone to come into contact with infectious waste, such as diarrhea

Epidemic – the rapid spread of disease to a large number of individuals

Fecal-oral route – means of transmission by which infected feces are directly or indirectly ingested

Flora – normal or pathologic bacteria or fungi found within or on an organ

Fungi – microorganisms that require an oxygen-rich environment to live and survive, including both yeasts and molds

Gastroenteritis – inflammation of the stomach and bowel that typically results in watery diarrhea, abdominal cramping, and vomiting

Gonorrhea – sexually transmitted disease caused by the bacteria *Neisseria gonorrhoeae*

Healthcare-associated infections – an infection acquired by any means of healthcare delivery in any setting, including home health, ambulatory services, and long-term facilities

Hemoptysis – coughing up blood

Hepatitis – inflammation of the liver

Hepatomegaly – enlargement of the liver

High-level chemical disinfectant – a disinfectant used to sterilize endocavity equipment

Histoplasmosis – an infection caused by breathing in spores of a fungus often found in bird and bat droppings

Human immunodeficiency virus – the virus responsible for acquired immune deficiency syndrome (AIDS)

Immunocompromised – a person with an impaired immune system

Indirect transmission – a means of disease transmission by a contaminated object termed a vector

Infection – a condition that results when microorganisms cause injury to a susceptible host

Infection control precautions – physical measures that are taken to restrain the transmission of infectious diseases

Infectious diseases – diseases that are spread from one person to another

Influenza – viral infection commonly known as the flu

Jaundice – the yellowing of the skin and whites (sclera) of the eyes

Kaposi sarcoma – a form of cancer associated with AIDS

Malaria – a mosquito-borne infectious disease of humans and other animals caused by parasitic protozoa

Measles – a highly contagious respiratory disease caused by the measles virus

Medical asepsis – the practices used to render an object or area free of pathogenic microorganisms

Methicillin-resistant *Staphylococcus aureus* (MRSA) – a type of antibiotic-resistant bacteria that easily colonizes on the skin and transmits from patient to patient by either direct or indirect contact

Microorganisms – living organisms that can only be seen with a microscope

Mode of transmission – the manner in which a microorganism can be transmitted

Mumps – a viral infection that primarily affects the parotid glands but can affect other organs

N95 respirator – respirator that can be worn to avoid contracting airborne pathogens such as tuberculosis

Nosocomial infections – hospital-acquired infections

Pandemic – an epidemic of an infectious disease that has spread to a large human population across a large region of the world

Parasite – an organism that lives in or on another organism from which it gathers its nourishment

Pathogenicity – the ability of an organism to cause disease

Pathogens – disease-causing organisms

Personal protective equipment – items that are worn by healthcare professionals to protect them from exposure or contact with infectious agents

Portal hypertension – hypertension in the portal venous system of the liver

Portal of entry – route for a pathogen to enter the body, such as a wound, mucous membranes, mouth, nose, and genitourinary tract of someone that is susceptible to infection

Portal of exit – route for a pathogen to exit the body, such as the nose, throat, mouth, ear, intestinal tract, urinary tract, or an open wound

Probe cover – a latex or non-latex drape in which the ultrasound transducer is placed before a sonographic examination

Pseudomembranous colitis – an infection of the large intestine caused by *Clostridium difficile* bacterium and resulting in infectious diarrhea

Pulmonary tuberculosis – tuberculosis found within the lungs and transmitted via airborne transmission

Purified protein derivative skin test – type of skin test used for detecting tuberculosis

Reservoir – a human or animal, plant, water, food, or any combination of organic material that can support the growth of a pathogen

Sanitization – the lowest level of infection control that includes the use of soap or detergent, warm water, and manual friction

Sepsis – a life-threatening immune response that is the result of a bacterial infection

Severe acute respiratory syndrome (SARS) – a life-threatening form of pneumonia that results from a virus

Splenomegaly – enlargement of the spleen

Spores – bacterial seeds that are resistant to many attempted forms of destruction and thus remain dormant for a long period of time until optimal growth situations arise

Standard precautions – measures for reducing the risk of microorganism transmission from both recognized and unrecognized sources

Sterilization – the complete destruction of all microorganisms, including spores, on inanimate objects

Streptococci – a group of bacteria that cause infection in some parts of the body and on the skin

Susceptible host – a person whose body cannot repel the pathogen

Tetanus – a bacterium found in soil, saliva, dust, and manure that causes a serious disease affecting the nervous system

Thrush – a yeast infection of the tongue, inner cheek, lip, or gums that causes white patches to develop within the mouth and on the tongue

Toxoplasmosis – a disease that results from an infection by a parasite that can be found in cat feces

Transmission-based precautions – precautions taken based on airborne, droplet, or contact transmission

Trichomoniasis – a sexually transmitted disease caused by a parasite that leads to foul-smelling vaginal discharge, genital itching, and painful urination

Tuberculosis – a bacterial infection that can affect many different organs of the body

Vancomycin-resistant *Enterococcus* (VRE) – an antibiotic-resistant bacterial infection found within the stool of patients who have been colonized

Vector – a contaminated object such as insects, food and water, drinking glasses, computer keyboards, infected medical equipment, etc.

Viral hepatitis – inflammation of the cells of the liver due to a viral infection

Viruses – the smallest organisms known to cause disease to humans

INTRODUCTION

We encounter pathogens every day, from those that may be on the handle on the grocery cart, to those that may be on the hands of a friendly handshake, and to those that may come from the sneeze of a stranger as he passes by. Fortunately, many of these **communicable** diseases can be combated with a healthy immune system. But for the healthcare worker, the risk is much higher, and the pathogens can be much more menacing. This chapter will provide you with an overview of infection control in the sonography department by offering some insight into the cycle of infection and what you can do to prevent the spread of infection. We work with many patients throughout the day—some who appear healthy and some who are already in a weak state. The optimal way to treat each patient equally is the practice of standard precautions, treating everyone as if they are carriers of hidden pathogenic microorganisms. Our duty as healthcare workers is to ensure that our patients do not leave us less healthy than when we first meet them. We can do this by using simple, routine infection control practices in our daily work as sonographers.

INFECTION

An **infection** is a condition that results when **microorganisms** cause injury to a **susceptible host**.[1] Microorganisms are living organisms that can only be seen with a microscope. Microorganisms that are known to cause diseases, such as **bacteria**, **fungi**, and **viruses**, may be referred to as **pathogens** or pathogenic microorganisms (Table 12-1). A **parasite** can also cause disease. This is an organism that lives in or on another organism and survives by drawing nourishment from the host.[2]

TABLE 12-1	Pathogen types	
Pathogen	**Description**	**Examples**
Bacteria	One-celled microorganisms of varying shapes that contain both DNA and RNA	**Methicillin-resistant *Staphylococcus aureus*** **Tuberculosis** **Streptococci** **Chlamydia** **Gonorrhea**
Fungi	Microorganisms that require an oxygen-rich environment to live and survive; includes both yeasts and molds	**Thrush** **Histoplasmosis** Athlete foot Jock itch Ringworm
Viruses	Smallest organisms known to cause disease to humans; genetic composition is either DNA or RNA, but never both; attach to a host cell that has a receptor site and invade the cell; can mutate.	Common cold **Influenza (flu)** **Mumps** **Measles** **Human immunodeficiency virus (HIV)** **Hepatitis**
Parasites	Organisms that live in or on another organism and draw nourishment from that host; microscopic and can enter the human body via contaminated water or food, person-to-person contact, or insect bite	**Malaria** **Toxoplasmosis** **Trichomoniasis** ***Echinococcus granulosus***

From Dutton AG, Linn-Watson TA, Torres LS. *Torres' Patient Care in Imaging Technology.* 8th ed. Philadelphia, PA: Lippincott Williams & Wilkins; 2013.[2]

Infectious diseases, which are also referred to as **contagious** diseases, communicable diseases, or community-acquired diseases, are spread from one person to another. We occasionally read or hear on the news about an **epidemic** of disease or a threatened **pandemic** of disease, such as the Ebola virus that ravaged parts of Africa beginning in 2014. The news of such a potentially fatal and highly contagious disease heightens our awareness and understandably frightens us. We should realize that even with our advances in science, humans have still not won the war against some lethal pathogens.

Because some microorganisms are helpful, the **pathogenicity** of a certain microorganism can depend upon many factors, including the number and location of it. For example, a small number of bacteria may not result in an infection, but if allowed to grow, an infection will more likely occur. Infection can also occur if certain beneficial microorganisms are reintroduced elsewhere. For example, when those bacteria found within the gastrointestinal tract are introduced into the urinary tract, they may cause a urinary tract infection.

Sound Off

We should realize that even with our advances in science, humans have still not won the war against some lethal pathogens.

Conditions that Favor the Growth of Pathogens

Several conditions provide an environment in which a number of pathogens can thrive. Most microorganisms require a certain amount of moisture or water to survive. However, some microorganisms, like bacteria, can produce **spores**, which are resistant to many attempted forms of destruction and thus remain dormant for a long period of time until optimal growth situations arise. Eventually, all microorganisms need nourishment to survive and continue to replicate.

Nourishment may be found on contaminated organic matter, such as food products, blood, or other body fluids, such as saliva. Pathogens also require the right temperature and darkness. Many pathogens that can be passed from direct contact among humans require normal body temperature to survive. Other more virulent pathogens may be capable of surviving at room temperatures, and some can even survive in extreme temperatures, such as freezing and boiling. Pathogens may be destroyed by bright light, so they typically prefer darkness. Lastly, most pathogens thrive in a neutral pH environment and one that provides them with plentiful oxygen. **Tetanus** and **botulism**, however, do not require oxygen to thrive.

The Cycle of Infection and Modes of Transmission

The cycle of infection is often pictured as links in a chain or succession of steps, which all begins with the presence of an invasive microorganism or pathogen such as a bacterium, virus, or fungus (Fig. 12-1). The first link in the cycle is the presence of a **reservoir**. This reservoir can be a human or animal, plant, water, food, or any combination of organic material that can support the growth of the pathogen. Recall from the previous section that each pathogenic microorganism has specific requirements that need to be met in order for it to survive.

In order to be transmitted from the reservoir, the pathogen requires a **portal of exit**. This exit provides an escape route for the pathogen, such as a nose, throat, mouth, ear, intestinal tract, urinary tract, or open wound. Once the pathogen has exited the host, it then requires a **mode of transmission**. This is where the sonographer can break the chain. Our hands, hospital equipment (e.g., transducers and bedrails), dishes, linens, and droplets (e.g., those from sneezing and coughing) are all means by which a pathogen can travel to another person. The modes of transmission are described as **contact transmission**, **droplet transmission**, and **airborne transmission** (Table 12-2). There are several common communicable diseases on which this chapter will not explicitly focus, such as mononucleosis and influenza, but that you may encounter in everyday sonographic practice (Table 12-3). Consequently,

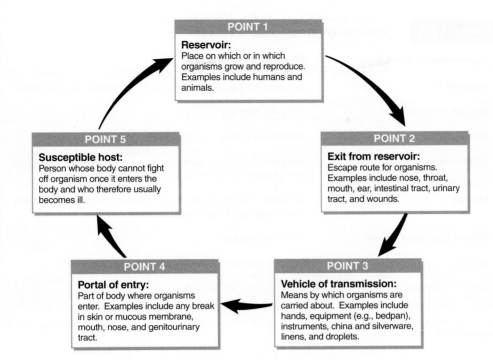

Figure 12-1. The cycle of infection.

certain precautions based on these modes of transmission can be put into place in the clinical setting to prevent the spread of infection (see the "Transmission-Based Precautions" section).

Direct means of transmission examples include when a person touches contaminated blood or another body fluid, inhales infected droplets from someone's sneeze, kisses or has sexual intercourse with an infected individual, or simply shakes someone's pathogen-saturated hands. It is important to

TABLE 12-2	Modes of pathogen transmission
Mode of Transmission	**Description**
Contact transmission	Direct—microorganisms are transmitted from an infected person to another person without the need of a contaminated intermediate object or person. Indirect—microorganisms are transferred by means of a contaminated intermediate object or person.
Droplet transmission	Respiratory droplets carrying infectious pathogens transmit infection when they travel directly from the respiratory tract of the infectious individual to susceptible mucosal surfaces, such as the nasal passages, of the recipient. Respiratory droplets are generated when an infected person coughs, sneezes, talks, or undergoes invasive procedures that require suctioning or airway intervention.
Airborne transmission	Transmission method of either airborne droplet nuclei or small particles that are small enough to be inhaled and that contain infectious agents that remain infective over time and distance, such as those that are moveable by air currents or in the case of face-to-face contact.

From 2007 Guidelines for Isolation Precautions: Preventing transmission of infectious agents in healthcare settings. Retrieved from http://www.cdc.gov/hicpac/pdf/isolation/Isolation2007.pdf.[3]

TABLE 12-3	Common communicable diseases
Communicable Disease	**Mode of Transmission**
Influenza (flu)	Airborne droplet or direct contact with contaminated object
Measles (rubeola)	Airborne droplets
Meningitis	Airborne droplets
Mononucleosis	Airborne droplets or direct contact with contaminated object containing saliva from host
Mumps	Airborne droplets or direct contact with contaminated object containing saliva from host
Rubella (German measles)	Airborne droplets
Tetanus	Direct contact with spores or infected animal feces
Varicella (chickenpox)	Direct contact or droplets

From Molle EA, Kronenberger J, West-Stack C. *Lippincott Williams and Wilkins' Clinical Medical Assisting.* 2nd ed. Philadelphia, PA: Lippincott Williams & Wilkins; 2005.[4]

note that simply because someone does not display signs of infection does not mean that he or she cannot transmit disease. Someone who appears to be **asymptomatic** may simply be a **carrier** of the pathogen—a mode of transmission. A carrier of an infection may be colonized by a pathogen but not physiologically affected by it. **Colonization** is a condition in which a person has been exposed and carries the pathogen but does not display any signs or symptoms of the infection. In this case, many pathogens can still be transmitted. **Indirect transmission** is often caused by a contaminated object termed a **vector** or fomite. Vectors include insects, food and water, drinking glasses, computer keyboards, infected medical equipment, and more (Fig. 12-2). Sonographers can break the cycle of infection at this point by practicing **medical asepsis** and using proper **disinfection** techniques discussed later in this chapter.

Sound Off

Simply because someone does not display signs of infection does not mean he or she cannot transmit disease.

The pathogen next needs a **portal of entry** into another person. The portal of entry can be a wound, mucous membrane, mouth, nose, or genitourinary tract of someone who is susceptible to infection. A susceptible host is a person whose body cannot repel the pathogen, such as someone who is **immunocompromised** or immunosuppressed, leading to the development of an infection. Other susceptible hosts include children with immature immune systems, cancer or diabetic patients, those who suffer from poor nutrition, and those who practice poor hygiene.[4] Once the pathogen enters the body, there are four stages of development: incubation, prodromal, full disease, and convalescent (Table 12-4).[2]

Sound Off

Sonographers can break the cycle of infection by practicing medical asepsis and using proper disinfection techniques.

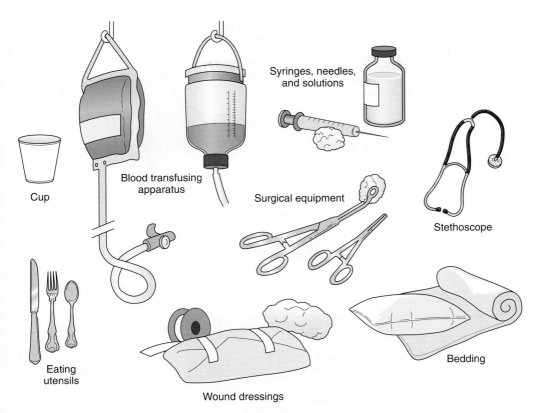

Figure 12-2. Vectors. Everyday use medical instruments or tools such as these may serve as vectors of infection.

Nosocomial and Healthcare-Associated Infections

As a critical part of the healthcare team, the sonographer has to do his or her part to prevent the spread of infection within the hospital. Because sonographers execute procedures during which they must touch the patient with their hands and a transducer, the spread of infection is highly likely if

TABLE 12-4	Stage of infection
Stages of Infection	**Explanation**
Stage 1: Incubation	Pathogen enters the body and becomes dormant. Eventually, the person may start to exhibit symptoms of the disease.
Stage 2: Prodromal	Explicit disease symptoms abound. The disease becomes highly infectious.
Stage 3: Full disease	Disease reaches full potential with distinct clinical features. However, some diseases may not produce symptoms while still producing damage. The disease remains very infectious.
Stage 4: Convalescent	Symptoms dissipate. However, some diseases, like herpes and tuberculosis, can go through a dormant period, only to return again to produce symptoms.

From Dutton AG, Linn-Watson TA, Torres LS. *Torres' Patient Care in Imaging Technology*. 8th ed. Philadelphia, PA: Lippincott Williams & Wilkins; 2013.[2]

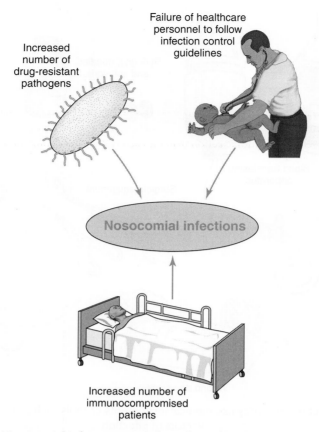

Increased
number of
drug-resistant
pathogens

Failure of healthcare
personnel to follow
infection control
guidelines

Nosocomial infections

Increased number of
immunocompromised
patients

Figure 12-3. Nosocomial infections result from these three major contributing factors.

proper infection control steps are not taken. Without them, patients may contract **nosocomial infections**, or hospital-acquired infections, as a result of a hospital stay. These infections are not present in the patient prior to entering the hospital and are unrelated to the initial admitting diagnosis. Nosocomial infections often result from the inability or noncompliance of healthcare workers to follow infection control guidelines, an increasing number of drug-resistant pathogens, and an increasing number of immunocompromised patients (Fig. 12-3).

Sound Off

Nosocomial infections are hospital-acquired infections. In other words, patients do not have these infections when they enter the hospital.

According to the **Centers for Disease Control and Prevention** (CDC), the most common nosocomial infections in the United States have been grouped under the heading of **healthcare-associated infections** (HAI). While the CDC defines nosocomial infections as strictly hospital-acquired infections, the term HAI is associated with infections acquired by any means of healthcare delivery in any setting, including home health, ambulatory services, and long-term facilities.[5]

The types of healthcare-associated infections include central line-associated bloodstream infections, ventilator-associated pneumonia, catheter-associated urinary tract infections, and surgical site infections.[5] Both ventilator-associated pneumonia and central line-associated bloodstream infections result in billions of dollars in treatment costs and thousands of preventable deaths each year in the United States.[5]

Urinary tract infections (UTIs) comprise the most common type of healthcare-associated infection reported.[6] UTIs are associated with long-term use of an indwelling urinary catheter and can occur as a result of improper care. Care for patients with urinary catheters was discussed in Chapter 10. Recall that urinary catheter bags should always be placed lower than the level of the urinary bladder to prevent retrograde flow of urine and bacteria into the urinary tract.

Surgical site infections can occur at the site of a surgical procedure or elsewhere in the body. These infections can quickly spread if not treated aggressively and appropriately. In response to healthcare-associated infections, the CDC, in conjunction with the Office of Disease Prevention and Health Promotion, has developed a national action plan for each type of infection. The action plan includes three phases that address prevention in the acute care hospital, outpatient setting, and long-term care facilities.[7] The next sections will address the role that the sonographer plays in reducing the spread of infection in the healthcare setting.

WORKPLACE EXPOSURE FOR THE SONOGRAPHER

Varied pathogens are commonly encountered in the sonographer's workplace, especially in the hospital setting. The CDC provides a long list of diseases and organism in the healthcare setting (www.cdc.org). The following section will provide an overview of several of the pathogens the sonographer will most likely encounter.

Methicillin-Resistant *Staphylococcus Aureus* (MRSA)

Staphylococcus aureus (staph) infections are a great malady in healthcare because some strains of the bacteria have become resistant to previously successful treatments. This bacterium was initially treated with penicillin, but eventually, it developed resistance to penicillin and other antibiotics, such as the commonly used amoxicillin. This type of staph bacteria easily colonizes the skin and is thus transmitted without difficulty from patient to patient by either direct or indirect contact. Patients who are prone to methicillin-resistant *Staphylococcus aureus* (MRSA) infections include those in nursing homes, on dialysis, in intensive care, and on extended hospital stays.[2] Patients who appear healthy and healthcare workers can spread MRSA easily.

According to the CDC, one in three people carry staph in their noses, though it typically does not result in infection, while two in 100 people carry MRSA.[8] The CDC estimates that a hemodialysis patient is 100 times more likely to contract MRSA infections in the bloodstream than other people.[9] Clinical signs of MRSA include fever and a wound that is pus-filled, warm, red, swollen, painful, and oozing (Fig. 12-4).[8] Vancomycin has been used in the past to treat patients with MRSA; however, this bacterium is at risk of soon becoming resistant, resulting in vancomycin-resistant *Staphylococcus aureus* (VRSA). For staph infections, the presence of the bacteria in the wound site or bloodstream leads to the diagnosis and resulting treatment method.

Sound Off

According to the CDC, one in three people carry staph in their noses, though it typically does not result in infection, while two in 100 people carry MRSA.

Vancomycin-Resistant *Enterococcus*

Enterococcus is a normal type of **flora**, or beneficial bacteria, found in the gastrointestinal tract and female genital tract.[2] However, if allowed to enter the blood, urine, or a wound, it can cause an infection.[2] Like MRSA, some strains of *Enterococcus* have become resistant to vancomycin treatment and are now **vancomycin-resistant** *Enterococcus* (VRE). VRE is the second most common microbe to cause nosocomial infections.[2] VRE is found within the stool of patients who have been colonized;

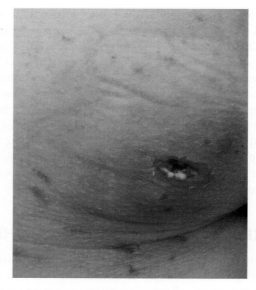

Figure 12-4. A staph infection on a patient's buttocks.

thus, patients on bed pans who have VRE can easily spread the bacteria if proper infection control is not maintained. Like MRSA, patients who are immunocompromised or have had surgical procedures and those who have been in the hospital for extended amounts of time are at increased risk for contracting VRE. In some situations, VRE may be resistant to normal hand-washing procedures, and thus special **contact precautions** must be adhered to with known VRE colonization and infection.[2]

Clostridium difficile

Clostridium difficile (*C. difficile*) is a spore-forming bacterium that releases toxins into the bowel. *C. difficile* is resistant to disinfectants and can be spread by means of casual contact via healthcare workers' hands. It can lead to **pseudomembranous colitis** and **gastroenteritis**, which can result in **sepsis**.[2] *C. difficile* can develop in patients who have been taking antibiotics for a long time. Long-term antibiotics eventually destroy the normal flora within the colon, increasing a patient's susceptibility to *C. difficile*. Patients with *C. difficile* often present with watery diarrhea for several days. The disease can progress to a more severe stage, resulting in bloody diarrhea, dehydration, abdominal cramping, fever, and leukocytosis.[10]

Tuberculosis

Tuberculosis (TB) is a chronic recurrent disease caused by the *Mycobacterium tuberculosis* and *Mycobacterium africanum* bacteria (Fig. 12-5).[2] Though most individuals know that TB can affect the lungs, referred to as **pulmonary tuberculosis**, it can also affect many other parts of the body, including the spleen and testicles. Pulmonary tuberculosis can be asymptomatic, also referred to as **clinically silent**, especially in the early stage of the disease. A person with a positive **purified protein derivative** (PPD) **skin test** does not necessarily have active disease and therefore may not be contagious.

Sound Off

Though most individuals know that TB can affect the lungs, it can also affect many other parts of the body, including the spleen and testicles.

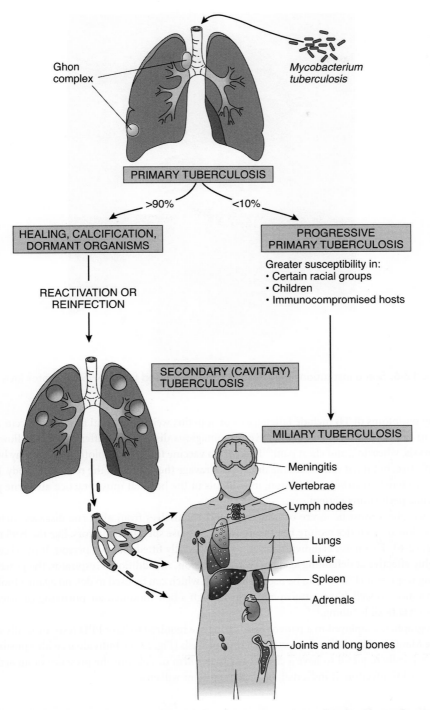

Figure 12-5. Stages of the tuberculosis. With primary tuberculosis, the person is infected, but there are no symptoms, and the person is unaware. Progressive primary tuberculosis develops in less than 10% of infected normal adults, but those who are more frequently affected include children and those who are immunosuppressed. Secondary tuberculosis, also referred to as cavitary, results from reactivation of dormant disease or reinfection with exogenous bacilli. With miliary tuberculosis, distant organs can be affected, manifesting in numerous, minute, yellow-white lesions.

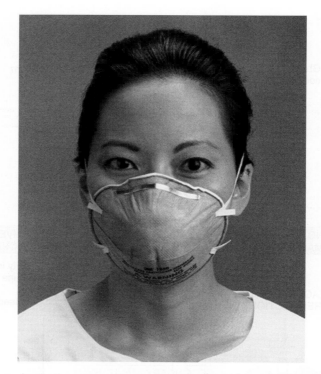

Figure 12-6. Some institutions may require you to be fitted for an N95 respirator face mask.

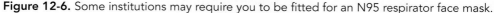

Early symptoms of TB include fatigue, loss of appetite, weight loss, and fevers that occur at night or late in the day.[2] Individuals with active or contagious disease can suffer from a shallow cough, **hemoptysis**, wheezing, and chest pain.[2] There is no vaccine for TB. Antibiotic therapy may be somewhat effective, but if left untreated, the disease can ravage the lungs and the rest of the body. Because TB is considered an airborne infection, individuals in the hospital must practice **airborne precautions** while performing patient care.

Sonographers must be aware of how to protect themselves from airborne diseases such as TB. Many healthcare facilities require healthcare workers to use special respirators, like the **N95 respirator** (Fig. 12-6). This mask is individualized, so it is specially fitted for each person. If fitted correctly, it is highly effective at defending against TB transmission. An additional respirator, the powered air-purifying respirator (PAPR), can be used. The PAPR, which can be used to defend against biohazardous substances as well, blows atmospheric air through a belt-mounted air-purifying canister to the face mask via flexible tubing.[1]

Sonographers employed in a patient care setting are required to have PPD tests, officially referred to as the Mantoux tuberculin skin tests, on a routine basis (Fig. 12-7). Individuals with a positive PPD test are typically required to have a chest x-ray to confirm or rule out the presence of an active and contagious TB infection. If indicated, medical treatment will ensue.

Bloodborne Pathogens

A **bloodborne pathogen** is a disease-causing microorganism contained within the human blood. According to the CDC, human immunodeficiency virus (HIV), hepatitis B (HBV), and hepatitis C (HCV) are the three most common bloodborne pathogens that put healthcare workers at risk.[11] Typical exposure for a healthcare worker is either via a percutaneous injury by a sharp object, such as a needlestick, or via direct contact with mucous membranes or non-intact skin with blood, tissue,

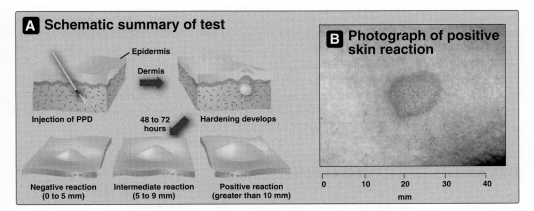

Figure 12-7. Mantoux skin test for tuberculosis.

or other potentially infectious bodily fluids.[11] The following section will provide an overview of each of these bloodborne pathogens.

Viral Hepatitis

Viral hepatitis is inflammation of the cells of the liver. Hepatitis may be in the form of hepatitis A (HAV), HBV, HCV, HDV, and HEV. HAV and HEV are transmitted via the **fecal-oral route**, while all of the other hepatitis viruses are transmitted via blood and other body fluids, such as via a healthcare worker's accidental needlestick exposure. The most common bloodborne infection in the United States is HCV.[2] It is important to note that hepatitis, specifically HBV, can live within pooled, dried blood for more than a week.[4]

Those with acute viral hepatitis demonstrate flu-like symptoms, such as a low-grade fever, muscle aches, and fatigue, as well as darkening of the urine.[2] If hepatitis is not treated aggressively, the liver can become quite enlarged (**hepatomegaly**), and the patient may have **jaundice**. While patients can suffer from recurrent bouts of inflammation that resolves, the long-standing effects of the disease— **chronic hepatitis**—can lead to permanent liver damage. HBV, HCV, and HDV can all lead to chronic hepatitis, which in turn increases the individual's likelihood of developing **cirrhosis, portal hypertension**, and liver cancer. The disease is communicable, even during the early incubation period, when symptoms may not be obvious. Vaccines are currently available for HAV and HBV. Most healthcare employers require workers to receive these vaccines prior to employment.

Sound Off

HBV can live within pooled, dried blood for more than a week.

HIV and AIDS

Though HIV and AIDS are not discussed as often as they were in the 1980s and 1990s, they are still critical health conditions that sonographers must understand. HIV is the virus that can lead to AIDS. It is a retrovirus, which means that it has a propensity to alter RNA to DNA, infect cells, and destroy the immune system of the carrier. Several diseases are associated with AIDS, such as *Pneumocystis carinii* (a form of pneumonia), **Kaposi sarcoma**, and AIDS dementia complex.[2]

There are five phases of symptoms for HIV. In the earlier phases, the person may demonstrate flu-like symptoms or show no signs of infection, though the virus can still be transmitted. The later phases may not manifest clinically for many years, though the immune system is gradually being degraded.[2] Specifically, the T lymphocytes or T cells, which are immune cells, are targeted by the virus and destroyed. As a result of this battle, the lymphatic system becomes reactive, causing enlargement of the spleen (**splenomegaly**) and other lymphatic organs.[2] In the final phases of the disease, the immune system is so weakened that the individual suffers from viral, protozoal, and bacterial infections easily, and possibly cancer as well. If the virus progresses to Phase 5, the person has a 90% chance to live only three more years.[2] There is no current vaccine or cure for HIV. However, several treatments are currently being used to decrease the viral load in the bloodstream.[2] Though the disease can be transmitted via sexual intercourse, the main concern for healthcare workers is accidental needlestick exposure or contact with infected body fluids.

BREAKING THE CYCLE OF INFECTION

The goal for the sonographer should be to attempt to break the cycle of infection. Sonographers can play an active role to prevent the spread of infection by taking **infection control precautions** to restrain the transmission of infectious diseases. The following section will provide an overview of **standard precautions**, **transmission-based precautions**, and the use of medical asepsis in the sonography department.

Standard Precautions

Standard precautions, formerly referred to as universal precautions, are measures for reducing the risk of microorganism transmission from both recognized and unrecognized sources (Fig. 12-8).[1] Sonographers are required to use standard precautions with every patient, regardless of whether or not the patient appears ill. Standard precautions include (1) hand hygiene, (2) use of **personal protective equipment** (PPE) (e.g., gloves, gowns, masks), (3) safe injection practices, (4) safe handling of potentially contaminated equipment or surfaces in the patient environment, and (5) respiratory hygiene/cough etiquette (Fig. 12-9).[12] Standard precautions apply to blood, non-intact skin, mucous membranes, contaminated equipment, and all body fluids and secretions, except for sweat. Essentially, a sonographer should treat all blood and body substances as if they contain disease-producing microorganisms.

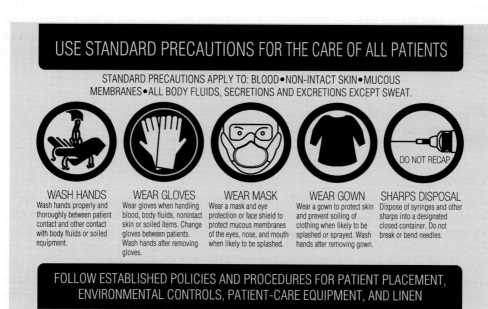

Figure 12-8. Remember to use standard precautions at all times.

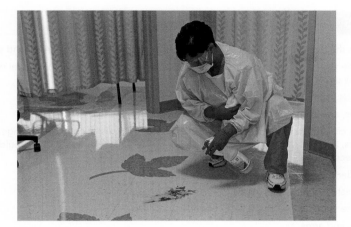

Figure 12-9. You should always use standard precautions, such as wearing personal protective equipment, whenever contact with blood or other body fluids is possible.

Sound Off

Sonographers are required to use standard precautions with every patient regardless of whether or not the patient appears ill.

Hand Hygiene (Appendix 3, Procedure 12-1)

Hand-washing has long been recognized as an effective means of preventing the spread of infection. The CDC recommends the use of alcohol-based hand rub (ABHR) as the primary mode of hand hygiene in the healthcare setting because it is effective at destroying a broad range of pathogens, easy to use, less of an irritant on hands, and quicker than washing the hands with water and soap (Fig. 12-10).[12] However, if the hands are visibly soiled or when caring for someone with known infectious diarrhea (e.g., *C. difficile*), the CDC does recommend hand-washing with soap and water.[12] The proper aseptic hand-washing technique can be found in Table 12-5 and is outlined in Appendix 3, Procedure 12-1.

A sonographer should consistently consider the need to wash his or her hands throughout the day, including before and after every instance of patient contact; after coming in contact with any blood or other body fluids; after coming in contact with suspected infectious material; after invasive procedures such as biopsies; after coughing, sneezing, or blowing one's nose; after using the restroom; and

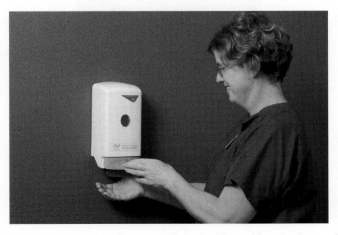

Figure 12-10. Typically, there are wall-mounted alcohol-based hand rubs available in patient care settings.

TABLE 12-5	Aseptic hand-washing technique

1. Approach the sink, but do not touch the sink with your clothes. Remove rings and your watch.
2. Turn on the tap to produce a warm, controlled flow of water. A clean paper towel may be used to turn the tap on, though some sinks have foot or knee controls.
3. Keep hands lower than forearms and elbows to allow drainage of water.
4. Wet hands, and apply a generous amount of soap.
5. With firm, circular, scrubbing motions, wash your palms, backs of hands, each finger, between the fingers, and the knuckles. Wash your wrists and forearms if needed. This should take at least 15 seconds.
6. Clean under fingernails with a brush if provided.
7. Repeat washing your hands.
8. Turn off the water with a clean paper towel.
9. Dry hands and arms.
10. Lotion may be required for your skin, because washing your hands can cause the skin to dry and crack.

From Dutton AG, Linn-Watson TA, Torres LS. *Torres' Patient Care in Imaging Technology*. 8th ed. Philadelphia, PA: Lippincott Williams & Wilkins; 2013.[2]

before going to lunch or break and leaving for the day. The aseptic hand-washing technique would be an optimal way to begin the workday and certainly should be utilized when appropriate. At minimum, proper hand-washing or the use of an ABHR should precede and follow each patient contact, regardless of whether or not gloves are worn.

Sound Off

Proper hand-washing or the use of an ABHR should precede and follow each patient contact regardless of whether or not gloves are worn.

Personal Protective Equipment

PPE is worn by healthcare professionals to protect them from exposure or contact with an infectious agent (Fig. 12-11). PPE includes gloves, masks, goggles, face shields, gowns, shoe covers, and respirators. The form of PPE chosen depends upon the patient interaction. For example, for an outpatient,

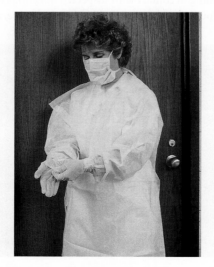

Figure 12-11. Personal protective equipment, such as a face mask, gown, and gloves, helps prevent the transmission of infectious microorganisms.

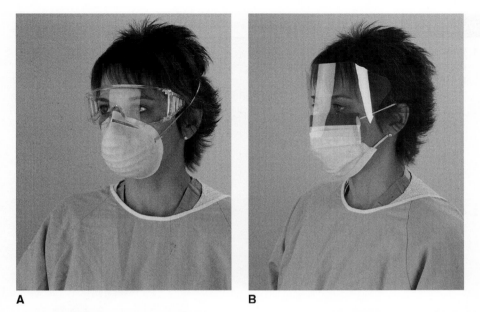

A   **B**

Figure 12-12. Mask and eye protection. A mask and eye protection can prevent splatter from reaching the sonographer's face. Along with a gown, the individual can wear goggles **(A)** or a mask with a solid eye shield **(B)**.

sonographers should wear a clean pair of gloves to perform an examination, while for an isolation patient, the sonographer may need to wear a gown or mask depending upon the isolation precautions recommended. Nonetheless, you should wear gloves, a gown, a mask, and eye protection if potential exposure from splatter of blood or other body fluids is possible (Fig. 12-12).

Gloving

After washing your hands or using an ABHR, you should always put on a pair of gloves before performing a sonogram even if the patient appears outwardly healthy. Gloving is a fundamental step that can be taken to prevent the spread of infection among you and your patients. Hospitals and other healthcare institutions should provide disposable, single-use gloves for those who may need to touch or interact with patients who may have communicable diseases. Latex gloves, although popular in the past, often caused the user to develop latex sensitivity with resulting focal latex allergies on the hands and also increased the likelihood of allergic reactions in patients. Most gloves used today come in some form of synthetic rubber material, such as nitrile, or a combination of other non-latex materials. After each examination, gloves should be removed, and your hands should be washed or cleaned with an ABHR. Table 12-6 provides the steps for removing dirty gloves.

Sound Off

After washing your hands or using an ABHR, you should always put on a pair of gloves before performing a sonogram even if the patient appears outwardly healthy.

Other Personal Protective Equipment (Appendix 3, Procedure 12-2)

Some invasive procedures, such as paracentesis and thoracentesis, may expose the sonographer to a splatter of body fluids. In these situations, it is best to wear a mask and eye protection. Masks that incorporate a face shield can be used (Fig. 12-12). Gowns, hair covers, and shoe covers are also means of protection. These PPEs should be worn when splatter may occur, there is potential for contact with infected body fluids, or contact isolation is recommended. For example, gowning is important to prevent contamination of your clothes and to protect the skin from contact with infectious

TABLE 12-6	Removing dirty gloves
1. With the gloved right hand, take hold of the upper, outside portion of the left glove, and pull it off, turning it inside out.	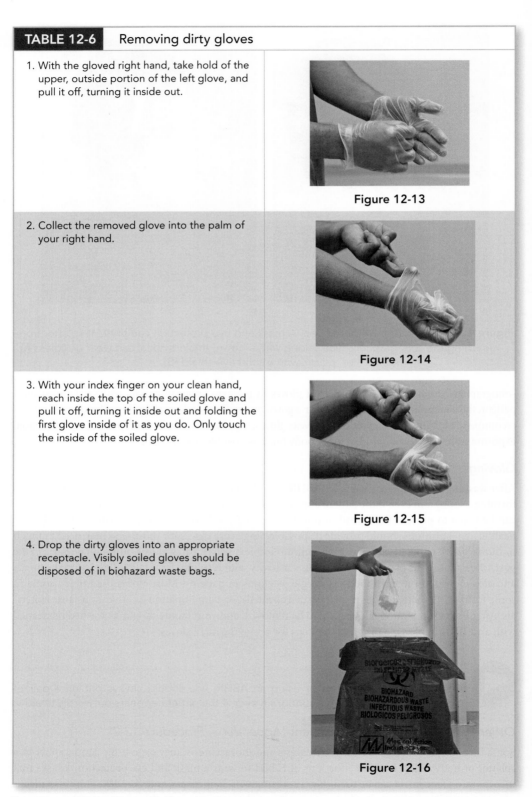**Figure 12-13**
2. Collect the removed glove into the palm of your right hand.	**Figure 12-14**
3. With your index finger on your clean hand, reach inside the top of the soiled glove and pull it off, turning it inside out and folding the first glove inside of it as you do. Only touch the inside of the soiled glove.	**Figure 12-15**
4. Drop the dirty gloves into an appropriate receptacle. Visibly soiled gloves should be disposed of in biohazard waste bags.	**Figure 12-16**

From Dutton AG, Linn-Watson TA, Torres LS. *Torres' Patient Care in Imaging Technology.* 8th ed. Philadelphia, PA: Lippincott Williams & Wilkins; 2013.[2]

TABLE 12-7	Gowning
1. Apply the gown by holding the gown with the opening toward you.	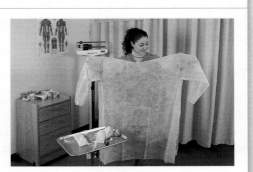 **Figure 12-17**
2. Slip your arms into the sleeves.	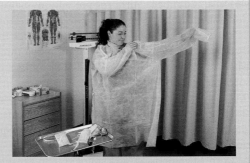 **Figure 12-18**
3. Tie or fasten the gown at the neck and the waist. Ask for help if assistance is needed.	 **Figure 12-19**
4. Obtain gloves, and place the gloves on your hands and over your wrists, covering the sleeve of the gown.	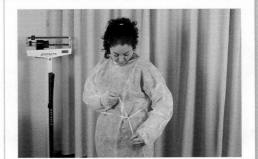 **Figure 12-20**

From Bedford DJ, Allen MM. *LWW's Visual Atlas of Medical Assisting.* Philadelphia, PA: Lippincott Williams & Wilkins; 2008.[13]

materials. Suggested steps for gowning are provided in Table 12-7. Removing PPEs should follow an orderly sequence as well (Appendix 3, Procedure 12-2). After removing gloves, as demonstrated in Table 12-6, you should wash your hands or apply an ABHR, remove your mask, remove the gown, and discard the items appropriately.

Transmission-Based Precautions

Transmission-based precautions, or isolation precautions, are measures used for controlling the spread of infection based on known transmission mechanisms for each disease (Fig. 12-21). Consequently, patients may be placed in isolation as a result of these precautions. There are three transmission-based precautions: airborne precautions, **droplet precautions**, and contact precautions.

Airborne precautions are taken to prevent the spread of pathogens through the air. Diseases that are spread in this manner include **severe acute respiratory syndrome** (SARS), smallpox, tuberculosis, varicella, and rubella. Airborne precautions may include a private room, negative air pressure ventilation, the use of an N95 respirator, or a surgical mask placed on the patient during transportation.[2]

Droplet precautions are measures that block the spread of pathogens within moist droplets larger than 5 μm.[1] These pathogens are transmitted through respiratory secretions via mucous membranes when a person coughs, sneezes, talks, or undergoes airway suctioning. Contact precautions are measures used to block the spread of pathogens by either direct or indirect contact as described earlier in this chapter. A specific form of contact precaution, **enteric precaution**, may also be advised in some situations, specifically for those patients with infectious waste, such as *C. difficile* and *E. coli*. In some circumstances, a gown and shoe covers may be required if the patient has infected diarrhea or is incontinent. It is your duty to be familiar with specific contact isolations and be aware of what PPE should be worn when performing a sonogram on isolation patients. When you travel to perform a portable sonogram on an isolation patient, *stop*, read the isolation signs, and, if needed, clarify with the patient's nurse about the isolation precautions that you should take prior to entering the patient's room.

Sound Off

When you travel to perform a portable sonogram on an isolation patient, *stop*, read the isolation signs, and, if needed, clarify with the patient's nurse about the isolation precautions that you should take prior to entering the patient's room.

Medical Asepsis in the Sonography Department

Medical asepsis does not mean the total elimination of all microorganisms from the workplace; rather, it refers to the practices used to render an object or area free of *pathogenic* microorganisms. Medical asepsis helps to prevent the spread of infection through effective hand-washing techniques; the use of soap, water, and friction; and the use of various chemical disinfectants to control the proliferation of microorganisms. Proper dress in the workplace, the cleaning of medical and ultrasound equipment, and the use of **probe covers** are all discussed in the following sections.

Personal Hygiene and Dress in the Workplace

Several simple work practices will reduce the likelihood of you becoming a carrier of microorganisms. For example, your fingernails should be kept short, and cracked or broken nails should be covered. Fingernail polish and acrylic nails should be discouraged, as they tend to harbor microorganisms. It is best to only wear a plain wedding band and minimal jewelry, and especially avoid dangling jewelry, as patients may inadvertently grab or become tangled in them. Maintaining a short hairstyle is best, as hair can also harbor microorganisms. Long hair should be worn up and away from clothing and patients.[2]

Sonographers are typically required to wear short-sleeved scrubs that are easily washed and worn only at work. These outfits, including any laboratory coats, should be washed daily with hot water

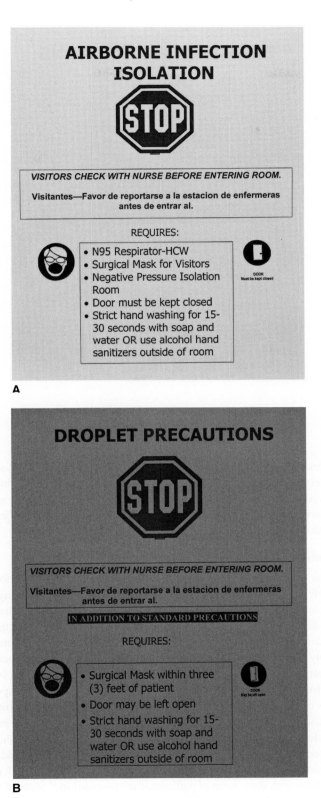

Figure 12-21. Category-specific isolation precautions. These are signs **(A, B, and C)** that you may see outside of an inpatient's room.

(continues)

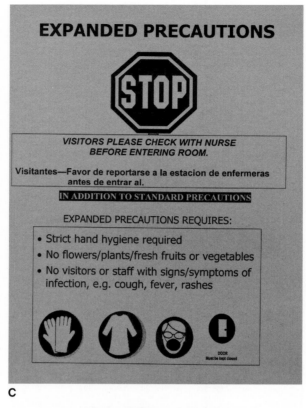

C

Figure 12-21. (*Continued*)

and detergent. Bleach can be used for overtly contaminated clothing. However, some facilities may provide cleaning services for your scrubs should they become obviously contaminated with blood or other body fluids. Also, your employer may suggest that you remove obviously soiled clothing and change into a clean set of employer-provided scrubs. Shoe requirements are different per employer, though typically no open-toed shoes should be worn in the healthcare setting.[2]

Cleaning Equipment

Sonographers must maintain a safe and clean environment for patients. Therefore, we are responsible for adequately cleaning all ultrasound and medical equipment, including stretchers, ultrasound machines, and transducers. There are three levels of infection control that the sonographer can conduct on a daily basis: **sanitization**, disinfection, and **sterilization**. Sanitization is the lowest level of infection control. It includes the use of soap or detergent, warm water, and manual friction. Sanitation of visibly dirty, dusty, or contaminated items should be performed routinely.

The next highest level of infection control includes the use of disinfectants, such as germicides, that inactivate virtually all recognized pathogenic microorganisms except for spores on inanimate objects.[4] Examples of disinfectants used in the hospital setting include bleach-based cleaners, alcohol-based cleaners, iodine, phenols, and hydrogen peroxide. Employers typically provide appropriate cleaning solutions for medical equipment such as stretchers and positioning cushions.

Transducers used externally—against any part of the patient's skin—should also be routinely cleaned with a disinfectant solution. One study demonstrated that out of 191 patients, 60% had infected the transducer with some form of pathogenic microorganism.[14] Some of the most common microorganisms transmitted are strains of *Staphylococcus aureus*, with one study finding that three out of every four transducers tested positive for MRSA.[14]

A common cleaner used to disinfect transducers between examinations is T-Spray II. This type of cleaner should be sprayed on the transducer and the cord. Some institutions may use disinfectant wipes for transducer cleaning. Follow the instructions offered by the manufacturers, and always clean transducers, including the transducer cords, before and after each sonographic examination. Gel bottles may harbor bacteria, especially on the tips.[14] In order to prevent the spread of contaminants from the gel bottle to the patient, some institutions have resolved to use individual gel packets for each examination.

Sound Off

Follow the instructions for probe cleaning offered by the manufacturers, and always clean transducers, including the transducer cords, before and after each sonographic examination.

Sterilization is the complete destruction of all microorganisms, including spores, on inanimate objects. Endocavity transducers must undergo sterilization, the highest level of infection control. Endocavity transducers include endovaginal (transvaginal), endorectal, and transesophageal transducers. Though all of these transducers require sterilization after each use, the manner in which the transducer is sterilized may vary per facility and is typically specific to manufacturer guidelines. Transducers can be damaged in an autoclave, which uses hot, high-pressure steam. Therefore, sterilization typically includes submerging the transducer in a **high-level chemical disinfectant** for a recommended amount of time. High-level chemical sterilization agents may have name brands such as Cidex OPA, Cidex Plus, and MetriCide, among many others. Some transducer cleaning devices are wall-mounted ultrasound transducer-soaking stations that are capable of sterilizing multiple transducers simultaneously (Fig. 12-22). These sterilization agents must be changed regularly and used for a minimal amount of time as prescribed by the manufacturer to be fully effective.

One of the obligations of the sonographer is to understand the importance of cleaning and sterilizing transducers effectively according to the manufacturer's recommendations. You should also wear suggested PPE equipment when handling and cleaning transducers, as some of the chemicals can elicit physical reactions, such as headaches and respiratory troubles. For this reason, these sterilization solutions should also be located in well-ventilated rooms, labeled properly, and handled with extreme caution.

Sound Off

You should wear suggested PPE equipment when handling and cleaning transducers.

Nonsterile Probe Covers

During an **endocavity sonogram**, a transducer or probe cover should be utilized. A probe cover is a latex or non-latex drape in which the ultrasound transducer is placed before a sonographic examination. Probe covers may be referred to as sheaths or condoms as well (Fig. 12-23). They should be used for all endovaginal and endorectal examinations and, in some cases, other examinations during which the transducer could potentially come in contact with blood or other body fluids, such as translabial or scrotal sonograms. Table 12-8 provides some steps on how to drape a transducer with a non-sterile probe cover. If latex probe covers are used, it is important to ask the patient if he or she has any history of latex allergy prior to the examination. If so, do not use a latex probe cover.

Before placing the probe cover on the transducer, ultrasound gel should be placed within the probe cover to prevent any artifacts caused by air. Some probe cover manufacturers have created

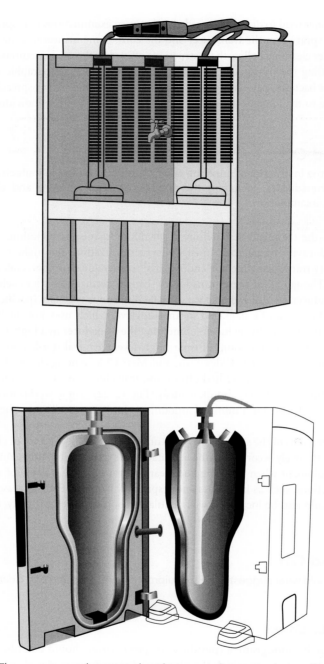

Figure 12-22. There are several means whereby a transducer may be sterilized, including a wall unit (**upper image**) and tabletop unit (**lower image**).

covers that include a small amount of gel within them. A lubricating gel should be placed on the outside of the probe cover over the end of the transducer before the transducer is inserted into the patient. Some institutions may require the use of sterile gel on the outside of the probe cover. This gel provides a lubricant to help ease patient discomfort during endocavity examinations. Probe covers have been known to fail.[15] Therefore, though a probe cover should be routinely utilized for endocavity imaging, the transducer must be sterilized anyway following the examination. Some studies have

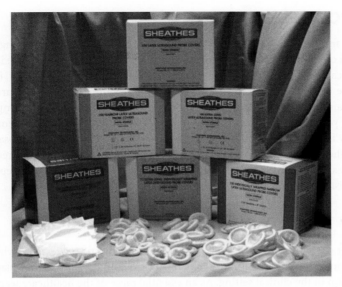

Figure 12-23. Image of varying types of transducer probe covers. Image used with permission from Sheathes.

shown that condoms are superior to commercially available probe covers for covering the transducer effectively.[15]

Sound Off

It is your obligation to familiarize yourself with infection control requirements at each clinical facility that you visit.

Proper Disposal of Examination Waste Items (Appendix 3, Procedure 12-3)

Cleaning up biohazard spills must be done carefully (Appendix 3, Procedure 12-3). All waste materials accumulated as a result of a sonographic examination, such as gloves, probe covers, paper towels, and cloth towels, should be placed in an appropriate container for disposal. Other non-reusable PPEs, such as masks and gowns, should also be disposed of according to the institution's guidelines. Items that are visually contaminated with blood or other body fluids must typically be placed in biohazard waste bags. Cloth towels soiled only by gel can be cleaned and should be placed in a dirty bin, while paper towels can be disposed of in a trash can.

TABLE 12-8	Steps for draping a transducer with a non-sterile probe cover

1. Put on a clean pair of non-sterile gloves.
2. Retrieve the sterilized transducer.
3. Obtain a probe cover, and visually inspect the probe cover for obvious tears. Do not use a damaged probe cover.
4. Squeeze a small amount of acoustic gel into the probe cover.
5. Place the probe cover over the transducer by gently rolling the cover down, being mindful to completely cover the transducer face with gel to prevent artifacts.
6. Stabilize the probe cover end near the transducer handle by holding it in place with a rubber band or provided means.

WHAT IF YOU ARE EXPOSED?

As you can see from the reading, healthcare workers are exposed to a wide range of pathogenic microorganisms on a daily basis. Sonographers and students must be aware of the infection control plan in the clinical setting. If you rotate to another clinical facility while in school, it is your obligation to be aware of how each clinical facility handles infection control. If you are exposed to an undocumented airborne disease, such as tuberculosis, it is the obligation of your employer or clinical facility to notify you. The facility will most likely want to monitor your health to ensure that you do not contract any illnesses as a result of the occurrence. The proper care and disposal of needles will be discussed in the following chapter, but for infection control purposes, if you receive an accidental needlestick, you should immediately report the occurrence to your clinical preceptor, sonography program administration, and employee health department of the facility.

SUMMARY

The sonographer certainly plays an important part in the diagnostic process. But while we are caring for patients, we must also be mindful of infection control and the part we can play to prevent the spread of infection in the clinical setting. As an essential piece of the healthcare team, our responsibility is to be aware of how pathogenic microorganisms are spread, how they are managed or eliminated, and how we can play a role in breaking the chain of infection. Although this chapter provided an overview of several pathogenic microorganisms you may encounter as a sonographer, you must be aware that you may be exposed to many other types of microorganisms in the workplace. Be cognizant of the basic practices used to prevent the spread of infection, and also be aware that the standards and protocols used to prevent the transmission of diseases are ever-evolving. Remember, always put patient safety first, and understand that fighting infections in the workplace is something that will impact your health and the health of your patients.

REFERENCES

1. Timby BK. *Fundamental Nursing Skills and Concepts*. 10th ed. Philadelphia, PA: Lippincott Williams & Wilkins; 2013.
2. Dutton AG, Linn-Watson TA, Torres LS. *Torres' Patient Care in Imaging Technology*. 8th ed. Philadelphia, PA: Lippincott Williams & Wilkins; 2013.
3. 2007 guidelines for isolation precautions: preventing transmission of infectious agents in healthcare settings. Retrieved from http://www.cdc.gov/hicpac/pdf/isolation/Isolation2007.pdf
4. Molle EA, Kronenberger J, West-Stack C. *Lippincott Williams and Wilkins' Clinical Medical Assisting*. 2nd ed. Philadelphia, PA: Lippincott Williams & Wilkins; 2005.
5. Center for Disease Control and Prevention. Types of healthcare-associated infections. Retrieved from http://www.cdc.gov/HAI/infectionTypes.html
6. Center for Disease Control and Prevention. Catheter-associated urinary tract infections. Retrieved from http://www.cdc.gov/HAI/ca_uti/uti.html
7. National action plan to prevent health care-associated infections: road map to elimination. Retrieved from http://www.health.gov/hai/prevent_hai.asp#hai_plan
8. Center for Disease Control and Prevention. General information about MRSA in healthcare settings. Retrieved from http://www.cdc.gov/mrsa/healthcare/index.html
9. CDC Vital Signs 2011. Making Health Care Safer. Retrieved from http://www.cdc.gov/vitalsigns/pdf/2011-03-vitalsigns.pdf
10. Mayo Clinic. *C. difficile* infection. Retrieved from http://www.mayoclinic.org/diseases-conditions/c-difficile/basics/definition/con-20029664
11. Center for Disease Control and Prevention. Stop sticks campaign. Retrieved from http://www.cdc.gov/niosh/stop-sticks/bloodborne.html
12. Guide to infection prevention for outpatient settings: minimum expectations for safe care. Retrieved from http://www.cdc.gov/HAI/settings/outpatient/outpatient-care-gl-standard-precautions.html

13. Bedford DJ, Allen MM. *LWW's Visual Atlas of Medical Assisting*. Philadelphia, PA: Lippincott Williams & Wilkins; 2008.

14. Ridge C. Sonographers and the fight against nosocomial infections: how are we doing? *Journal of Diagnostic Medical Sonography* 2005;21(7):7–11.

15. Guidelines for disinfection and sterilization in healthcare facilities; 2008. Retrieved from http://www.cdc.gov/hicpac/pdf/Disinfection_Sterilization/Pages17_21Disinfection_Nov_2008.pdf

Thinking Critically

1. Inquire at your clinical facility about the institution's infection control plan, and document how infection control is conducted. Read the plan, and understand what to do if you are exposed to infection.

2. How are transducer cleaning and sterilization performed in your clinical facility? Understand the steps in the process of sterilization.

3. Locate personal protective equipment provided in your clinical facility. Practice putting on gloves, gown, mask, hair covering, and shoe covers in preparation for cleaning up biohazard spills.

Chapter 12
Review Questions

1. **Which of the following is associated with hemoptysis?**
   a. HIV
   b. Hepatitis
   c. TB
   d. HBV

2. **Which of the following is associated with the clinical finding of jaundice?**
   a. HIV
   b. Hepatitis
   c. *C. difficile*
   d. MRSA

3. **Which of the following is the smallest known organism that can cause disease in humans?**
   a. Virus
   b. Parasite
   c. Bacterium
   d. Fungus

4. **Which of the following is the first link in the cycle of infection?**
   a. Mode of transmission
   b. Portal of entry
   c. Portal of exit
   d. Reservoir

5. **At what time would an alcohol-based hand rub be suboptimal?**
   a. Before performing a sonogram
   b. After performing a sonogram
   c. When your hands are visibly soiled
   d. After removing gloves

6. Which of the following modes of transmission is based on physically touching an infected person?
   a. Direct contact
   b. Indirect contact
   c. Droplet
   d. Airborne

7. Which of the following would not be considered a portal of entry?
   a. Nose
   b. Mouth
   c. Wound
   d. Hands

8. Which of the following patients would most likely be in an immunocompromised state?
   a. An athlete
   b. Middle-aged male
   c. Child undergoing chemotherapy
   d. Pregnant female

9. Which of the following would be the least likely healthcare-associated infection?
   a. Urinary tract infection
   b. HIV
   c. MRSA
   d. Ventilator-associated infections

10. Which of the following is transmitted via an airborne fashion?
    a. MRSA
    b. Malaria
    c. Tuberculosis
    d. Chlamydia

11. Which of the following is not a virus?
    a. Hepatitis
    b. Influenza
    c. Toxoplasmosis
    d. Measles

12. Which of the following is a sexually transmitted disease?
    a. Chlamydia
    b. Mumps
    c. Toxoplasmosis
    d. Thrush

13. What is the most likely manner by which a healthcare worker would be exposed to HBV?
    a. Needle
    b. Airborne
    c. Droplet
    d. Enteric

14. **Enteric precaution is a form of**
    a. airborne precaution
    b. contact precaution
    c. droplet precaution
    d. foodborne precaution

15. **Which of the following personal care issues would be an appropriate means to decrease the likelihood of passing an infectious microorganism to a patient?**
    a. Limiting jewelry to a solitary wedding band
    b. Putting on acrylic nails to prevent spreading infection
    c. Wearing the same pair of gloves all day
    d. Wearing the same labcoat every day and leaving it at work

16. **In which situation would a non-sterile probe cover need to be utilized?**
    a. Right upper quadrant sonogram
    b. Obstetric sonogram
    c. Endovaginal sonogram
    d. Transthoracic echocardiogram

17. **Transducer sterilization is best defined as the**
    a. scrubbing of a transducer with alcohol-based sanitizers to destroy most pathogenic organisms.
    b. germicidal disinfecting of a transducer to remove most pathogenic organisms.
    c. cleaning of a transducer to sanitize all external components, including the cord.
    d. complete destruction of all microorganisms, including spores, on the transducer.

18. **Which of the following is a bacterium that releases toxins into the bowel?**
    a. MRSA
    b. VRE
    c. Tuberculosis
    d. *C. difficile*

19. **Which of the following is defined as the practices that are used to render objects or areas free of pathogenic organisms?**
    a. Medical asepsis
    b. Surgical asepsis
    c. Disinfection
    d. Colonization

20. **Which of the following is not a bloodborne pathogen?**
    a. HCV
    b. Tuberculosis
    c. HIV
    d. HBV

Invasive Procedures and Surgical Asepsis

CHAPTER OBJECTIVES

- Understand the rules of surgical asepsis for invasive procedures.
- Comprehend the importance of maintaining a sterile field.
- Be capable of correctly opening a sterile tray.
- Be skilled at establishing a sterile field and correctly donning sterile personal equipment.
- Appreciate the sonographer's role as part of the team in the surgical suite.

KEY TERMS

Amniocentesis – a surgical procedure in which amniotic fluid is extracted for genetic testing or removed when there is an accumulation of excessive amniotic fluid

Ascites – a collection of abdominal fluid within the peritoneal cavity

Basic metabolic panel – a blood test that provides information concerning the glucose level, electrolytes and fluid balance, and kidney function

Complete blood count – blood test that provides information about the number and types of cells in the blood

Colostomy – a surgical opening in the abdomen that allows the colon to empty into an attached bag

Fenestrated drape – a sterile drape with an opening that is placed over the sterile surgical site

Ileostomy – a surgical opening in the abdomen that allows the ileum to empty into an attached bag

International normalized ratio – a calculation made to standardize prothrombin time

Invasive procedures – medical procedures that involve penetration of body tissues

Needle guide – a sterile device placed on the transducer to aid in needle placement during an invasive procedure

Paracentesis – an invasive procedure that uses a needle to drain abdominal fluid for either diagnostic or therapeutic reasons

Partial thromboplastin time – a blood test that looks at how long it takes for blood to clot

Pericardiocentesis – surgical procedure that utilizes a needle and catheter to drain fluid around the heart

Pleural effusion – the abnormal accumulation of fluid in the pleural space

Prothrombin time – a blood test that measures the time it takes for the liquid portion (plasma) of the blood to clot

Sharps container – a specified container in which to place sharp objects, like needles, in order to prevent needlesticks

Skin preparation – procedure to remove microorganisms by mechanical and chemical means to reduce the likelihood of infection

Sterile – free from living germs and microorganisms

Sterile field – a special area that is free of microorganisms

Sterile gel – ultrasound gel that is pre-packed and considered free of microorganisms

Sterile gloves – gloves that are pre-packed and free of microorganisms

Surgical asepsis – the complete removal of microorganisms and their spores from the surface of an object

Surgical hand antisepsis – the complete removal of microorganisms from the hands and arms

Surgical scrub – see surgical hand antisepsis

Surgical suite – a group of one or more operating rooms and adjacent rooms

Thoracentesis – an invasive procedure that uses a needle to drain fluid from the pleural cavity for either diagnostic or therapeutic reasons

INTRODUCTION

The sonographer plays an important role before and during invasive procedures. These procedures require the sonographer to be proficient at establishing a sterile field, donning sterile gear, and maintaining a sterile environment. This chapter will provide an overview of surgical asepsis, the establishment of a sterile field for invasive procedures, and sonography in the operating room. The use of sonography during invasive procedures is vital because it provides the physician with a non-ionizing, realtime demonstration of anatomy. Our readily available and easy-to-use technology ultimately instills in the physician more confidence during biopsies and other invasive procedures. This confidence will lead to a sufficient course of action and in the end provide the patient with valuable therapy and/or an accurate diagnosis.

SURGICAL ASEPSIS

Several systems or parts of the body are considered **sterile**, including the blood, brain, bone, heart, and vascular system. **Surgical asepsis**, or sterile technique, is the complete removal of microorganisms and their spores from the surface of an object. It applies to all **invasive procedures** performed within the sonography department and surgical procedures performed in the operating room that require a **sterile field**. Invasive procedures are medical procedures that involve penetration of body tissues.[1] Examples of invasive procedures include **amniocentesis, paracentesis, thoracentesis, pericardiocentesis**, intravascular ultrasound, joint injections, line placement guidance, mass biopsies, and organ biopsies (Table 13-1).

Surgical asepsis is also required for the sonographer to perform minimal wound care, though this is typically beyond the scope of practice for a sonographer. Also, for patients who have surgical, wound, or burn bandages, or have an ostomy, like a **colostomy** or **ileostomy**, the sonographer should attempt to examine the area adjacent to the surgical bandages without disrupting them if possible in order to prevent the spread of infection to the area. However, if you must remove surgical bandages to perform the sonogram, always follow the institution's guidelines for the sonographer. You should never remove surgical bandages or replace bandages without the direct permission and supervision of the patient's physician. Care should also be taken if wound drainage equipment is encountered. Be careful to not dislodge drains and tubing as you scan or assist your patient into varying positions. Surgical asepsis must be maintained throughout the exam if you are required to scan open wounds.

TABLE 13-1	Invasive procedures commonly performed in the sonography department	
Common Invasive Procedure	**Explanation**	**Figure**
Amniocentesis	This procedure requires the use of a needle and catheter guided by sonography to sample amniotic fluid around the fetus for genetic testing or to relieve the buildup of excess fluid.	Figure 13-1
Paracentesis	Sonography is used to evaluate for excessive abdominal fluid (**ascites**) and provide guidance for needle and catheter placement for drainage.	Figure 13-2
Thoracentesis	Sonography is used to evaluate for excessive pleural fluid (**pleural effusion**) and provide guidance for needle and catheter placement for drainage.	Figure 13-3
Mass biopsy	Focal masses, such as breast or thyroid masses, are biopsied with the use of sonographic guidance.	Figure 13-4
Organ biopsy	An organ biopsy, such as a liver or renal biopsy, may be performed using sonography to evaluate the function of the organ and to sample for disease.	Figure 13-5

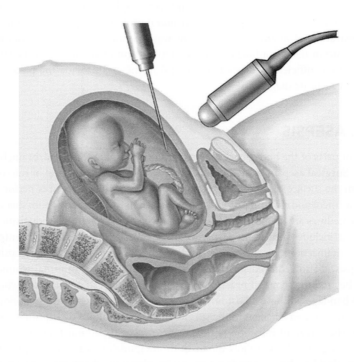

Figure 13-1. Amniocentesis. An amniocentesis can be performed for various reasons under ultrasound guidance. The amniotic fluid can be removed for therapeutic reasons or for diagnostic genetic screening. In some cases, fluid can also be instilled into the amniotic cavity if the fluid around the baby is too low.

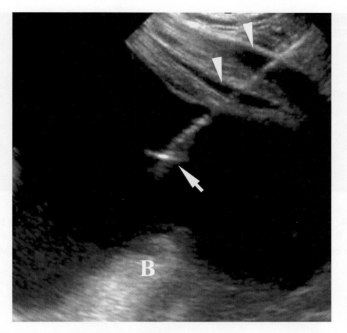

Figure 13-2. Paracentesis. This sonogram demonstrates the needle (*arrow*) passing through the skin (*arrowheads*) and into the abdominal fluid, which is often referred to as ascites. When performing the paracentesis, the physician will try to avoid puncturing the bowel (B). A paracentesis is often performed for both diagnostic and therapeutic reasons.

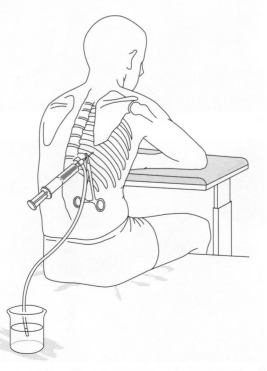

Figure 13-3. Thoracentesis. The patient often sits upright on the side of the stretcher and rests against a table for a thoracentesis. A needle and catheter are inserted into the pleural fluid space, and the fluid is extracted into a collecting container, and in many cases, a small amount of fluid is obtained for diagnostic purposes.

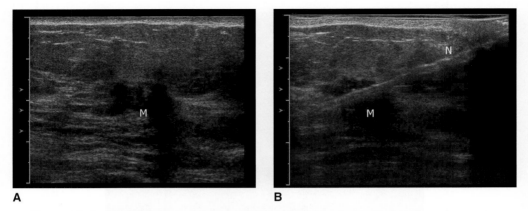

A   **B**

Figure 13-4. Core biopsy. **A.** A sonogram is performed prior to the biopsy to locate the mass (M). **B.** Under sonographic guidance, a core biopsy of the mass is performed. The needle can be seen (N) passing through the tissue and through the mass (M). The tissue is removed for testing.

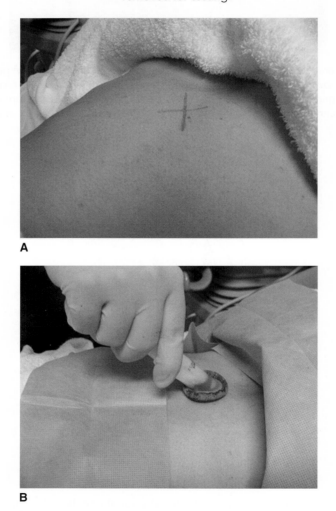

A

B

Figure 13-5. Liver biopsy. **A.** Sonography is used. An "X" is placed over the best location for sampling. **B.** A sterile setup is performed, and the area is then cleaned with an antiseptic solution and covered with sterile drapes.

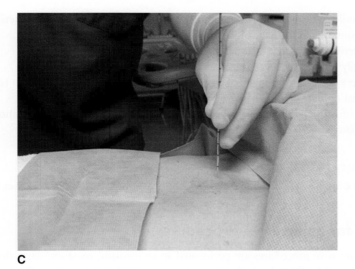

C

Figure 13-5. (*Continued*) **C.** The biopsy gun is lined up with the "X" before beginning the biopsy. The patient is typically asked to cease breathing temporarily.

The Rules of Surgical Asepsis

Several rules of surgical asepsis apply whenever an invasive procedure or sterile procedure is performed[1,2]:

1. Always know which areas and items are sterile and which are not.
2. If the sterility of an object is questionable, the object is considered non-sterile.
3. Always keep sterile objects and persons away from those that are non-sterile.
4. If you recognize that an item has become non-sterile, act immediately.
5. A sterile drape must be placed on a non-sterile tabletop to initialize a sterile field.
6. To be considered sterile, a person must don sterile gloves and a sterile gown.
7. Any sterile instrument or sterile area that touches a non-sterile object or person is considered contaminated and removed from the sterile field.
8. A sterile field must be created just prior to use, and the sterile field must not be left unattended. If a sterile field is left unattended, it is considered non-sterile.
9. A non-sterile person does not reach across a sterile field.
10. A sterile person should not lean across a sterile field.
11. A sterile field ends at the level of the tabletop or at the waist of the sterile person's gown. Anything that drops below the tabletop or the sterile person's waistline is considered non-sterile.
12. The only parts of the sterile gown considered sterile are the areas from the waist to the shoulders in the front and the sleeves from 2 in above the elbow to the cuffs.
13. Cuffs of a sterile gown are non-sterile, and therefore, they must always be covered by sterile gloves.
14. The edges of a sterile wrapper are not considered sterile.
15. Sterile drapes are placed by a sterile person. The sterile person places the drapes on the area closest to him or her first to protect the sterile gown.
16. A sterile person must remain within the sterile area.
17. If one sterile person must pass another, they must pass back to back.
18. The sterile person faces the sterile field and keeps sterile gloves above the waist in front of the chest.
19. Any sterile material or pack that becomes damp or wet is considered non-sterile.
20. When pouring sterile solution onto a sterile field, pour off a small amount of solution (perhaps in a trashcan) before the remainder is poured into the sterile container or onto the tray.

21. When a sterile solution is to be poured into a container on a sterile field, a sterile person must place the container at the edge of the sterile field.
22. Preserve sterility of an item by touching it only with another sterile item.
23. Any partially unwrapped sterile package is considered non-sterile.
24. Always check the expiration date of items. A commercially packed sterile item is only sterile up to its expiration date.
25. Coughing, sneezing, or excessive talking over a sterile filed leads to contamination and the field must be changed.

Sound Off

If an object's sterility is in question, then you must assume the object is not sterile.

Preparing for an Invasive Procedure

Though some invasive procedures are performed spontaneously, most are scheduled days or even weeks in advance. This allows for both patient and sonographer preparation. The patient may have unique preparation provisions prior to an invasive procedure, including the temporary cessation of blood thinners and other medications. Laboratory tests are often required prior to an invasive procedure, including a **complete blood count** (CBC), **prothrombin time** (PT), **international normalized ratio** (INR), **partial thromboplastin time** (PTT), and **basic metabolic panel** (BMP). These blood tests provide a good analysis of the patient's general health and, in the case of PT, PTT, and INR, assess the patient's ability to stop bleeding during and after the procedure.

Sonographers are often asked to gather information, including the aforementioned laboratory results, prior to the invasive procedure. Sonographers may also be required to gather a clinical history and complete a patient questionnaire prior to the examination. At some facilities, the sonographer may be required to perform a baseline analysis of the patient's overall health, including blood pressure, pulse, and respirations (see Chapter 10). Documentation is a vital part of an invasive procedure. The physician completes an informed consent form with the patient, providing him or her with an explanation of the procedure, the possible side effects during the procedure, and any potential future complications that may result from the procedure. Though sonographers do not typically provide the informed consent, they may be asked to witness the signing of an informed consent document prior to the examination. Sonographers are involved with room preparation and may be required to perform a sonogram prior to the procedure. The following sections will provide some insight into skin preparation, sterile packs and field, sterile gloving, draping the transducer with a sterile probe cover, and needle care and disposal.

Sound Off

Before an invasive procedure, the sonographer may be asked to perform a basic assessment of the patient's vital signs, including pulse, respirations, and blood pressure.

Skin Preparation and Draping (Appendix 3, Procedure 13-1)

Occasionally, sonographers may be responsible for cleaning a surgical site prior to an invasive procedure. Patient skin preparation for invasive procedures includes the possibility of scrubbing the skin and shaving the surgical area to remove hair. The purpose of this **skin preparation** is to remove microorganisms by mechanical and chemical means to reduce the likelihood of infection.[1] In many cases, especially if shaving is required, the physician or a nurse may perform skin prep. Procedure 13-1 in Appendix 3 provides the steps for skin preparation for a sterile procedure (Fig. 13-6).

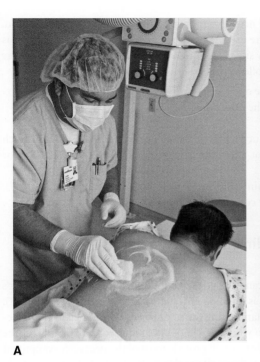

A

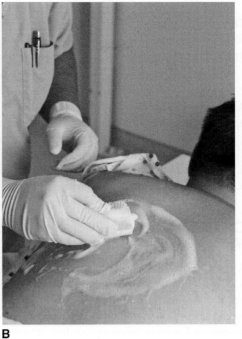

B

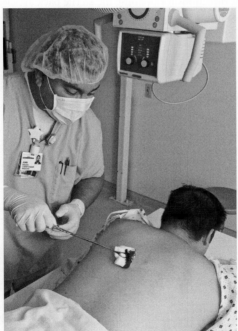

C

Figure 13-6. Sonographers may have to perform skin preparation **(A, B, and C)** prior to an invasive procedure. See Appendix 3, Procedure 13-1, for detailed instructions.

Following skin preparation, sterile drapes may need to be applied to provide a barrier to infection. Though drapes vary, typically single-use drapes are used. Sometimes, a **fenestrated drape**, which has an opening, is used around the surgical or biopsy site. If a sonographer must place sterile drapes, he or she obtains the drapes and sterile gloves and follows these steps:

1. Place the pack of sterile drapes on a table to be opened.
2. Open the pack of sterile drapes according to the directions.
3. Put on sterile gloves.
4. Pick up the first drape, holding the drape in such a manner that your sterile gloves do not touch any potentially contaminated objects. Do not allow the drape to fall below the waist level or touch your uniform.
5. Drop the drape in place, and do not move it again as the underside is now contaminated (Fig. 13-7).
6. Add additional drapes as needed. Remove any contaminated drapes.

Opening a Sterile Pack and Adding Items to a Sterile Field (Appendix 3, Procedure 13-2)

A sterile field is a microorganism-free area that can hold sterile supplies.[3] One of the sonographer's fundamental jobs prior to an invasive procedure is opening a sterile pack or sterile tray (Fig. 13-8). The primary goal is to open the pack without contaminating the sterile field. Commercially manufactured sterile packs are unique to the procedure, so you must choose the required pack or tray for the procedure. For most invasive procedures, the sterile tray will provide most of the necessary equipment for the procedure. Typically, directions for opening the sterile pack are clearly printed on the outside of the pack. However, Procedure 13-2 in Appendix 3 provides the steps for opening a sterile pack.

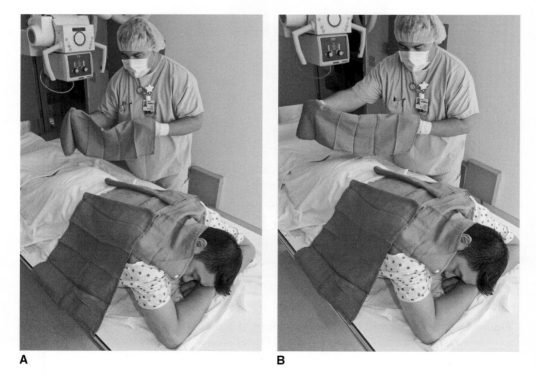

A   **B**

Figure 13-7. Draping a sterile field. Sonographers may have to perform draping of a sterile field prior to an invasive procedure. **A.** Folds of sterile towels must face operative site. **B.** Pick up first drape, holding it to protect sterile gloves.

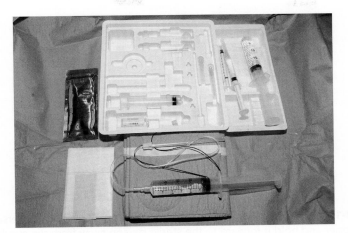

Figure 13-8. A sterile tray that includes a pack of sterile gel (top left of image).

Sonographers will often have to add items to a sterile field or a sterile tray, such as a sterile probe cover or additional needles. To complete this task, follow these steps:

1. Open the package as directed in Procedure 13-2 in Appendix 3.
2. Take the item to the sterile field, and from a distance, drop or flip it onto the field (Fig. 13-9). Do not touch the sterile field, and do not let the wrapper touch the field.
3. To pass a sterile object to a sterile person, grasp the underside of the wrapper and hold it forward to the sterile person so that he or she may grasp it without touching the outside of the wrapper. Do this away from the field, so that the item will not fall into the field (Fig. 13-10).
4. To add a liquid such as Betadine or sterile water to a sterile tray, you should open the container, empty a small amount into a trashcan, and then squeeze some into the sterile field where needed (Fig. 13-11).

Sound Off
One of the sonographer's fundamental jobs prior to an invasive procedure is opening a sterile pack or sterile tray.

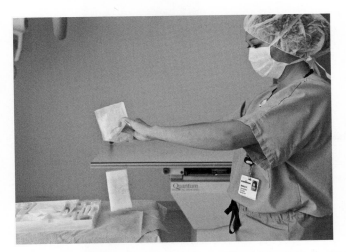

Figure 13-9. Once the packet is open containing the sterile object, take the item to the sterile field and drop it on sterile field from a distance, being careful to not let the wrapper come in contact with the sterile field.

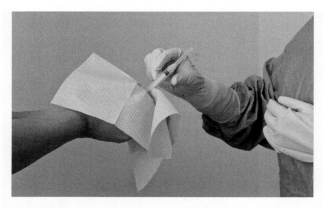

Figure 13-10. To pass a sterile object to a sterile person, grasp the underside of the wrapper and hold it forward to the sterile person away from the sterile field.

Sterile Gloving

Sonographers may be required to put on **sterile gloves** during an invasive procedure. In these situations, sonographers typically are not required to put on a sterile gown also. The sonographer should wash his or her hands and follow these steps[1]:

1. Open the wrapper as directed for opening sterile packs (see the "Opening a Sterile Pack" section). Sterile gloves are packed folded down at the cuff and powdered so they may be put on easily.
2. Glove the dominant hand first. Assuming that the left hand is dominant, pick up the left glove with the right hand at the folded cuff and slide the left hand into the glove, leaving the cuff folded down (Fig. 13-12).
3. When the glove is over the hand, leave it and pick up the right glove with the gloved left hand under the fold (Fig. 13-13).
4. Pull the glove over your hand and over the cuff of the gown (if you are wearing one) (Fig. 13-14).
5. Place the fingers of the gloved right hand under the cuff of the left glove and pull it over the cuff of the gown if you are wearing one (Fig. 13-15).[1]

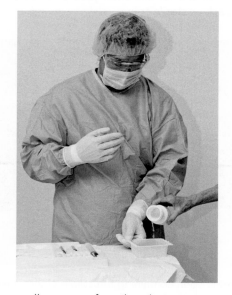

Figure 13-11. Empty a small amount of sterile solution into a trashcan, and then, dispense some into the sterile field where needed.

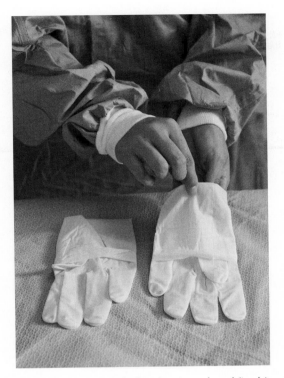

Figure 13-12. Pick up the folded glove with the dominant hand (in this case, the left), leaving cuff folded.

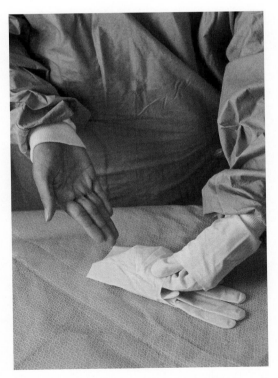

Figure 13-13. When the glove is over the hand, leave it and pick up the other glove with the gloved hand under the fold.

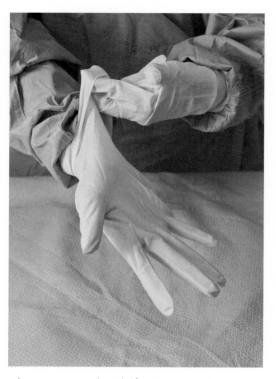

Figure 13-14. Pull the glove over your hand. If you are wearing a gown, the cuff of the gown should be covered by the glove as well.

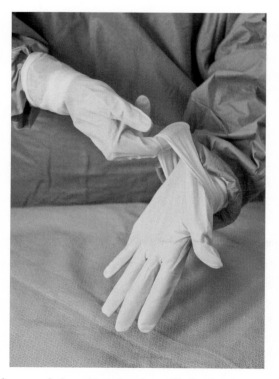

Figure 13-15. Place fingers of gloved hand under cuff of right glove, and pull it over the cuff of the gown also (if wearing one).

Sound Off

You should practice how to don sterile gloves in preparation for a sterile procedure. Sterile gloves come in different sizes, so find out which size works best for you.

Draping a Transducer with a Sterile Probe Cover and Needle Guide

The previous chapter discussed the importance of utilizing a non-sterile probe cover for endocavity sonograms. For invasive procedures in which surgical asepsis is required, a sterile probe cover should be used (Fig. 13-16). Sterile probe covers are pre-packed and can easily be added to a sterile field (see the "Opening a Sterile Pack and Adding Items to a Sterile Field" section). Draping the transducer with a sterile probe cover requires two people: a sterile and a non-sterile person. The steps are as follows:

1. The sterile person must obtain the sterile probe cover that has been placed in the sterile field by the non-sterile person.
2. He or she must then unroll the probe cover slightly. **Sterile gel** or non-sterile gel will need to be placed into the probe cover to prevent artifacts.
3. The non-sterile person must grab the transducer by the cord, slightly away from the base of the transducer.
4. Having the sterile person hold the probe cover down, the non-sterile person places the transducer into the probe cover, not allowing the transducer to touch the sterile person's gloves. Some individuals may prefer to unroll the probe cover over their sterile glove, inside out, and then grab the transducer.
5. The sterile individual can grab the covered transducer once it is completely covered and continue to roll down the cover over the cord as needed. The non-sterile person does not drop the rest of the cord until instructed by the sterile person.
6. The sterile probe cover is typically held in place with provided tape fasteners or a sterile rubber band.
7. A sterile **needle guide** may need to be placed on the outside of the sterile probe cover over the transducer (Fig. 13-17).

Sound Off

Sterile probe covers are used in the sonography department and in the operating room.

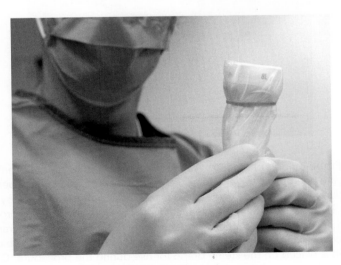

Figure 13-16. Sterile probe cover.

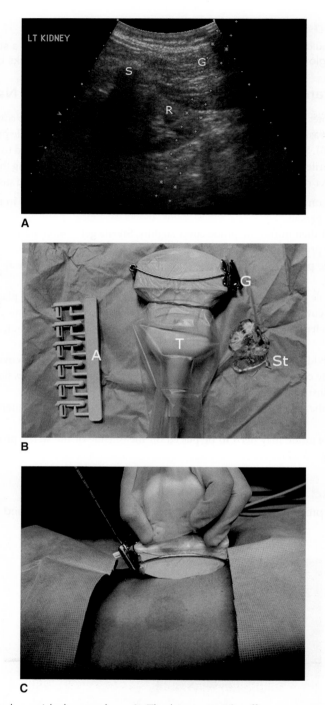

Figure 13-17. Probe-guided procedure. **A.** The biopsy guide offers a representative pathway by which the needle will travel during the procedure. Occasionally, depending upon the procedure, inverting the image and transducer facilitates many biopsy procedures. R, kidney; S, rib shadow. **B.** The transducer (T) is covered with a sterile probe cover for the procedure. The reusable sterile biopsy bracket (G) is placed on the transducer over the sterile cover. The disposable sterile needle guides (A) clips onto the biopsy bracket. Sterile gel (St) is placed on the sterile drape for use during the procedure. **C.** The needle is inserted through the needle guide, into the organ, and a biopsy of the tissue is obtained.

Syringe Assistance and Needle Disposal

Physicians may require assistance when local anesthesia administration is needed or if another liquid such as saline is required to be drawn into a syringe. Most often, a sterile syringe and needle are provided within the sterile pack or tray. Regardless of the fluid needed for the procedure, always show the physician the label of the fluid on the vial before you assist in filling a syringe. If the fluid is located outside of the sterile field, you should open the vial and clean the top with an alcohol swab. Hold the vial steady in one hand while supporting it at the wrist with the other hand. Hold it at an angle so that the physician can insert the needle into the center of the vial and draw the required amount of liquid into the syringe (Fig. 13-18).[4] Sonographers may also be required to obtain needles for biopsies. The gauge of the needle indicates the size of the lumen of the needle. As the gauge number increases, the actual diameter of the needle decreases. Typically, higher-gauge needles are utilized for thyroid biopsies and small structures, while lower-gauge needles are used for large organ biopsies, such as renal and liver biopsies.

Following invasive procedures, it is the duty of the sonographer to dispose of sharp objects, like syringes with needles and scalpels, appropriately. Used needles should not be recapped but rather discarded in a red biohazard **sharps container** (Fig. 13-19). The sterile tray will have many unused instruments and accessories that should be placed in the sharps container, such as broken vials, needles, and scalpels. Never toss sharps into a trashcan. All blood-soiled gauze and instruments should be discarded in a biohazard bag or container.

Sound Off

Used needles should not be recapped but rather discarded in a red biohazard sharps container.

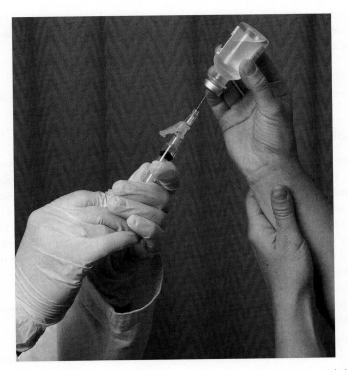

Figure 13-18. The sonographer should first allow the physician to read the vial then hold the vial containing the liquid downward, supporting that wrist with the other hand. Hold the vial steadily and firmly so the physician can insert the needle and withdraw the fluid.

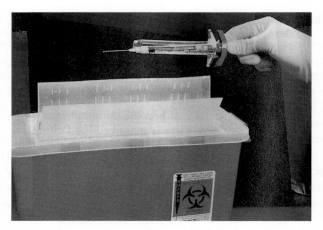

Figure 13-19. Sharps disposal. All sharps, whether used or unused, should be disposed of properly after the procedure by placing them in a plastic puncture-resistant sharps container like this one. There will always be a biohazard symbol on the sharps container.

SONOGRAPHY IN THE OPERATING ROOM

Sonography is occasionally performed in the operating room, so awareness of surgical asepsis is vital in preventing contamination and disruption to the surgical process. The **surgical suite** has three zones that typically are clearly marked[1]:

Zone 1: Unrestricted zone. No special clothing requirements.

Zone 2: Persons must be dressed in scrub dress with hair and shoes covered.

Zone 3: Restricted zone that requires persons to wear surgical clothing (provided by the employer), shoe covers, and masks. Doors are kept closed. Those directly involved in the surgery must wear sterile gowns and sterile gloves. This is referred to as "being scrubbed."

Sound Off

Remember to practice strict surgical asepsis in the operating room at all times.

The Surgical Scrub (Appendix 3, Procedure 13-4)

The sonographer is typically not the sterile individual involved in an invasive procedure or in the operating room. However, you should be capable of performing a **surgical scrub**, also referred to as **surgical hand antisepsis**, in case the circumstances call for it. Before entering the surgical suite, the sonographer must change into surgical scrubs, hair covering, shoe coverings, and a mask. The mask should cover the nose and mouth, while the hair covering should completely cover the hair and ears. All rings must be removed for surgical scrubbing. In some special situations, like entering the intensive care nursery, extensive hand and arm scrubbing may be necessary as well. For the sonographer, the procedure is slightly different, because your hands will perform the sonogram. Never forget to clean your transducer and the cord between patients.

Though the procedure and requirements may differ slightly between institutions, the following steps will most likely be adequate[2]:

1. Place a sterile glove, gown, and towel packet close by within a sterile field.
2. Approach the sink. With the provided knee or foot controls, adjust the water temperature and water flow.
3. Obtain a scrub brush packet. Many brushes have prefilled antimicrobial soap within them.
4. The hands and forearms should be wet to approximately 2 in above the elbow. Hands should be held up to allow the water to drain downward toward the elbow. This allows the water to drain from the cleanest to dirtiest area. Apply the soap.

5. Scrub hands and arms using a firm, rotary motion. Fingers, hands, and arms should be cleaned on all four sides. Begin with the thumb, and then proceed to the other fingers. Next, thoroughly scrub the back side of the hand, the wrist, and all the way up the arm, ending at about 2 in above the elbow. Utilize the orange pick or device to thoroughly clean under the fingernails. The antisepsis will be required to last between two and six minutes, depending upon the type of soap used.

6. Rinse the soap from the hands and arms, and then repeat procedure.

7. When the scrub is complete, dispose of the brush in the provided receptacle. Hold hands up above the waist and higher than the elbows during the surgical scrub.

8. Proceed to obtain the aforementioned sterile towel, sterile gown, and sterile gloves.

9. Pick up the towel, which should be folded on top of the sterile gown, by one corner, and let it drop and unfold in front of you at waist level. Never let the sterile towel touch your clothing.

10. Dry one hand and one arm with each end of the towel. Do not return to areas that have already been dried.

11. When your arms and hands are dry, dispose of the towel in a receptacle. Keep your hands above your waist.

STERILE GOWNING

After the surgical scrub, you may need to put on a sterile gown. The sterile gown should be opened and placed into a sterile field prior to the surgical scrub. To put it on, follow these directions[2]:

1. Grasp the gown and step away from the sterile field.

2. Hold the gown away from the body and allow it to unfold lengthwise. Do not let it come in contact with the floor.

3. Open the gown, and hold it by the shoulder seams. Place both arms into the armholes and wait for a non-sterile person to assist you (Fig. 13-20).

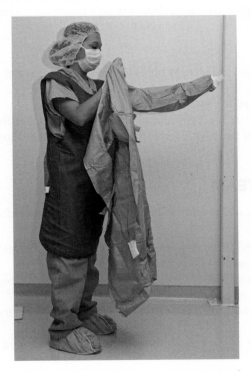

Figure 13-20. Place one arm at a time into the armholes, and wait for a non-sterile person to assist you.

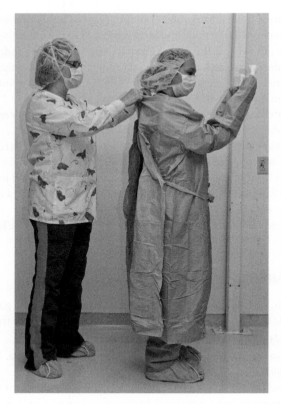

Figure 13-21. He or she will fasten the back of the gown and tie it for you as well and will then pull the gown over shoulders until your hands are exposed. Sterile gloves will be put on last.

4. The non-sterile person will fasten the upper part of the gown first and then the waist ties for you (Fig. 13-21).
5. The gown should be pulled until both hands are exposed.
6. Put on sterile gloves (see the "Sterile Gloving" section). Remember, the sterile gloves should be pulled over the cuff of the gown, because the cuff is not considered sterile.

THE SURGICAL TEAM

In the operating room, the sonographer will encounter various health professionals with unique jobs. They are as follows[1]:

Surgeon: The physician who performs the procedures and who is in charge

Surgical assistant: May be another surgeon or surgical student

Anesthesiologist: Physician in charge of anesthesia who makes decisions about dose and type of anesthesia required for the surgery

Nurse anesthetist: Nurse who administers prescribed anesthesia and monitors the patient throughout the surgery

Circulating nurse: Nurse who oversees the safety of the patient and maintains the surgical environment

Scrub nurse or technician: Assists the surgeon during the procedure and maintains the surgical environment

The role of the sonographer will vary according to the surgery being performed. Prior to entering the room, the sonographer should thoroughly clean the ultrasound machine and transducers using medical asepsis techniques. The sonographer must wear provided surgical scrubs, hair cover, shoe covers, and mask.

Though the sonographer may perform some imaging during surgery, many times, the surgeon performs the scanning. However, the sonographer must be capable of manipulating the machine controls and assisting in the sterile draping of the transducer. Therefore, the sonographer may need to provide sterile gel and a sterile probe cover. All measures must be taken to avoid coming in contact with the sterile field. Occasionally, a radiologist or other physician may accompany the sonographer to the operating room as well.

Sound Off

Have your supplies ready, and prior to entering the operating room, you should thoroughly clean the ultrasound machine and transducers using medical asepsis techniques.

SUMMARY

Every clinical experience is different. Each facility may have differing requirements for the sonographer before and during an invasive procedure. As a student, it is your obligation to discover those requirements and be capable of carrying them out. The need for the sonographer to understand and be capable of practicing surgical asepsis is part of the infection control process in the clinical setting. This chapter provided easy-to-remember steps for several common tasks performed by sonographers. Take the time now to learn the correct process so that in the future you are prepared to execute the vital role that the sonographer plays in invasive and other surgical procedures.

REFERENCES

1. Dutton AG, Linn-Watson TA, Torres LS. *Torres' Patient Care in Imaging Technology*. 8th ed. Philadelphia, PA: Lippincott Williams & Wilkins; 2013.
2. Timby BK. *Fundamental Nursing Skills and Concepts*. 10th ed. Philadelphia, PA: Lippincott Williams & Wilkins; 2013.
3. Adler AM, Carlton RR. *Introduction to Radiologic Sciences and Patient Care*. 4th ed. St Louis, MO: Saunders Elsevier; 2007.
4. Molle EA, Kronenberger J, West-Stack C. *Lippincott Williams & Wilkins' Clinical Medical Assisting*. 2nd ed. Philadelphia, PA: Lippincott Williams & Wilkins; 2005.

Thinking Critically

1. What invasive procedures are performed at your clinical facility? Observe the sonographer as he or she establishes a sterile field for a procedure.
2. Locate the sterile supplies and all necessary supplies for an invasive procedure. Be able to provide assistance to the sonographer and the physician during an invasive procedure.
3. Have someone show you the process for entering the surgical suite at your clinical facility. Explore the requirements for how to prepare to enter the operating room.
4. Practice the surgical hand scrub and donning sterile gloves and sterile gown.

Chapter 13
Review Questions

1. Which of the following is an invasive procedure in which ascites is removed from a patient's abdomen?
   a. Thoracentesis
   b. Paracentesis
   c. Organ biopsy
   d. Pericardiocentesis

2. Which of the following is the complete removal of microorganisms and their spores?
   a. Surgical asepsis
   b. Medical asepsis
   c. Medical antisepsis
   d. Disinfection

3. Which of the following would typically not be needed prior to an invasive procedure?
   a. CBC
   b. PTT
   c. PT
   d. AFP

4. Which of the following is not normally a part of the sonographer's duties during or before an invasive procedure?
   a. To prepare a sterile tray prior to the procedure
   b. To perform a sonogram prior to the procedure
   c. To inject numbing medicine in the surgical site prior to the procedure
   d. To obtain vital signs prior to the procedure

5. Which of the following procedures would not necessitate the use of a sterile probe cover?
   a. Amniocentesis
   b. Endocavity sonogram
   c. Paracentesis
   d. Pericardiocentesis

6. The complete removal of microorganisms from the hands and arms describes
   a. hand asepsis.
   b. medical asepsis.
   c. hand-washing.
   d. surgical hand antisepsis.

7. Which of the following is a blood test that provides information about the number and types of cells found within the patient's blood?
   a. Complete blood count
   b. PTT
   c. Basic metabolic panel
   d. Prothrombin time

8. A device used during an invasive ultrasound procedure that is attached to the transducer to assist in needle placement is referred to as a
   a. needle placer.
   b. needle guide.
   c. transducer lead.
   d. transducer supplanter.

9. Which of the following is described as a medical procedure that involves penetration of body tissues?
   a. Surgical procedure
   b. Invasive procedure
   c. Infiltrative procedure
   d. Therapeutic procedure

10. Fluid that collects within the abdominal cavity is referred to as:
    a. Parafluid
    b. Pleural fluid
    c. Ascites
    d. Amniotic fluid

11. Fluid that collects outside of the lungs in the pleural space is referred to as
    a. pleural fluid.
    b. ascites.
    c. amniotic fluid.
    d. parafluid

12. Which of the following is not a rule of surgical asepsis?
    a. Always know what is sterile and what is not.
    b. Sterile objects must be kept separate from non-sterile objects.
    c. A sterile field may be left alone in the room for no more than five minutes before use.
    d. Any sterile object that comes in contact with a non-sterile object is considered contaminated.

13. Which of the following needle gauges is the largest size?
    a. 12
    b. 24
    c. 26
    d. 10

14. Which of the following would not need to be worn in the operating room by a sonographer?
    a. Hair cover
    b. Sterile gown
    c. Shoe covers
    d. Mask

15. Which part of the sterile gown is not considered sterile?
    a. The gown at the level of the chest
    b. The front of the gown above the waist
    c. The arms of the gown
    d. The cuffs of the gown

16. **Which of the following is true concerning surgical asepsis?**
    a. A sterile field can be left uncovered for no more than three hours.
    b. Personnel must wear sterile masks to be considered sterile.
    c. If the sterility of an object is under question, the object is considered sterile.
    d. A non-sterile person does not reach over a sterile field.

17. **A blood test that provides information concerning glucose level, electrolytes, fluid balance, and kidney function is the**
    a. complete blood count.
    b. PTT.
    c. basic metabolic panel.
    d. prothrombin time.

18. **A surgical procedure in which fluid is collected from around a fetus is referred to as**
    a. amniocentesis.
    b. thoracentesis.
    c. paracentesis.
    d. pericardiocentesis.

19. **Which of the following is not true of zone 3 in the surgical suite?**
    a. Doors are kept opened.
    b. Mask is required.
    c. Surgical clothing is required.
    d. Shoe covers are required.

20. **Which blood test is used to measure the time it takes for plasma to clot?**
    a. PTT
    b. PT
    c. INR
    d. CBC

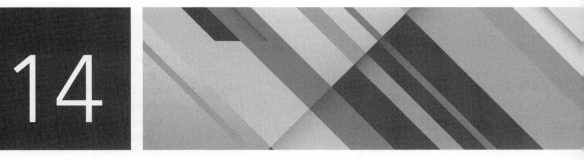

14

Sonographic Examination and Guidelines

CHAPTER OBJECTIVES

■ Appreciate the importance of a quality assurance program.

■ Provide the novice with an overview of many of the suggested requirements that are typically included in various routine sonographic examination.

■ Appreciate the variations required to standard protocols in the everyday practice of sonography.

KEY TERMS

ACR Breast Imaging Reporting and Data System – an organized system that uses sonography to categorize breast lesions by size, shape, orientation, margin, echogenicity, lesion boundary, attenuation, special cases, vascularity, and surrounding tissue

Adnexa – the areas located posterior to the broad ligaments adjacent to the uterus

AIUM 100-mm test object – older test object used to evaluate realtime scanning transducers

Amnionicity – the number of amniotic sacs

Anastomosis – surgical connection between two structures

Ankle-brachial index – test used to evaluate for peripheral artery disease that establishes a ratio of the blood pressure in the lower legs to the blood pressure in the arms

Bifurcation – the splitting of a vessel into two

Chorionicity – the number of placentas

Crown-rump length – the measurement of the fetus from the crown to the rump

Cul-de-sacs – peritoneal spaces found within the pelvis where fluid may collect

Doppler phantom – flow phantom that evaluates the parameter of Doppler systems

Extrauterine pregnancy – a pregnancy located outside of the uterus; also referred to as an ectopic pregnancy

Focused abdominal sonography for trauma (FAST) – sonographic exam that can be used to evaluate the patient for evidence of peritoneal fluid in cases of trauma

Hypercalcemia – elevated serum calcium

Hyperemia – increased blood flow to an organ or area

Hypertrophy – enlargement of an organ or structure

Lumen – opening or inside of a structure

Lymphadenopathy – abnormality of a lymph node or lymph nodes

Murphy sign – sonographic sign of pain with probe pressure over the gallbladder; often used to assess for cholecystitis

Native organs – the organs with which one is born

Orthogonal – lying perpendicular

Parenchyma – the functional tissue of an organ

Quality assurance program – a program that assesses all ultrasound system components, provides repairs, performs preventative

maintenance on ultrasound equipment, and keep records of all assessments

Thrombosis – formation of a blood clot

Tissue equivalent phantom – a phantom that has sonographic features similar to that of the soft tissue of the body; used to evaluate transducer sensitivity and grayscale characteristics

Torsion – twisting

Valsalva maneuver – the maneuver that requires the patient to forcibly exhale while keeping the mouth and nose closed; it is used in many sonographic specialties for vascular assessment

INTRODUCTION

The following chapter will provide an overview of the American Institute of Ultrasound in Medicine (AIUM) guidelines and guidelines from other professional organizations suggested for individual sonographic examinations. Each section will be divided into a main section for each specialty examination, including patient preparation and exam specifications, both prescribed by the AIUM in conjunction with many other professional medical organizations. The AIUM or other cited organization provides this information to all interested parties. The information has been paraphrased and placed in this text for student convenience. For a more extensive explanation of guidelines, please inspect the reference section at the end of this chapter for provided web links. Indications for many of these examinations can be found in Chapter 3 of this text. Keep in mind that protocols vary per institution. It is your responsibility to obtain protocol information and adjust your scanning to meet both institutional and national standards.

QUALITY ASSURANCE

Every sonography department should have a **quality assurance program**. Quality assurance programs assess all ultrasound system components, provide repairs, perform preventative maintenance on ultrasound equipment, and keep records of all assessments.[1] The primary goals of these programs are to maintain the highest function of all sonography-related equipment, to detect any gradual degradation of sonographic images, to minimize potential downtime of equipment, and to protect patients from overexposure by reducing the necessity for repeat procedures secondary to poor equipment function.[1]

Most sonography departments have engineer specialists who perform routine analyses of all equipment. There are several instruments that are used to assess the function of the ultrasound machine, including the **AIUM 100-mm test object**, the **tissue equivalent phantom**, a **Doppler phantom**, and the beam profile/slice thickness phantom.[1] Though the role of the sonographer may be minimal in the quality assurance official assessment in many departments, the sonographer should continually monitor equipment for proper function.

Though a detailed explanation of how to use the ultrasound phantoms is beyond the scope of this book, as a sonography student, you will eventually learn more about quality assurance in your ultrasound physics courses. Keep in mind, quality assurance information, especially how to use the ultrasound phantoms, is found on the physics certification examinations. In general, if you observe cracks in the transducer housing, tears in the ultrasound wiring, or general degradation of the image, you should report these to management. If you accidentally drop a transducer or if you cross over the wires with the machine, examine them closely for detectable flaws. Since patient safety should be placed first, it is best to let someone know as well.

AS LOW AS REASONABLY ACHIEVABLE

In conjunction with thorough protocols and quality assurance, all sonographic examinations should be conducted with the ALARA (as low as reasonably achievable) principle in mind. The potential benefits and risks of each examination should be considered. And though ultrasound has been proven to be safe at diagnostic ranges, minimal exposure to the patient should always be practiced. Further details on ALARA may be found in the AIUM publication *Medical Ultrasound Safety, Second Edition*, and the organization's official statement.[2]

ABDOMINAL AND SMALL PART SONOGRAPHY

Abdominal sonographic imaging typically requires the patient to fast prior to the examination. Though this requirement can vary for each provider, six to eight hours is optimal, but in some cases, especially emergent situations, only four hours may be recommended. In fact, in some emergent situations, immediate action is required and NPO standards are bypassed to expedite care. The reason for fasting is to allow the gallbladder to be thoroughly distended and to inhibit the accumulation of bowel gas after eating. For renal examinations, the patient may need to be fully hydrated as well. Specifics of patient preparation may vary by facility.[3]

Liver

According to the AIUM, the liver should be evaluated in longitudinal and transverse scanning planes. The **parenchyma** of the liver, the functional components, should be examined for any focal or diffuse abnormalities. Typically, the echogenicity and sonographic texture of the liver is also compared to adjacent organs, especially the right kidney. Within the liver, the hepatic vessels, including the portal veins and branches, hepatic veins, and the inferior vena cava (IVC), should be evaluated and imaged.[3]

The three major lobes of the liver, the right, left, and caudate, should be evaluated. If possible, the right diaphragm should be imaged to look for evidence of a pleural effusion.[3] If the patient has had a liver transplant, extensive assessment of the transplant, including Doppler evaluation of the **anastomosis** of vessels, should be performed. Various other specific images may be required of the liver according to the institution. In order to meet these standards, obtain a copy of the protocol requirements for your records.

Gallbladder and Biliary Tract

The gallbladder and biliary tract is often imaged in conjunction with the entire right upper quadrant. The gallbladder should be evaluated in longitudinal and transverse views in the supine position initially. Other positions may be used as well, including left lateral decubitus, upright, and even prone. These positions help the sonographer evaluate the gallbladder for evidence of intraluminal objects, like gallstones. The gallbladder wall measurement and the length and width may be assessed with sonography and thus may be required by some institutions. Furthermore, probe pressure over the gallbladder may be required in order to assess for a painful gallbladder; this is termed **Murphy sign**.[3]

The biliary tree can readily be evaluated with sonography. The intrahepatic and extrahepatic ducts should be evaluated for dilatation, wall thickening, and for the presence of gallstones and other pathology.[3] The entire length of the duct should be imaged if possible from the porta hepatis to the pancreatic head. Various other specific images may be required of the gallbladder and biliary tract according to the institution. In order to meet these standards, obtain a copy of the protocol requirements for your records.

Pancreas

The pancreas is an organ that can be difficult to image in some patients. It is typically included in an abdominal or right upper quadrant sonogram. The pancreas is often imaged via a transverse plane to the patient, though oblique imaging may be useful in some patients. All portions, including the head, uncinate process, body, and tail, should be identified when technically feasible. Occasionally, a small amount of ingested water can be used as a contrast agent to outline the pancreatic head. Also, upright imaging can be helpful.[3]

The pancreas should be assessed for parenchymal abnormalities, ductal dilatations, and echotexture alterations. When the main pancreatic duct is seen, a quick measurement can be taken to evaluate for enlargement. Also, the distal common bile duct should be evaluated in the head of the pancreas for enlargement. The peripancreatic region should be assessed for fluid and adenopathy.[3] Lastly, some institutions may require longitudinal imaging of the pancreas and measurements of the organ as well. Various other specific images may be required of the pancreas according to the institution. In order to meet these standards, obtain a copy of the protocol requirements for your records.

Spleen

The spleen should be viewed in the longitudinal and transverse projections. The spleen may be examined solitarily, as in cases that require follow-up after trauma. The splenic length can be measured to assess for enlargement, though other measurements may be helpful as well. The echogenicity of the spleen is often compared to the left kidney. The left diaphragm should be evaluated for pleural effusion as well. Various other specific images may be required of the spleen according to the institution. In order to meet these standards, obtain a copy of the protocol requirements for your records.[3]

Bowel

The various sections of the small and large intestines can be evaluated for wall thickening, dilation, muscular **hypertrophy**, masses, **hyperemia** (identified with color Doppler), and other abnormalities. Patients can be examined for infantile pyloric stenosis and intussusception. For pyloric stenosis, the infant is often given fluid to drink, such as Pedialyte, to better visualize the pyloric region of the stomach.[3] For other bowel pathologies, like intussusceptions and appendicitis, sonographers often utilize graded compression. These structures should be evaluated in at least two perpendicular scanning planes. Various other specific images may be required of bowel segments according to the institution. In order to meet these standards, obtain a copy of the protocol requirements for your records.[3]

Peritoneal Fluid

Within the abdomen, evidence of peritoneal fluid or ascites should be documented. The location and extent of the fluid should be offered. In emergency situations, a **focused abdominal sonography for trauma** (FAST) exam can be performed. The objective of the abdominal portion of the FAST exam can be used to evaluate the patient for evidence of peritoneal fluid in cases of trauma.[3]

Longitudinal and transverse plane images should be obtained of the right upper quadrant through the area of the liver with attention to fluid collections adjacent to the liver and in the subhepatic spaces. Longitudinal and transverse plane images should be obtained in the left upper quadrant through the area of the spleen with attention to fluid collections adjacent to the spleen. Longitudinal and transverse images should be obtained at the periphery of the left and right abdomen in the areas of the left and right paracolic gutters for evidence of free fluid. Longitudinal and transverse midline images of the pelvis should be obtained to evaluate for free pelvic fluid in the **cul-de-sacs** and **adnexa**.[3] Analysis through a fluid-filled bladder may help in evaluation of the pelvis. If necessary, the bladder can be filled through a Foley catheter when possible. Various other specific images may be required for fluid searches according to the institution. In order to meet these standards, obtain a copy of the protocol requirements for your records.

Abdominal Wall

Abdominal wall imaging is performed in the location of the symptoms or signs. The relationship of any identified mass with the peritoneum should be demonstrated, and any defect in the peritoneum should be documented. The surrounding musculature should also be evaluated. The defect should be evaluated for the presence of bowel, fluid, or other tissues located within the abdominal wall defect.[3] Occasionally, the **Valsalva maneuver** and having the patient sit upright (or simply change position) may allow for improved visualization of abdominal wall defects. Color Doppler may be used to identify vessels within the defect as well.[3] Various other specific images may be required for abdominal wall imaging according to the institution. In order to meet these standards, obtain a copy of the protocol requirements for your records.[3]

Kidneys and Urinary Bladder (Renal Sonogram)

Sonography of the kidneys, often referred to as a renal sonogram, includes the examination of the **native organs** and in some cases transplanted kidneys in both longitudinal and transverse scanning planes. The kidneys are often scanned with the patient supine, though upright and decubitus position can help. The cortices, renal pelvis, and echogenicity of each kidney should be assessed. The echogenicity of the right and left kidneys should be examined in relationship to the liver and spleen, respectively. The maximum renal length should be recorded, and some institutions may require other measurements, including the anteroposterior dimension and transverse diameter.[3]

The perirenal area should also be evaluated, and the right and left adrenal gland areas can be readily examined in the adult, though the adrenal gland itself may not be seen.[3] When possible, usually in the neonate or young infant, longitudinal and transverse images of the adrenal glands may be obtained.

The urinary bladder should also be imaged in the transverse and longitudinal scanning planes along with the kidneys. The bladder wall should be evaluated for thickening and masses. The intraluminal contents should also be examined for signs of debris. Dilatation or other distal ureteral abnormalities should be documented. Transverse and longitudinal scans may be used to demonstrate any postvoid residual, which may be quantitated and reported.[3] Various other specific images may be required for a renal sonogram according to the institution. In order to meet these standards, obtain a copy of the protocol requirements for your records.

Renal Vascular Assessment

For a vascular examination of native kidneys or transplanted kidneys, Doppler imaging can be used for several purposes. Renal Doppler may be used to assess renal arterial and venous patency. It is also useful in evaluating suspected renal artery stenosis. For this application, angle-adjusted measurements of the peak systolic velocity should be made proximally, centrally, and distally in the extrarenal portion of the main renal arteries when possible. The peak systolic velocity of the adjacent aorta should also be documented for calculating the renal-to-aortic peak systolic velocity ratio.[3] Spectral Doppler evaluation of the intrarenal arteries may be of value as indirect evidence of proximal stenosis in the main renal artery. For vascular examinations of transplanted kidneys, Doppler evaluation should be used to document vascular patency and blood flow characteristics. The structures that may be examined include the main renal artery and vein, arterial and venous anastomoses, the iliac artery and vein, and the intrarenal arteries.[3] Though a renal duplex examination is beyond the scope of this chapter, information can be found on the AIUM website. Various other specific images may be required for renal vascular assessment according to the institution. In order to meet these standards, obtain a copy of the protocol requirements for your records.[3]

Abdominal Aorta and Inferior Vena Cava (IVC)

An abdominal aorta sonogram can be ordered as a separate sonographic examination. However, the abdominal aorta is also typically included in an abdominal sonogram or a renal sonogram.

The abdominal aorta should be imaged in the longitudinal and transverse scan planes, including the proximal, mid, and distal segments. The **bifurcation** area of the aorta and the proximal common iliac arteries should also be imaged in both longitudinal and transverse planes.[4]

The greatest dimension of the different segment of the aorta (proximal, mid, and distal) and the proximal common iliac vessels should be obtained. This dimension is from outer edge to other outer edge of the vessel. If an aneurysm is discovered, the maximum size and location of the aneurysm should be documented and recorded. The relationship of the aneurysm to the renal arteries and to the aortic bifurcation should be determined if possible.[4] Color Doppler and/or spectral Doppler imaging with waveform analysis of the aorta and iliac arteries may provide additional information. After endoluminal graft placement, color (or power) Doppler imaging and spectral Doppler imaging are required to document the presence or absence of endoleaks.[4]

The IVC is typically included in a sonogram of the abdomen or right upper quadrant. Representative images of the IVC should be obtained. Patency and abnormalities may be evaluated with Doppler imaging. Vena cava filters, interruption devices, and catheters may need to be localized with respect to the hepatic and/or renal veins.[4] Various other specific images may be required for an abdominal aorta or IVC sonogram according to the institution. In order to meet these standards, obtain a copy of the protocol requirements for your records.

BREAST SONOGRAPHY

There is typically no patient preparation for a breast sonogram. A breast sonogram should be correlated with clinical signs and/or symptoms and with mammographic and other appropriate breast imaging studies. If sonography has been performed previously, the current examination should be compared with prior sonograms as appropriate. A lesion or any area of the breast being studied should be viewed in two perpendicular projections. Some institutions require longitudinal and transverse imaging, while others may prefer radial and antiradial views. Realtime scanning by the interpreter is encouraged.[5]

The size of a lesion should be determined by recording its maximal dimensions in at least two **orthogonal** planes. At least one set of images of a lesion should be obtained without calipers. The images should be labeled as to right or left breast, location of lesions, and orientation of the transducer with respect to the breast (e.g., transverse or longitudinal, radial or antiradial). The location of the lesion should be recorded using clock-face notation and distance from the nipple, and/or shown on a diagram of the breast.[5] The length of the transducer face (footprint), usually between 3.5 and 5 cm, or other measuring devices can be used to estimate the distance from the nipple.[5]

Sonographic features are helpful in characterizing breast masses. These feature categories and their descriptors are listed and exemplified in the **ACR Breast Imaging Reporting and Data System** (BI-RADS). The BI-RADS sonographic categories include size, shape, orientation, margin, echogenicity, lesion boundary, attenuation (e.g., shadowing or enhancement), special cases, vascularity, and surrounding tissue.[5]

Elastography, or tissue stiffness assessment, may be used by some institutions. To minimize errors in communication or interpretation, if elastography is performed, the color scales should be annotated to denote hardness or softness.

Mass characterization with sonography is highly dependent on technical factors. Breast sonography should be performed with a high-resolution transducer, such as a linear array.[5] All settings should be optimized. The patient should be positioned to minimize the thickness of the portion of the breast being evaluated. For evaluation of lesions in, on, or just beneath the skin, a stand-off device or thick layer of gel may be helpful. Various other specific images may be required for a breast sonogram according to the institution. In order to meet these standards, obtain a copy of the protocol requirements for your records.

SCROTAL SONOGRAPHY

There is typically no patient preparation for a scrotal sonogram. The patient should be positioned so that both testicles can be imaged simultaneously in order to evaluate disparity in echotexture and vascularity, as seen in cases of testicular **torsion** and orchitis. A rolled towel placed between the legs may be used. The testicles are placed on the towel, and the penis is placed on the belly. The testicles are examined in both the longitudinal and transverse scanning planes. Longitudinally, images should be obtained in the center of each testicle, and the medial and lateral portions. Transversely, the superior, mid, and inferior portions should be imaged.[6]

All parts of the epididymis (head, body, tail) should be evaluated. Also the size of each testicle and epididymis should be obtained and compared. Side-by-side transverse or dual images can be obtained to compare the echogenicity and vasculature (color Doppler) of the testicles. The scrotal wall thickness and any focal palpable masses should also be examined. Imaging using the Valsalva maneuver may be used to better demonstrate varicoceles. Upright imaging may be helpful as well.[6]

Color and spectral Doppler should be employed to evaluate the vascularity of both testicles. Doppler setting should be set to identify low flow, though flow parameters should not be altered between testicular analyses with Doppler in order to identify discrepancies of flow between the testicles.[6] Various other specific images may be required for a scrotal sonogram according to the institution. In order to meet these standards, obtain a copy of the protocol requirements for your records.

THYROID, CERVICAL LYMPH NODE, AND PARATHYROID SONOGRAPHY

There is typically no patient preparation required for a thyroid or neck sonogram. The patient is positioned supine, and the neck is hyperextended, which may be facilitated with the use of rolled cloth towels placed under the neck or shoulders. The right and left lobes of the thyroid gland should be imaged in longitudinal and transverse planes. Images of the superior, mid, and inferior portions of both lobes are suggested in transverse. While in the longitudinal position, the central, medial, and lateral aspects of the thyroid should be imaged. The thyroid isthmus should be imaged in transverse.[7]

Each lobe should be measured in three dimensions—length, width, and height (anteroposterior). The thickness of the thyroid isthmus should also be measured in the anteroposterior dimension for signs of enlargement. Color Doppler imaging can be employed when masses are identified or to assess the overall vascularity of each lobe or the entire gland. Focal lesions are measured in three dimensions.[7]

A general assessment of the neck may be required for patients with palpable lesions outside of the thyroid gland, as in the case of thyroglossal duct cysts. For this reason, the lateral neck on both sides is often included with thyroid sonography in order to assess for signs of lymphadenopathy, especially in those patients with a history of thyroid carcinoma. If visualized, prominent lymph nodes should be measured in three dimensions and can be evaluated with color Doppler as well. In patients who have had a thyroidectomy, the entire thyroid area should still be imaged in both longitudinal and transverse scan planes. The neck can also be examined with sonography for cervical **lymphadenopathy** without including the thyroid gland, as in cases of palpable nodes. However, a demonstration of the relationship to the vasculature within the neck and the thyroid gland may be helpful for surgical intervention.[7]

Patient positioning for a parathyroid sonogram is the same as for a thyroid sonogram. For parathyroid sonography, patients may have palpable lesions, such as a parathyroid adenoma, in which case they will have clinical signs and symptoms of **hypercalcemia**.[7] However, the adenoma may not be palpable. Therefore, the sonographer should search the common locations of the parathyroid glands in the neck in both longitudinal and transverse scan planes, including a thorough assessment from the carotid bulb superiorly to the thoracic inlet inferiorly on both sides of the neck.[7] Scanning techniques such as having the patient swallow and the use of color Doppler may be helpful.

When seen, parathyroid glands and/or parathyroid pathology should be demonstrated in relationship to the thyroid gland if possible. Various other specific images may be required for the sonographic evaluation of the neck according to the institution. In order to meet these standards, obtain a copy of the protocol requirements for your records.

MUSCULOSKELETAL SONOGRAPHY

Shoulder Examination

Though the AIUM offers examination specifications for other joints, the shoulder joint is the most common joint analyzed with sonography. For other musculoskeletal examination specifications, such as the elbow, wrist, hand, hip, ankle, foot, and knee, visit www.aium.org.[8]

There is typically no preparation required for a shoulder sonogram. The examination is performed with a high-frequency transducer. Depending upon the practitioner, however, a rotating chair may be needed to perform the sonogram.[8] The shoulder is imaged according to the structure examined, with long-axis and short-axis views obtained and with some oblique orientation to specific structure required. Images are obtained of the joint spaces, the long head of the biceps tendon, and all of the structures of the rotator cuff. Dynamic imaging is performed with the patient moving the arm into different positions throughout the examination to obtain optimal visualization of certain structures. Therefore, the shoulder is scanned through the full range of internal to external rotation.[8] Color Doppler may be employed to demonstrate hyperemia as well. Also, a comparison of the contralateral side may be helpful. The bones of the shoulder may also be examined for signs of fracture. This is not an extensive list for shoulder analysis, as multiple images are typically required for the sonographic evaluation of the shoulder. In order to meet these standards, obtain a copy of the protocol requirements for your institution for your records.

GYNECOLOGIC SONOGRAPHY

Patient preparation for a transabdominal pelvic sonogram requires that the patient's urinary bladder be distended with urine. Typically, this requires that the patient drink at least 32 oz of water an hour before the examination. However, in emergency situations, the urinary bladder can be retro-filled with saline solution through a Foley catheter. Over-distention of the bladder should be avoided. During the examination, the urinary bladder can also be evaluated for abnormalities as well. Transabdominal imaging is performed using the highest-frequency curved transducer that provides the best penetration without sacrificing resolution.[9]

There is typically no patient preparation required for a transvaginal sonogram. Insertion of the transducer can be performed by the physician, a sonographer, or the patient. A chaperone should be considered for transvaginal imaging.[9] The uterus is examined in longitudinal and transverse scan planes. The uterine shape, orientations, myometrium, endometrium, and the cervix are evaluated. The size of the uterus should also be obtained. Longitudinally, the length and anteroposterior measurement is taken, while transversely (or coronally), the uterine width is obtained. The endometrium should also be measured in the anteroposterior dimension in the longitudinal plane, measuring the thickness from basal layer (echogenic border) to the opposite basal layer (other echogenic border). The adjacent hypoechoic myometrium should not be included in this measurement.[9] Furthermore, intracavitary abnormalities, including fluid, should be excluded from this measurement. However, they can be measured separately and should be documented. Any abnormalities of the uterus should be located, characterized sonographically, and measured. If an intrauterine device is noted, its location should be demonstrated. Sonohysterography and three-dimensional imaging can provide further analysis of the uterus.

The ovaries should be evaluated and the depth, length, and width measured in at least two orthogonal planes. When an adnexal mass is identified, demonstration of the mass in regard to the location of the ipsilateral ovary should be performed when possible. The adnexa should be evaluated for fluid, dilated tubes, and masses. All pathology should be measured and characterized sonographically. The cul-de-sacs should also be evaluated for fluid. When fluid is noted, a general assessment of the fluid should be performed in regard to amount and sonographic appearance. Spectral, color, and/or power Doppler ultrasound may be useful in evaluating the vascular characteristics of pelvic lesions.[9] Various other specific images may be required for the sonographic evaluation of the female pelvis according to the institution. In order to meet these standards, obtain a copy of the protocol requirements for your records.

Sonohysterography

Patient preparation for a sonohysterogram may vary according to the institution. A nurse or the physician may perform an initial pelvic examination, including the preparation of the site using aseptic technique. Saline solution or water is used for the procedure. Precatheterization images should be obtained and recorded in at least two planes to show normal and abnormal findings.[10] These images should include the thickest bilayer endometrial measurement on a sagittal image when possible. Once the uterine cavity is filled with fluid, a complete survey of the uterine cavity should be performed and representative images obtained to document normal and abnormal findings. If a balloon catheter is used for the examination, images should be obtained at the end of the procedure with the balloon deflated to fully evaluate the endometrial cavity, particularly the cervical canal and lower portion of the endometrial cavity.[10] Additional techniques such as color Doppler and three-dimensional imaging may be helpful in evaluating both normal and abnormal findings. Various other specific images may be required for sonohysterography according to the institution. In order to meet these standards, obtain a copy of the protocol requirements for your records.[10]

OBSTETRIC SONOGRAPHY

First Trimester

For a transabdominal first-trimester sonogram, the patient should have a distended bladder. If transvaginal scanning is performed, the bladder should be emptied. Keep in mind that in some situations when abnormalities are detected, a more detailed examination may be warranted.[11]

The maternal uterus should be evaluated as if performing a pelvic sonogram (see the "Gynecologic Sonography" section). In the early pregnancy, the endometrium should be thoroughly analyzed for signs of a gestational sac. Once a yolk sac or an embryo with cardiac activity is visualized within the gestational sac, an intrauterine pregnancy (IUP) can be confirmed. If clinical correlation is suggestive of an IUP and it is not identified, the pelvis should be thoroughly examined for signs of an **extrauterine pregnancy** or ectopic pregnancy.[11]

If an IUP is identified, the crown-rump length is a more accurate indicator of gestational (menstrual) age than is the mean gestational sac diameter (MSD). However, the MSD may be recorded when an embryo is not identified. The MSD measurements are made in at least two orthogonal planes (length, width, depth). The **crown-rump length** is obtained at the longest axis of the embryo/fetus. If an embryo/fetus is identified, cardiac activity can be demonstrated using M-mode and/or a video clip. The yolk sac should also be evaluated, and some institutions may require a measurement.[11]

Amnionicity and **chorionicity** should be documented for all multiple gestations when possible. Embryonic/fetal anatomy appropriate for the first trimester should be assessed and documented. For those patients desiring to assess their individual risk of fetal aneuploidy, a specific measurement of the nuchal translucency (NT) during a specific age interval is necessary as determined by the laboratory used.[11] NT measurements should be used in conjunction with serum biochemistry to determine the risk of having a fetus with aneuploidy or other anatomic abnormalities, such as heart defects.[11] There are specific standards for performing an accurate NT measurement, though the fetal neck can be examined for signs of a cystic hygroma during a routine first-trimester sonogram. Various other specific images may be required for a first-trimester sonogram according to the institution. In order to meet these standards, obtain a copy of the protocol requirements for your records.

Second and Third Trimesters

There is no patient preparation typically warranted in the second and third trimesters. However, if the cervix needs to be further evaluated with transvaginal or translabial scanning, the bladder may require emptying.[11] Fetal number, fetal cardiac activity, including abnormal heart rate or rhythm, and presentation should be documented. For multiple gestations, the documentation of additional information such as chorionicity, amnionicity, comparison of fetal sizes, estimation of amniotic fluid volume (increased, decreased, or normal) in each gestational sac, and fetal genitalia (when visualized) is suggested.[11]

An assessment of the amniotic fluid volume should be performed. For some institutions, this requires the performance of an amniotic fluid index, single-pocket measurement, or other method. The location and appearance of the placenta should be assessed. The location of the placenta in regard to the internal os of the cervix should be evaluated.[11] Translabial or transvaginal imaging may help to visualize the internal os, especially in cases of suspected placenta previa or cervical incompetence. The umbilical cord should be evaluated for the presence of two arteries and one vein, and its insertion into the placenta should also be evaluated when technically feasible.[11]

Biometric parameters, such as biparietal diameter, abdominal circumference, and femoral diaphysis length, can be used to estimate gestational (menstrual) age. Fetal weight can be estimated by obtaining these measurements as well. The maternal adnexa and cul-de-sacs should be evaluated when technically feasible, though it is not always possible to image the normal maternal ovaries during the second and third trimesters.[11] Table 14-1 provides the anatomy to include

TABLE 14-1	Basic fetal anatomy survey in the second- and third-trimester sonogram

- Head, face, and neck:
  - Lateral cerebral ventricles
  - Choroid plexus
  - Midline falx
  - Cavum septi pellucidi
  - Cerebellum
  - Cistern magna
  - Upper lip
  - A measurement of the nuchal fold may be helpful during a specific age interval to assess the risk of aneuploidy
- Chest, heart:
  - Four-chamber view
  - Left ventricular outflow tract
  - Right ventricular outflow tract
- Abdomen:
  - Stomach (presence, size, and situs)
  - Kidneys
  - Urinary bladder
  - Umbilical cord insertion site into the fetal abdomen
  - Umbilical cord vessel number
- Spine: Cervical, thoracic, lumbar, and sacral spine
- Extremities: Legs and arms
- Sex: In multiple gestations and when medically indicated

AIUM Practice Guideline for the Performance of Obstetric Ultrasound Examinations. Retrieved from http://www.aium.org/resources/guidelines/obstetric.pdf.

in a basic fetal anatomy survey. A more detailed fetal anatomic examination may be necessary if an abnormality or suspected abnormality is found on the standard examination. Various other specific images may be required for a second- or third-trimester sonogram according to the institution. In order to meet these standards, obtain a copy of the protocol requirements for your records.

VASCULAR SONOGRAPHY

Carotid Sonogram

There is no patient preparation for a carotid sonogram. Extracranial cerebrovascular ultrasound evaluation consists of assessment of the common and internal carotid arteries and basic assessment of the external carotid and vertebral arteries.[12] All arteries should be scanned using appropriate grayscale and Doppler techniques and proper patient positioning. Grayscale imaging of the common carotid artery, the bifurcation, and both of the internal and external carotid arteries should be performed in longitudinal and transverse planes.[12] The internal carotid and common carotid arteries should be imaged completely from just above the clavicle to the level of the mandible.[12]

Color Doppler imaging should be used to detect areas of narrowing and abnormal flow to select areas for Doppler spectral analysis. Power Doppler evaluation may be helpful in searching for a narrow channel of residual flow with suspected pathology within the vessels. Spectral Doppler imaging with angle-corrected blood flow velocity measurements should be obtained at representative sites in the vessels.[12] Additionally, scanning in areas of stenosis or suspected stenosis must be adequate to determine the maximal peak systolic velocity associated with the stenosis and to document disturbances in the waveform distal to the stenosis.[12]

All angle-corrected spectral Doppler waveforms must be obtained from longitudinal images. Angle correction should be applied in a consistent manner for all measurements. The angle between the direction of flowing blood and the applied Doppler ultrasound signal should not exceed 60 degrees.[12] Gain setting should be appropriate and consistent. Also, many specific images may be required for a carotid sonogram according to the institution. In order to meet these standards, obtain a copy of the protocol requirements for your records.

Peripheral Venous Sonography

No patient preparation is required for a peripheral vasculature sonography. For a lower extremity venous sonogram, compression sonography is utilized to investigate for **thrombosis**.[13] All vessels are examined in the longitudinal and transverse scan planes. Venous compression is applied in the transverse plane with adequate pressure on the skin to completely obliterate the normal vein **lumen**.[13] At a minimum, right and left common femoral or right and left external iliac venous spectral Doppler waveforms should be recorded.[13] Though protocols may vary, abnormal findings generally require additional images to document the complete extent of the abnormalities. Anatomic variations, such as duplications, should be noted. Augmentation and duplex sonography is utilized to evaluate the veins for venous insufficiency or reflux. When evaluating for venous insufficiency, the location and duration of reversed blood flow should be determined during the performance of accepted maneuvers. For example, the Valsalva maneuver can be used at the groin level. All spectral Doppler waveforms should be obtained from the long axis.[13] Other pathology should be recorded. Also, various other specific images may be required for a lower extremity venous sonogram according to the institution. In order to meet these standards, obtain a copy of the protocol requirements for your records. Generally, veins in the superficial and deep systems should be evaluated.

Upper Extremity Venous Sonogram

There is no preparation for an upper extremity venous sonogram. Upper extremity duplex evaluation consists of grayscale and Doppler evaluation of all portions of the subclavian, innominate, internal jugular veins, and axillary veins, as well as the brachial, basilica, and cephalic veins using compression sonography.[13] Compression is typically performed in the transverse plane to the vessel. Specific images may be required for an upper extremity venous sonogram according to the institution. In order to meet these standards, obtain a copy of the protocol requirements for your records.[13]

Peripheral Arterial

There is no patient preparation for a peripheral arterial sonogram. Physiologic tests of the arterial system such as the **ankle brachial index** (ABI), segmental pressure, and waveform analysis are frequently the initial examinations performed to determine the presence of arterial disease.[14] Essentially, the ABI is used to evaluate for the hemodynamic consequences of lower extremity arterial disease.[14]

The sonographic examination of the peripheral arteries consists of grayscale/color Doppler imaging and spectral Doppler waveforms in the appropriate arterial segments. Color Doppler imaging should be used to improve detection of arterial lesions by identifying visual narrowing and changes in color and to guide placement of the sample volume for spectral Doppler assessment.[14] Velocity measurements are obtained from angle-corrected longitudinal spectral Doppler images.[14] The angle created by the direction of blood flow and the direction of the ultrasound beam should be maintained at 60 degrees or less.[14]

TRANSTHORACIC ADULT ECHOCARDIOGRAPHY

There is typically no patient preparation for an adult echocardiographic examination, though institutional requirements may vary. Table 14-2 contains some suggested structures to evaluate routinely. Guidelines for pediatric and fetal echocardiography can be found at http://www.asecho.org/files/Guidelines/pediatricechoguidelines.pdf and http://www.aium.org/resources/guidelines/fetalEcho.pdf, respectively. Protocol requirements can vary per institution. Obtain a copy of your institution's protocol, and keep it for your records and use.[15]

TABLE 14-2	Transthoracic echocardiography basic assessment

Two-dimensional and/or M-mode numerical data for transthoracic echocardiograms must include but not be limited to (except where technically unobtainable):
- Measurements of the left ventricular internal dimension at end-diastole
- Left ventricular internal dimension at end-systole
- Left ventricular posterobasal free wall thickness at end-diastole
- Ventricular septal thickness at end-diastole
- Left atrial (LA) dimension at end-systole or indexed LA volume
- Aortic root dimension at end-diastole or ascending aorta

A report of the Doppler evaluation must include but not be limited to:
- Evaluation of peak and mean gradients (if stenotic)
- Valve area (if stenotic)
- Degree of regurgitation
- Right ventricular systolic pressure value reported when tricuspid regurgitation is present
- Other pathology as noted

IAC Standards and Guidelines for Adult Echocardiography Accreditation. Retrieved from http://www.intersocietal.org/echo/standards/IACAdultEchoStandardsJuly2014.pdf.

SUMMARY

The information found in this chapter is not exhaustive and may not be the most current recommendations for each examination, as recommendations may change after the publication of this book. One vital task for the sonographer is to maintain an awareness of the ever-changing environment in which we work. New additions to protocols and suggested guidelines can happen at any time. Therefore, you can be aware by being vigilant of the changes in your profession and routinely visiting the AIUM and other organizations' websites for updates. By maintaining continuing medical education and joining professional organizations, like the AIUM and the Society of Diagnostic Medical Sonographers, we can preserve the high-quality care that our patients deserve, while at the same time actively pursuing professional development and participation.

REFERENCES

1. Edelman SK. *Understanding Ultrasound Physics*. 3rd ed. Woodland, TX: ESP, Inc.; 2005.
2. Medical Ultrasound Safety and As Low As Reasonably Achievable. Retrieved from http://www.aium.org/sound-Waves/article.aspx?aId=390&iId=20110915 Note: Document requires AIUM membership. Official statement can be found at http://www.aium.org/officialStatements/39
3. AIUM Practice Guidelines for the Performance of an Ultrasound Examination of the Abdomen and/or Retroperitoneum. Retrieved from http://www.aium.org/resources/guidelines/abdominal.pdf
4. AIUM Practice Guideline for the Performance of Diagnostic and Screening Ultrasound Examinations of the Abdominal Aorta in Adults. Retrieved from http://www.aium.org/resources/guidelines/abdominalAorta.pdf
5. ACR Practice Parameter for the Performance of a Breast Ultrasound Examination. Retrieved from http://www.acr.org/~/media/ACR/Documents/PGTS/guidelines/US_Breast.pdf
6. AIUM Practice Guideline for the Performance of Scrotal Ultrasound Examinations. Retrieved from http://www.aium.org/resources/guidelines/scrotal.pdf
7. AIUM Practice Guideline for the Performance of a Thyroid and Parathyroid Ultrasound Examination. Retrieved from http://www.aium.org/resources/guidelines/thyroid.pdf
8. AIUM Practice Guideline for the Performance of a Musculoskeletal Ultrasound Examination. Retrieved from http://www.aium.org/resources/guidelines/musculoskeletal.pdf
9. AIUM Practice Guideline for the Performance of Ultrasound of the Female Pelvis. Retrieved from http://www.aium.org/resources/guidelines/femalePelvis.pdf
10. AIUM Practice Guideline for the Performance of Sonohysterography. Retrieved from http://www.aium.org/resources/guidelines/sonohysterography.pdf
11. AIUM Practice Guideline for the Performance of Obstetric Ultrasound Examinations. Retrieved from http://www.aium.org/resources/guidelines/obstetric.pdf
12. AIUM Practice Guideline for the Performance of an Ultrasound Examination of the Extracranial Cerebrovascular System. Retrieved from http://www.aium.org/resources/guidelines/extracranial.pdf
13. Practice Guideline for the Performance of Peripheral Venous Ultrasound Examinations. Retrieved from http://www.aium.org/resources/guidelines/peripheralVenous.pdf
14. AIUM Practice Guideline for the Performance of Peripheral Arterial Ultrasound Examinations Using Color and Spectral Doppler Imaging. Retrieved from http://www.aium.org/resources/guidelines/peripheralArterial.pdf
15. IAC Standards and Guidelines for Adult Echocardiography Accreditation. Retrieved from http://www.intersocietal.org/echo/standards/IACAdultEchoStandardsJuly2014.pdf

Thinking Critically

1. How does your clinical facility undergo quality assurance? Who performs the quality assurance tasks?
2. Research your clinical facility's requirement for each examination performed. Most institutions have a protocol book. Find out how it established the protocol and what guidelines the department used.

3. Are there any different requirements between clinical facilities that you have visited? Why do you think that institutional protocols and guidelines vary?
4. As a sonographer, how can you stay abreast of new changes to national standards and guidelines?

Chapter 14
Review Questions

1. Which of the following is described as enlargement of an organ or structure?
   a. Hypertrophy
   b. Distilment
   c. Megaly
   d. Augmentation

2. What test is used to evaluate for peripheral artery disease that establishes a ratio of the blood pressure in the lower legs to the blood pressure in the arms?
   a. Ankle-brain index
   b. Ankle-brachial index
   c. Angle-bifid index
   d. Arterial-branchial index

3. What is the patient preparation for a transvaginal sonogram?
   a. There is no patient preparation required.
   b. NPO for six to eight hours prior to the exam.
   c. Enema and NPO for three hours prior to the exam.
   d. Drink 32 oz of water one hour prior to the exam.

4. In the first trimester of pregnancy, the fetal neck may be examined with sonography and a measurement obtained. What is this measurement called?
   a. Neck fold
   b. Crown-rump length
   c. Mean sac diameter
   d. Nuchal translucency

5. What contrast solution is typically used in sonohysterography?
   a. Barium
   b. Helium
   c. Saline
   d. Betadine

6. What term relates to increased vascularity in an organ or structure?
   a. Hypertrophy
   b. Enlargement
   c. Hyperemia
   d. Hyperextensive

7. What is the surgical connection between two structures?
   a. Fissure
   b. Staple
   c. Anastomosis
   d. Stent

8. **The formation of blood clot is termed**
   a. embolism
   b. thrombosis
   c. stenosis
   d. compaction

9. **What is another word for perpendicular?**
   a. Orthogonal
   b. Dipolar
   c. Hexagonal
   d. Analogous

10. **What is the name for areas located outside of the uterus posterior to the broad ligaments?**
    a. Cul-de-sacs
    b. Adnexas
    c. Morrison pouches
    d. Paracolic gutters

11. **Which of the following evaluates tissue stiffness?**
    a. Elastography
    b. Sonohysterography
    c. Valsalva technique
    d. Murphy sign

12. **Which of the following would most likely employ the Valsalva technique?**
    a. Breast sonography
    b. Echocardiography
    c. Gallbladder sonography
    d. Lower venous sonography

13. **Which quality assurance phantom would be most likely used to evaluate the transducers effectiveness at identifying liver masses?**
    a. AIUM test phantom
    b. Dead zone object
    c. Doppler phantom
    d. Tissue equivalent phantom

14. **The FAST exam would most likely be used in what setting?**
    a. Obstetric suite
    b. Outpatient clinic
    c. Emergency room
    d. Gynecologic office

15. **What is the medical term for twisting?**
    a. Orthogonal
    b. Torsion
    c. Augment
    d. Claudicate

16. **What should you do if you observe a crack in a transducer before a sonographic examination?**
    a. Perform the examination, and then tell someone.
    b. Ignore it and assume someone else already knows.
    c. Place tape over the crack.
    d. Tell someone in charge immediately.

17. **What is the term for abnormal lymph nodes?**
    a. Lymphadenopathy
    b. Lymphedema
    c. Lymphoma
    d. Lymphitis

18. **What is the first measurement of the embryo called in the first trimester?**
    a. Mean sac diameter
    b. Crown-rump length
    c. Gestational sac
    d. Yolk sac

19. **The splitting of one vessel into two vessels is termed a(n)**
    a. bifurcation.
    b. conjunction.
    c. intersection.
    d. dividend.

20. **If you roll the ultrasound machine over the transducer wire and notice damage, what should you do?**
    a. Report the damage immediately, and do not use the transducer.
    b. Nothing; it happens all the time.
    c. Apply bandage tape to the damaged area.
    d. Continue to use the transducer to see if the damage will affect image quality.

Appendix 1
Medical Terminology

Prefixes

a(n) – without
ab – away from
ad – toward
ambi – both sides
ante – before, forward
anti – against
aut(o) – self
bi – two
diplo – double
dys – difficult, painful
ec – out of
end(o) – inward
ex – outside
hetero – other, different
hyper – above, beyond
infra – beneath
intra – within, into
juxta – near
macr(o) – large, long
mal – bad
mega – great, large
micro – small
mono – one
morph(o) – shape
multi – many
olig(o) – few, little
par(a) – near, beside, accessory to
peri – around
poly – much, many
post – behind, after
pre – before, in front
pseudo – false
re – back, contrary
retro – backward
semi – half
sub – under
super – above
supra – above, upon
tetra – four
trans – across, through

Root Words

abdomen(o) – abdomen
acr(o) – extremity
aden(o) – gland
adipo – fat

alb – white
andr(o) – male
angi(o) – vessel
ankyl – crooked, fusion
bili – bile
blast (or -blast) – embryonic state
brachi(o) – arm
brady – slow
carcin(o) – cancer
cardi(o) – heart
caud – tail
cephal(o) – head
cerebr(o) – brain
cerv(i)(o) – neck
chol(e) – bile
chondr(o) – cartilage
col(i)(o) – colon
cost(o) – rib
cut – skin
cyan(o) – blue
cyst(i)(o) – bladder
cyt(o) – cell
dactyl – fingers or toes
derm (or -derm) – skin
dors(i)(o) – back
encephal – brain
enter(o) – intestine
fasci – bundle
galact(o) – milk
gastro – stomach
gest – carry
gloss(o) – tongue
gyn(o) – women, female reproductive organs
heme or hemato – blood
hepat(o) – liver
hist(i)(o) – tissue
hydro – water
hyster – uterus
ile(o) – ileum
ili(o) – ilium
ischi(o) – hip
jejun(o) – jejunum
kine(t)(o) – movement
labio – lips
lact(o) – milk
laryng(o) – larynx
latero – side

leuk(o) – white
lip(o) – fat
lith(o) – stone
mamm(o) – breast
mast(o) – breast
meno – menses
my(o) – muscle
myel(o) – marrow, spinal cord
myx – mucus
nas(o) – nose
nephr(o) – kidney
ocul(o) – eye
opthalm(o) – eye
orchi(o) – testes
oss or oste(o) – bone
path(o) – disease
ped(o) – child
pharyng(o) – pharynx
phleb(o) – vein
pleur(o) – pleura, rib, side
pneum(o) – lung
proct(o) – rectum
psych(o) – mind
pulmo(n) – lung
pyel(o) – kidney
pyr(o) – heart
ren(o) – kidney
sarc(o) – flesh
scler(o) – hard
scolio – crooked
sten(o) – narrow
tachy – rapid, swift
therm(o) – heat
thorac(o) – chest
thromb(o) – clot
toxi(o) – poison
trache(o) – trachea
ur(o) – urinary, urine
vas(o) – vessel
ven(i)(o) – vein
vesic(o) – bladder

Suffixes

-algia	pain
-ectomy	surgical removal
-itis	inflammation
-lys	breakdown
-oma	tumor
-osis	condition
-plasia	growth
-plasty	surgical repair
-plegia	paralysis
-pnea	breathing
-poiesis	production
-rrhea	fluid discharge
-scope	observe
-stomy	opening
-taxis	movement
-tripsy	crushing
-trophy	growth

Common Medical Abbreviations

AAA = abdominal aortic aneurysm
Ab = abortion
abd = abdomen
ABI = ankle-brachial index
AC = abdominal circumference
ACA = anterior cerebral artery
ACAD = atherosclerotic carotid artery disease
ACG = angiocardiography
ACL = anterior cruciate ligament
ACS = acute coronary syndrome
ADPKD = autosomal dominant polycystic kidney disease
AED = automated external defibrillator
AFI = amniotic fluid index
AFP = alpha-fetoprotein
AFV = amniotic fluid volume
AI = aortic insufficiency
AIDS = acquired immunodeficiency syndrome
ALARA = as low as reasonably achievable
ALK PHOS = alkaline phosphatase
ALT = alanine aminotransferase
AML = angiomyolipoma; acute monocytic leukemia
A-mode = amplitude mode; amplitude modulation scan
ant = anterior
AO = aorta
AP = anterior-posterior; anteroposterior
APC = atrial premature contraction
ARDS = acute respiratory distress syndrome; adult
    respiratory distress syndrome
ARPKD = autosomal recessive polycystic kidney disease
ART = assisted reproductive therapy
AS = aortic stenosis
ASAP = as soon as possible
ASCVD = arteriosclerotic cardiovascular disease
ASD = atrial septal defect
ASHD = arteriosclerotic heart disease
AST = aspartate aminotransferase
ATN = acute tubular necrosis
AVSD = atrioventricular septal defect
b.i.d. = twice a day
BD = binocular distance
BE = barium enema
BI-RADS = breast imaging and reporting system
BLS = basic life support
biVAD = biventricular assist device
B-mode = brightness modulation
BP = blood pressure
BPD = biparietal diameter
BPH = benign prostatic hypertrophy
BPM = beats per minute
BPP = biophysical profile
BUN = blood urea nitrogen
Bx = biopsy
C = Celsius
c = with
c/o = complains of
CA = cancer
ca = cancer
Ca = calcium
CABG = coronary artery bypass graft

CABS = coronary artery bypass surgery

CAD = coronary artery disease; computer-aided diagnosis

CAT or CT (scan) = computed axial tomography or computed tomography

CBC = complete blood count

CBD = common bile duct

cc = cubic centimeter

CCA = common carotid artery

CCU = cardiac care unit

CD = common duct

CDI = color Doppler imaging

CES = contrast-enhanced sonography

CFA = common femoral artery

CFD = color flow Doppler

CFI = color flow imaging

CFM = color flow mapping

CHB = complete heart block

CHD = congenital heart disease; congestive heart disease; common hepatic duct

CI = cephalic index; cardiac index

cm = centimeter

CMR = cardiovascular magnetic resonance; congenital mitral regurgitation

CNS = central nervous system

COPD = chronic obstructive pulmonary disease

CPR = cardiopulmonary resuscitation

Cr = creatinine

CRL = crown-rump length

CRT = cardiac resynchronization therapy; cathode ray tube

CSF = cerebrospinal fluid

CSP = cavum septum pellucidum

CST = contraction stress test

CTA = computed tomographic angiography

CTSU = cardiothoracic stepdown unit

CVA = cardiovascular accident; cerebrovascular accident

CVD = cardiovascular disease

CVS = chorionic villi sampling

Cvx = cervix

CW = continuous wave

Cx = cancelled

D&C = dilatation and curettage

D&E = dilatation and evacuation

D/C = discontinue

dB = decibel

DFV = deep femoral vein

DGC = depth gain compensation

DICOM = Digital Imaging and Communications in Medicine

DOB = date of birth

DORV = double-outlet right ventricle

DJD = degenerative joint disease

DTI = Doppler tissue imaging

DUS = duplex ultrasonography

DVT = deep venous thrombosis

Dx = diagnosis

ECA = external carotid artery

ECG or EKG = electrocardiogram

EDC = estimated date of confinement

EDD = estimated due date

EEG = electroencephalogram; echoencephalogram

EFW = estimated fetal weight

EFOV = extended field of view

EJV = external jugular vein

ERCP = endoscopic retrograde cholangiopancreatography

ERUS = endorectal ultrasound

ESP = early systolic peak; end-systolic pressure

EtOH = ethanol; alcohol

EUP = extrauterine pregnancy

EUS = endoscopic ultrasound

EVS or EVUS = endovaginal sonography or endovaginal ultrasound

F = Fahrenheit

F/U = follow-up

FAST = focal assessment by sonography in trauma

FBM = fetal breathing movement

FFT = fast Fourier transform

FHT = fetal heart tones

FL = femur length

FNA = fine needle aspiration

FNH = focal nodular hyperplasia

FSH = follicle-stimulating hormone

FSV = forward stroke volume

FUO = fever of unknown origin

Fx = fracture

G = gravid

GA = gestational age

GB = gallbladder

GERD = gastroesophageal reflux disease

GI = gastrointestinal

GIFT = gamete intrafallopian transfer

gm = gram

GS = gestational sac

GSV = greater saphenous vein

GTD = gestational trophoblastic disease

GU = genitourinary

GYN = gynecology

HC = head circumference

HC/AC = head circumference to abdominal circumference ratio

HCC = hepatocellular carcinoma

hCG = human chorionic gonadotropin

hct = hematocrit

HCVD = hypertensive cardiovascular disease

HF = heart failure

Hg = mercury

Hgb = hemoglobin

HIFU = high-intensity focused ultrasound

HIV = human immunodeficiency virus

HLHS = hypoplastic left heart syndrome

HPS = hypertrophic pyloric stenosis

HRHS = hypoplastic right heart syndrome

HVD = hypertensive vascular disease

HVL = half value layer

Hx = history

Hydro = hydronephrosis; hydrocephalus

Hz = Hertz

IAS = interatrial septum

IBS = irritable bowel syndrome
ICA = internal carotid artery
ICD = implantable cardioverter-defibrillator
ICE = intracardiac echocardiography
ICU = intensive care unit
IDDM = insulin-dependent diabetes mellitus
IJV = internal jugular vein
IM = intramuscular
IMA = inferior mesenteric artery
IOD = inner ocular diameter
IOS = intraoperative sonography
IRP = International Reference Preparation;
    interventional reference point
IUD or IUCD = intrauterine device or intrauterine
    contraceptive device
IUGR = intrauterine growth restriction
IUP = intrauterine pregnancy
IV = intravenous
IVC = inferior vena cava
IVF = in vitro fertilization
IVH = intraventricular hemorrhage
IVP = intravenous pyelogram
IVSD = interventricular septal defect
IVUS = intravascular ultrasound
JODM = juvenile onset diabetes mellitus
K = potassium
kg = kilogram
kHz = kilohertz
L/S (ratio) = lecithin-sphingomyelin
LA = left atrium
LAO = left anterior oblique
lat = lateral
LBBB = left bundle-branch block
LFT = liver function test
LH = luteinizing hormone
LHV = left hepatic vein
LIQ = lower inner quadrant
LK = left kidney
LLE = left lower extremity
LLQ = left lower quadrant
LMP = last menstrual period
LNMP = last normal menstrual period
LOQ = lower outer quadrant
LP = lumbar puncture
LPA = left pulmonary artery
LPO = left posterior oblique
LPV = left portal vein; left pulmonary vein
LRA = left renal artery
LRV = left renal vein
Lt = left
LUE = left upper extremity
LUQ = left upper quadrant
LUS = lower uterine segment
LV = left ventricular
LVD = left ventricular dysfunction
LVAD = left ventricular assist device
LVOT = left ventricular outflow tract
MCA = middle cerebral artery
MCDK = multicystic dysplastic kidney disease
MCL = medial collateral ligament

MET = estimated metabolic equivalents of exercise
mg = milligram
MHV = middle hepatic vein
MHz = megahertz
MI = myocardial infarction
MIS = mitral insufficiency
ML = midline
ml or mL = milliliter (1 ml = 1 cc)
mm = millimeter
M-mode = motion mode
MPA = main portal artery
MPV = main portal vein
MR = magnetic resonance imaging; mitral regurgitation
MRA = magnetic resonance angiography
MRCP = magnetic resonance cholangiopancreatography
MRI = magnetic resonance imaging
mrn = medical record number
MS = mitral stenosis; multiple sclerosis
MSD = mean sac diameter
MSI = musculoskeletal injury
MSK = musculoskeletal
MVP = mitral valve prolapsed
MVS = mitral valve stenosis
Na = sodium
Neuro = neurology; neurosurgery
NG = nasogastric
NICU = neonatal intensive care unit
NKDA = no known drug allergies
NPO = nothing by mouth
NT = nuchal translucency
NTD = neural tube defect
Ob = obstetrics
OCG = oral cholecystogram
OD = ocular diameter
OFD = occipital-frontal diameter
OR = operating room
Ortho = orthopedic
oz = ounce
PA = popliteal artery; popliteal aneurysm
PACS = picture archival communication system
PACU = postanesthesia care unit
PAH = pulmonary arterial hypertension
Para = number of full-term pregnancies, premature
    births, abortions, living children
PCA = posterior cerebral artery
PCI = percutaneous coronary intervention
PCOD = polycystic ovarian disease
PCOS or POS = polycystic ovarian syndrome
PDA = patent ductus arteriosus
PE = pericardial effusion; pulmonary embolus;
    pleural effusion
PET = positron emission tomography
PFO = patent foramen ovale
PI = pulsatility index
PID = pelvic inflammatory disease
post = posterior
PMV = prolapsed mitral valve
PMVL = posterior mitral valve leaflet
PPD = tuberculosis skin test
prep = preparation

PR = pulmonary regurgitation
PROM = premature rupture of membranes
PSA = prostate-specific antigen
Psych = psychology; psychiatric
pt = patient
PT = physical therapy; prothrombin time
PTT = partial thromboplastin time
PUBS = percutaneous umbilical cord sampling
PV = pulmonary valve
PVD = peripheral vascular disease
PVL = periventricular leukomalacia
PVR = peripheral vascular resistance
PVT = portal vein thrombosis
q = every
q.i.d. = four times a day
QA = quality assurance
qd = every day
QRS = electrocardiographic wave
R = right
R/O = rule out
RA = right atrium
RAD = reactive airway disease
RAO = right anterior oblique
RBC = red blood cell
RCC = renal cell carcinoma
RHV = right hepatic vein
RI = resistive index
RK = right kidney
RLE = right lower extremity
RLQ = right lower quadrant
RNI = radionuclide imaging
ROI = region of interest
RPO = right posterior oblique
RPOC = retained products of conception
RPA = right pulmonary artery
RPV = right portal vein; right pulmonary vein
Rt = right
RUQ = right upper quadrant
RV = right ventricle
RVOT = right ventricular outflow tract
Rx = prescription
s = without
s/p = status post
SD = standard deviation
SFA = superficial femoral artery
SHG = sonohysterography
SICU = surgical intensive care unit
SIS = saline infusion sonohysterography
SLN = sentinel lymph node
SMA = superior mesenteric artery
SMV = superior mesenteric vein
SOB = short of breath
SPECT = single-photon emission computed tomography
STAT = immediately
STD = sexually transmitted disease
Surg = surgery or surgical
SCV = superior vena cava
SVT = supraventricular tachycardia
TB = tuberculosis
t.i.d = three times a day

TCC = transitional cell carcinoma
TCD = transcranial Doppler
TE = transesophageal
TEE = transesophageal echocardiography
TGC or TCG = time gain compensation or time-compensated gain
THI = tissue harmonics imaging
TIA = transient ischemic attack
TIMI = thrombolysis in myocardial infarction
TIPS = transjugular intrahepatic portosystemic shunt
TOA = tubo-ovarian abscess
TOF = tetralogy of Fallot
TPN = total parenteral nutrition
Tr = transverse
tsp = teaspoon
TSH = thyroid-stimulating hormone
TTE = transthoracic echocardiogram
TTTS = twin-to-twin transfusion syndrome
TURP = transurethral resection of the prostate
TVS or TVUS = transvaginal sonography or transvaginal ultrasound
UA = urinalysis
UAE = uterine artery embolization
UE = upper extremity
UGI = upper gastrointestinal series
UIQ = upper inner quadrant
UPJ or PUJ = ureteropelvic junction or pelvic-ureteral junction
UOQ = upper outer quadrant
URI = upper respiratory infection
US = ultrasonography
UTI = urinary tract infection
UVJ = ureterovesical junction
VACTERL = vertebral, anal, cardiac, tracheal, esophageal, renal, limb
vag = vaginal or vagina
VATER = vertebral, anal, tracheal, esophageal, renal
VCUG = voiding cystourethrogram
VPC = ventricular premature contraction
VT = ventricular tachycardia
W/C = wheelchair
WBC = white blood cell; white blood count
WES = wall-echo-shadow
WNL = within normal limits
YS = yolk sac

Commonly Used Symbols

>	greater than
<	less than
=	equal to
≥	greater than or equal to
≤	less than or equal to
≠	not equal to
≈	approximately equal to
↑	increased
↓	decreased
°	degree
♀	female
♂	male
xx	female

xy	male	#	number or pound
@	at	:	ratio
+	positive	%	percent
−	negative	▲	change
×	times		

Bibliography

Stedman's Radiology Words: Includes Nuclear Medicine & Other Imaging. 6th ed. Baltimore, MA: Lippincott Williams & Wilkins; 2009.

Medical Terminology Made Incredibly Easy. 2nd ed. Ambler, PA: Lippincott Williams & Wilkins; 2004.

Appendix 2
Translation Resources and English-to-Spanish Phrases*

Helpful Free Internet Translation Resources	
FreeTranslation.com	http://www.freetranslation.com/
Google Translate	https://translate.google.com/
SpanishDict.com	http://www.spanishdict.com/translation
WorldLingo.com	http://www.worldlingo.com/en/products_services/worldlingo_translator.html

Review of English-to-Spanish Terminology†

Basic Phrases		
English	**Spanish**	**Phonetic Spelling**
Please	Por favor	por fah-vor
Thank you	Gracias	grah-see-ahs
Good morning	Buenos días	bway-nos dee-ahs
Good afternoon	Buenas tardes	bway-nas tar-days
Good evening	Buenas noches	bway-nas noh-chays
My name is _____.	Mi nombre es _____.	me nohm-bray ays
Yes	Sí	see
No	No	no
What is your name?	¿Cómo te llamas? ¿Cuál es tu nombre?	koh-moh tay jah-mahs kwal ays too nohm-bray
How old are you?	¿Cuántos años tienes?	kwan-tohs ahn-yos tee-aynjays
Do you understand me?	¿Me entiendes?	me ayn-tee-ayn-days
Speak slower please.	Hablar más despacio por favor.	ah-blahr mahs days-pah-see-oh por fah-vor
How do you feel?	¿Cómo te sientes?	koh-moh tay see-ayn-tays
Good	Bueno	bway-noh
Bad	Mal; malo	mahl; mahlo
Hello	Hola	o-la
Goodbye	Adiós	ah-dee-os

---

*In order to provide optimal patient care, the best practice is to obtain the assistance of a certified medical interpreter.
†This review section is provided for those who are already familiar with Spanish phraseology and correct diction.

General Words		
English	**Spanish**	**Phonetic Spelling**
Zero	Cero	se-roh
One	Uno	oo-noh
Two	Dos	dohs
Three	Tres	trays
Four	Cuatro	kwah-troh
Five	Cinco	sin-koh
Six	Seis	says
Seven	Siete	see-ay-tay
Eight	Ocho	oh-choh
Nine	Nueve	new-ay-vay
Ten	Diez	dee-ays
Hundred	Cien	see-en
Sunday	Domingo	doh-min-goh
Monday	Lunes	loo-nays
Tuesday	Martes	mar-tays
Wednesday	Miércoles	mee-er-cohl-ays
Thursday	Jueves	hway-vays
Friday	Viernes	vee-ayr-nays
Today	Hoy	oy
Tomorrow	Mañana	mah-nyah-nah
Last night	Anoche	ah-noh-chay
Yesterday	Ayer	ai-yer
Last week	La semana pasada	la say-may-nah pa-sa-da
Right	Derecho	day-ray-cho
Left	Izquierdo	eez-kee-ayr-doh
Girl	Chica	chee-ka
Boy	Niño	neen-yo

Anatomy Terms	
English	**Spanish**
Blood	Sangre
Blood vessel	Vaso sanguíneo
Stool	Taburete
The abdomen	El abdomen
The aorta	La aorta
The arm	El brazo
The back	La espalda
The bones	Los huesos
The bowel	El intestino
The brain	El cerebro
The carotid	La carótida
The chest	El pecho
The ears	Los oidos
The eye	El ojo
The foot	El pie
The gallbladder	La vesícula biliar
The hand	La mano
The head	La cabeza
The heart	El corazón
The kidneys	Los riñones
The leg	La pierna
The liver	El hígado
The mouth	La boca
The neck	El cuello
The nose	La nariz
The ovary	El ovario
The pancreas	El páncreas
The penis	El pene
The skin	La piel
The spleen	El bazo
The stomach	El estómago
The testicle	El testículo
The thyroid	La tiroides
The tongue	La lengua
The urinary bladder	La vejiga urinaria
The uterus	El útero
The vagina	La vagina
Urine	Orina
Vomit	Vómito

| Sonographic Examination Instructions ||
English	Spanish
Ultrasound gel	Gel de ultrasonido
Ultrasound transducer	Transductor de ultrasonido
Ultrasound machine	Máquina de ultrasonido
Wheelchair	Silla de ruedas
Stretcher	Camilla
Intravenous bag	Goteo intravenoso
Blanket	Manta
Please take in a deep breath.	Por favor, tome una respiración profunda.
Please hold your breath.	Por favor, mantenga la respiración.
Please roll over on your left side.	Por favor, darse la vuelta sobre su lado izquierdo.
Please roll over on your right side.	Por favor, darse la vuelta sobre su lado derecho.
Please sit up.	Por favor, siéntese.
Please stand up.	Por favor ponerse de pie.
Please empty your urinary bladder.	Por favor, vacíe la vejiga urinaria.
Please fill your urinary bladder.	Por favor, llene la vejiga urinaria.
Please lie on your back.	Por favor, acostarse boca arriba.
Please remove your clothes from the waist up.	Por favor, quítese la ropa de cintura para arriba.
Please remove your clothes from the waist down.	Por favor, quítese la ropa de la cintura para abajo.
Please lift your arm over your head.	Por favor, levante el brazo sobre la cabeza.
Please hold your breath.	Por favor, mantenga la respiración.
Please empty your bladder.	Por favor, vacíe la vejiga.
This may be uncomfortable.	Esto puede ser incómodo.
Take in a deep breath and hold it.	Tome una respiración profunda y mantenerla.
I am finished.	Estoy acabado.
I will be back soon.	Estaré de vuelta pronto.
Please stay here.	Por favor, quédate aquí.
Please sit here.	Por favor, siéntate aquí.
You may get dressed now.	Puede vestirse ahora.
Your doctor will give you the results of this test.	Su médico le dará los resultados de esta prueba.

Clinical History Questions	
English	**Spanish**
Are you comfortable?	¿Se siente cómodo?
Are you having vaginal bleeding?	¿Tiene sangrado vaginal?
Are you pregnant?	¿Está embarazada?
Do you feel dizzy?	¿Se siente mareado?
Do you have a fever?	¿Tiene fiebre?
Do you have pain?	¿Tiene dolor?
Do you have any difficulty breathing?	¿Tiene usted alguna dificultad para respirar?
Have you had an ultrasound before?	¿Ha tenido una ecografía antes?
How do you feel?	¿Cómo te sientes?
How long have you felt this way?	¿Cuánto tiempo has sentido así?
How many children do you have?	¿Cuántos hijos tienes?
How many times have you been pregnant?	¿Cuántas veces ha estado embarazada?
How much water have you had to drink?	¿Cuánta agua ha tenido que beber?
What was the date of your last menstrual period?	¿Cuál fue la fecha de su último período menstrual?
When is your due date?	¿Cuándo es la fecha de vencimiento?
When was the last time you had something to eat or drink?	¿Cuándo fue la última vez que tuvo algo de comer o beber?
Where is your pain?	¿Dónde está tu dolor?

Bibliography

Google Translate. Accessed December 29, 2014 from https://translate.google.com/

Molle EA, Kronenberger J, West-Stack C. *Lippincott Williams and Wilkins' Clinical Medical Assisting.* 2nd ed. Philadelphia: Lippincott, Williams, & Wilkins; 2005.

Appendix 3
Patient Care Procedures

Procedure 10-1 Measuring a Radial Pulse[1]

- Wash your hands, and put on gloves.
- Position the patient with the arm relaxed and supported either on the patient's lap or a table.
- Have the patient place his or her palm up.
- With the index finger, middle finger, and ring finger of your dominant hand, press with your fingertips firmly enough to feel the pulse on the wrist's thumb side (Fig. A3-1).

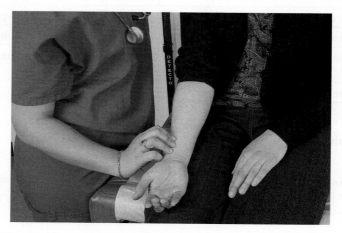

Figure A3-1. Press with your fingertips firmly enough to feel the pulse on the wrist's thumb side.

- Be gentle to avoid compressing the artery.
- If the pulse seems regular, count for 30 seconds, watching the second hand of your watch or a clock. Multiply that number by 2 to obtain the beats per minute. If the pulse is irregular, watch for an entire minute.
- Document the rate as required.
- Also note the rhythm of the pulse.
- Remove your gloves, and wash your hands.

Procedure 10-2 Measuring a Blood Pressure[1,2]

- Wash your hands, and put on gloves.
- Position the patient with the arm to be used supported with the forearm on the lap or a table and slightly flexed with the palm upward. The arm should be at the level of the patient's heart.
- The patient's arm should not be covered.
- Palpate the brachial pulse and center the cuff directly over the brachial artery (Fig. A3-2).

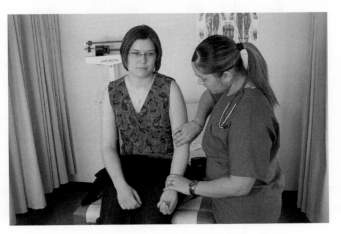

Figure A3-2. Palpate the brachial pulse.

- Wrap the cuff around the arm (Fig. A3-3).

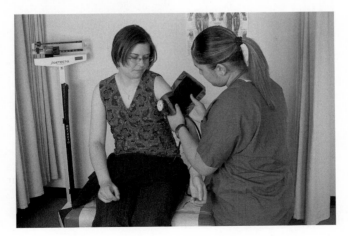

Figure A3-3. Wrap the cuff around the arm.

(*Continued*)

- Make sure the gauge can be clearly seen.
- Palpate the brachial pulse, and position the stethoscope over the brachial artery, holding it in position with two fingers (Fig. A3-4).

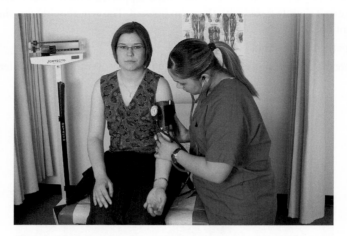

Figure A3-4. Position the stethoscope over the brachial artery.

- Tighten the screw valve on the bulb. Do not tighten it too much, however.
- Inflate the cuff smoothly and quickly to peak inflation level (Fig. A3-5).

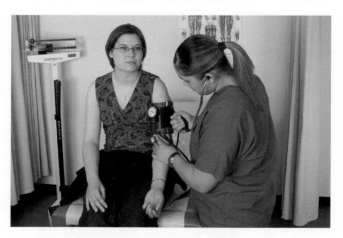

Figure A3-5. Inflate the cuff smoothly and quickly.

- Place the diaphragm of the stethoscope over the brachial artery.
- Loosen the screw valve carefully.

- Slowly deflate the cuff at 2 to 4 mm Hg per second (Fig. A3-6).

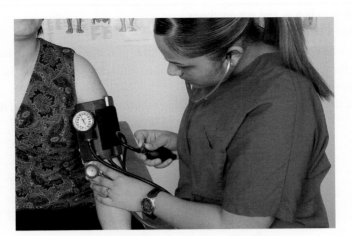

Figure A3-6. Slowly deflate the cuff, making note of the first and last beat that you can hear.

- Listen for the first beat (Korotkoff phase I), noting when it appears. This is the top number in the patient's blood pressure or the systolic pressure.
- Continue to listen to the beats, noting the point at which all sound disappears (Korotkoff phase V). This is the bottom number in the patient's blood pressure or the diastolic pressure.
- Continue to deflate the cuff.
- Remove the cuff.
- Document the blood pressure as required.
- Remove your gloves, and wash your hands.
- Remember to clean all used medical equipment.

Procedure 10-3 Measuring Respirations
<ul><li>If possible, have the patient sit upright to obtain the respiratory rate.</li><li>Without the patient's knowledge, count each respiration by observing his or her chest rise and fall.</li><li>One respiration, or breathing sequence, is equal to one inhalation and subsequent exhalation.</li><li>Count respiration for at least 30 seconds.</li><li>Multiply that number by 2 to obtain a full minute of respirations.</li><li>If rate, rhythm, or depth is obviously abnormal, count for a complete minute.</li><li>Document respirations as required.</li></ul>

Procedure 10-4 Sheet Transfer[3]

- Wash your hands, and put on gloves.
- Obtain a heavy sheet, and fold it in half.
- Have one person stand on each side of the table or bed at the patient's side.
- Roll the patient on to his or her side opposite to the direction that the patient needs to be moved.
- Place the sheet on the table with the fold against the patient's body (Fig. A3-7).

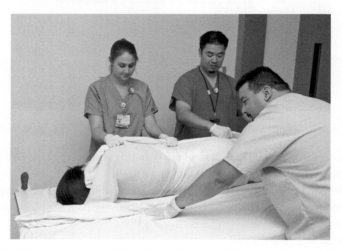

Figure A3-7. Roll the patient on to his or her side opposite to the direction that the patient needs to be moved.

- Roll the top half of the sheet as close to the patient's back as possible (Fig. A3-8).

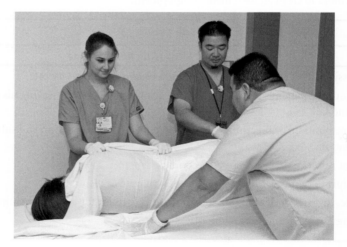

Figure A3-8. Roll the top half of the sheet as close to the patient's back as possible.

- Turn the patient toward the side of the move, and have your assistant straighten the sheet away from the patient. Return the patient to the supine position. The sheet should be accessible under the patient (Fig. A3-9).

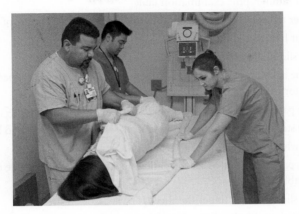

Figure A3-9. Turn the patient toward the side of the move, and have your assistant straighten the sheet away from the patient.

- To transfer the patient, obtain the assistance of three other individuals.
- Ensure that all tubing (intravenous line, catheter tubes, etc.) is stable for the move.
- Have two people at the shoulder level of the patient and two at the upper legs of the patient across from each other. One person will need to support the patient's head.
- Grasping the unrolled transfer sheet from under the patient in unison counting to three, the team transfers the patient onto the new surface.
- Remove your gloves, and wash your hands.

Procedure 10-5 Log Roll[3]

- Log roll is a method of transferring trauma patients who may have spinal injuries. This method is used to prevent any further damage to the spine. The goal is to maintain spinal alignment. At least three people are required or a log roll transfer.
- Wash your hands, and put on gloves.
- One person must hold the patient's head.
- Two people must support the chest, abdomen, and lower limbs.
- The patient should be told to lie still and to not try to move using his or her own strength.
- Ensure that all tubing (intravenous line, catheter tubes, etc.) is stable for the move.
- The patient's arm that is away from the side of the intended move must be placed on his or her chest or extended along his or her chest and abdomen.
- Place a pillow between the patient's legs.
- One individual on the side of the patient supports the patient's upper body by placing one hand on the shoulders and the other hand around the patient's thighs.
- The other individual supports the patient's abdomen and lower extremities by overlapping with the first individual's arm to place on the hand under the patient's lower back and the other over the patient's lower legs.
- The individual holding the patient's head directs the transfer.
- Once the sheet is placed under the patient (as noted in Procedure 10-4), the transfer can take place.
- Remove your gloves, and wash your hands.

Procedure 10-6 Sliding Board Transfer[3]

- A smooth sliding board may be used to move a sonography patient to another surface, perhaps a radiographic examination table.
- Remember to keep the side rails of the stretcher up until the time of the move.
- Wash your hands, and put on gloves.
- Obtain a sliding board.
- Obtain the assistance of at least one other person, though several people may be required for moving larger patients.
- Move the patient to the edge of the stretcher.
- Move the stretcher to the edge of the table to which the patient is to be transferred.
- Lock the wheels to the stretcher.
- Using the patient's sheet, assist the patient to turn on his or her side away from the transfer table.
- Place the sliding board under the sheet partway.
- Create a bridge with the sliding board between the stretcher and the table (Fig. A3-10).

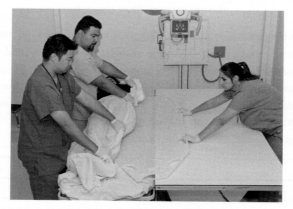

Figure A3-10. Create a bridge with the sliding board between the stretcher and the table.

- Ensure that the patient's sheet is over the board while allowing the patient to slowly lie down on the board.
- With one person on the side of the table and the other at the side of the stretcher, slide the patient over the board and onto the table using the patient's sheet (Fig. A3-11).

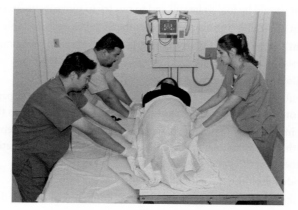

Figure A3-11. Slide the patient over the board and onto the table using the patient's sheet.

- To remove the board completely, have the patient roll on his or her side (Fig. A3-12).

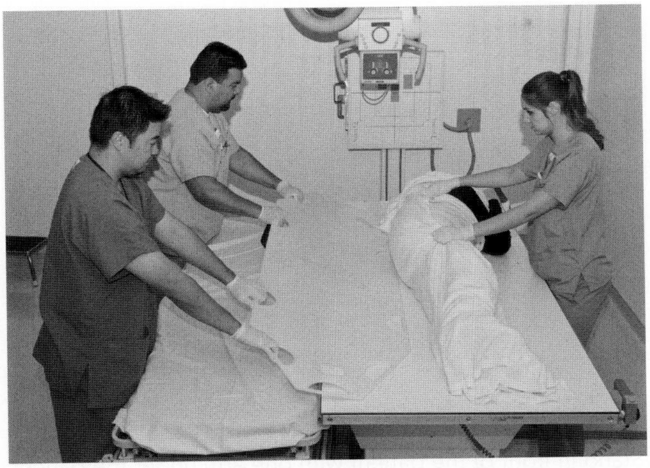

Figure A3-12. To remove the board completely, have the patient roll on his or her side.

- Once the board is removed, ensure that the patient is securely on the table before removing the stretcher.
- Remove your gloves, and wash your hands.

Procedure 10-7 Wheelchair Transfer[3]

- Occasionally, patients may visit the sonography department in a wheelchair, thus requiring that they be assisted from the wheelchair to the sonography stretcher.
- Wash your hands, and put on gloves.
- From the wheelchair to the stretcher:
  - Lower the stretcher or table to the lowest position.
  - Place the wheelchair near the stretcher.
  - Engage the brakes on the wheelchair, and open the footrests.
  - Assist the patient to the standing position.
  - Allow the patient to obtain his or her balance before walking.
  - Provide the patient with a stool if necessary.
  - Help the patient to the table.
  - Ask him or her to turn around, and assist him or her to the sitting position.
- From the supine position to the wheelchair:
  - Ask the patient or assist the patient on to his or her side facing you.
  - Ask the patient to flex his or her knees.

(*Continued*)

- ○ Stand in front of the patient with one arm under the patient's shoulder and the other across the knees (Fig. A3-13).

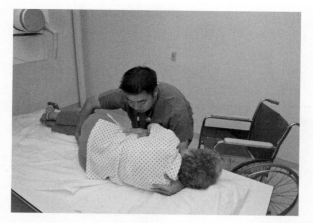

Figure A3-13. Stand in front of the patient with one arm under the patient's shoulder and the other across the knees.

- ○ If the patient can help, allow him or her to push with the upper arm.
- ○ On the count of three, move or help the patient to a sitting position.
- ○ Allow the patient to obtain his or her balance.
- ○ Obtain a stool or lower the stretcher until the patient's feet touch the floor.
- ○ If the patient needs minimal assistance, stand at the side of the stretcher, and help the patient stand.
- ○ Ensure that the wheelchair is placed close to the stretcher and that the brakes are engaged completely.
- ○ Open the footrests so that patient can approach the wheelchair safely.
- ○ Stand at the patient's side, and assist him or her to the wheelchair (Fig. A3-14).
- ○ Once the patient is near the wheelchair, have him or her turn around and sit down slowly. It is best to have someone hold the wheelchair steady for the patient as he or she sits down.

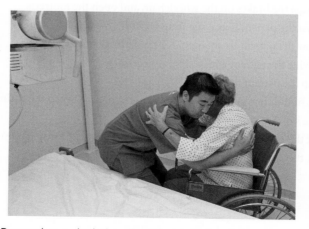

Figure A3-14. Remember to lock the wheelchair's brakes first. Assist him or her to the sitting position in the wheelchair.

- Transport the patient as needed.
- Once the wheelchair is no longer required, clean it thoroughly.
- Remove your gloves, and wash your hands.

Procedure 12-1 Hand Hygiene[1]

- Remove all rings and your wristwatch.
- Stand close to the sink without touching it.
- Turn the faucet on, and adjust the temperature so that it is warm.
- Wet your hands and wrists under the warm water, and apply liquid soap (Fig. A3-15).

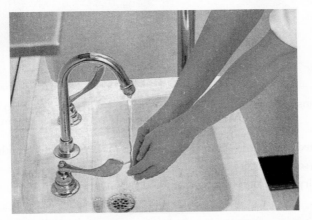

Figure A3-15. Wet your hands and wrists under the warm water, and apply liquid soap.

- Rub your palms together.
- Clean between your fingers at least 10 times.
- Scrub the palm of one hand with the fingertips of the other using a circular motion (Fig. A3-16).

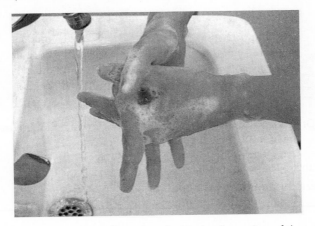

Figure A3-16. Scrub the palm of one hand with the fingertips of the other using a circular motion.

(Continued)

- Work the soap under your fingernails.
- Reverse the process for the other hand.
- Rinse hands thoroughly under running warm water, holding your hands lower than your elbows to allow the water to drain from them (Fig. A3-17).

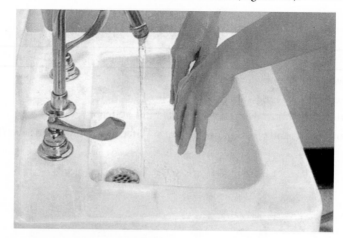

Figure A3-17. Rinse hands thoroughly under running warm water, holding your hands lower than your elbows to allow the water to drain from them.

- If supplied, use the orangewood stick to clean under each nail on both hands.
- Reapply soap, and wash and dry hands in the same manner as above.
- Gently dry your hands with a paper towel (Fig. A3-18).

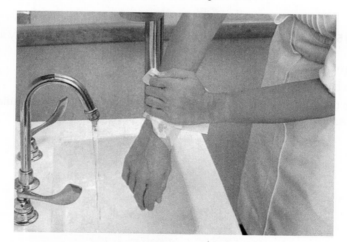

Figure A3-18. Dry your hands thoroughly with a paper towel and then use another paper towel to turn off the sink.

- Discard the soiled paper towels.
- Use a clean dry towel to turn off the faucet.

Procedure 12-2 Removing Personal Protective Equipment[4]

- After removing gloves.
- Remove any head or face coverings like masks first (Fig. A3-19).

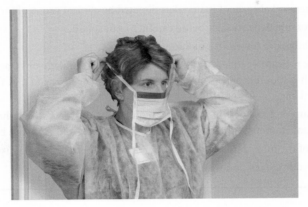

Figure A3-19. Remove your head and face covering first after removing your gloves.

- To remove the mask, touch only the ties or elastic bands and discard the mask in a receptacle.
- To remove a soiled gown, unfasten the neck and then back closure of the gown.
- Remove the gown by inserting your fingers into the upper sleeve near your shoulder (Fig. A3-20).

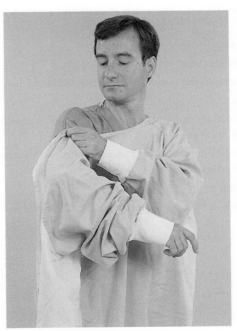

Figure A3-20. Roll the gown forward, keeping the soiled outer part inside and covered.

- Roll the gown forward, keeping the soiled outer part inside and covered.
- Once the gown is off, roll it up, and place it in the appropriate receptacle.
- Wash your hands.

Procedure 12-3 Cleaning Biohazardous Spills[1]

- Put on gloves.
- Wear any other necessary PPEs, such as a gown or eyewear, if you anticipate splatter.
- Apply chemical absorbent material as directed by clinical protocol for your facility.
- Use disposable paper towels, being careful to not splash.
- Dispose all paper towels in a biohazard (red) bag.
- Spray the previously soiled area with a commercial germicide or bleach solution and wipe with disposable paper towels, remembering to again dispose of these towels in the biohazard bag.
- Remove any reusable personal protective equipment and place in a biohazard laundry bag. Remove any nonreusable personal protective equipment and place in a biohazard bag.
- Discard of the biohazard bag as recommended by your clinical facility.
- Remove your gloves, and wash your hands.

Procedure 13-1 Skin Preparation[3]

- Supplies that you may need include (but are not limited to):
  - Sterile gloves
  - Sterile preparation tray
  - A flask of sterile water and a flask of antiseptic solution as recommended by the physician
  - A sterile towel
- Explain to the patient what you are about to do.
- Pour sterile water into one basin and antiseptic solution into another.
- Don sterile gloves.
- Examine the skin in the applicable area for any visual scars, open wounds, or other skin abnormalities. If none are seen, you may proceed.
- Pick up the sponge from the tray that is permeated with antiseptic soap and dampen it in the basin of sterile water.
- Scrub in the center of the area to be cleaned.
- Using an area of 6 to 10 in is an appropriate size for cleaning for most biopsies.

- Work around in an outward circular motion, using a firm stroke to remove microorganisms from the skin (Fig. A3-21).

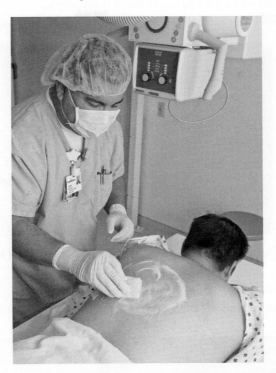

Figure A3-21. Work around in an outward circular motion, using a firm stroke to remove microorganisms from the skin.

- Do not overlap the area that has already been clean, but rather make progressively larger circles as you move away from the center.
- When the area has been covered, drop the sponge into the trash, and repeat the cleaning process with another sponge.
- Following the scrub, either rinse the area with sterile water, or remove the cleaning solution in the manner in which your institution suggests.
- Blot the skin dry with a sterile towel.
- Following the initial scrub, the area is typically cleaned with an antiseptic solution, such as chlorhexidine or hexachlorophene. This scrub is performed in a similar manner as above.

Procedure 13-2 Opening a Sterile Pack[3]

- Check the date on the pack to ensure that it is still usable.
- Place the pack on a clean tabletop with the sealed side toward you (Fig. A3-22).

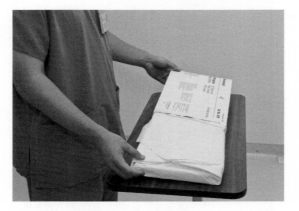

Figure A3-22. Place the pack on a clean tabletop with the sealed side toward you.

- Remove the outer plastic, and place the sealed end toward you.
- Open the first corner back and away (Fig. A3-23).

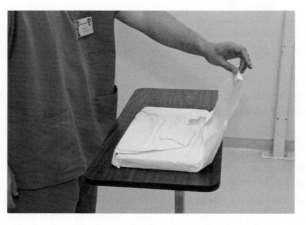

Figure A3-23. Open the first corner back and away.

- Open Corners 2 and 3 (Fig. A3-24).

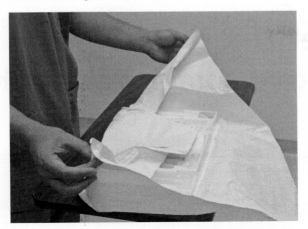

Figure A3-24. Open corners 2 and 3.

- Open Corner 4, and drop it toward you (Fig. A3-25).

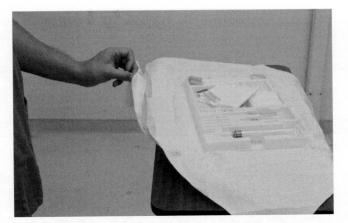

Figure A3-25. Open Corner 4, and drop it toward you.

- Do not leave the sterile pack unassisted or allow anything to come in contact with it.

References

1. Molle EA, Kronenberger J, West-Stack C. *Lippincott Williams and Wilkins' Clinical Medical Assisting*. 2nd ed. Philadelphia, PA: Lippincott Williams & Wilkins; 2005.
2. Bedford DJ, Allen MM. *LWW's Visual Atlas of Medical Assisting Skills*. Philadelphia, PA: Lippincott Williams & Wilkins; 2008.
3. Dutton AG, Linn-Watson TA, Torres LS. *Torres' Patient Care in Imaging Technology*. 8th ed. Philadelphia, PA: Lippincott Williams & Wilkins; 2013.
4. Timby BK. *Fundamental Nursing Skills and Concepts*. 10th ed. Philadelphia, PA: Lippincott Williams & Wilkins; 2013.

Appendix 4
Electrocardiographic Dysrhythmias[1]

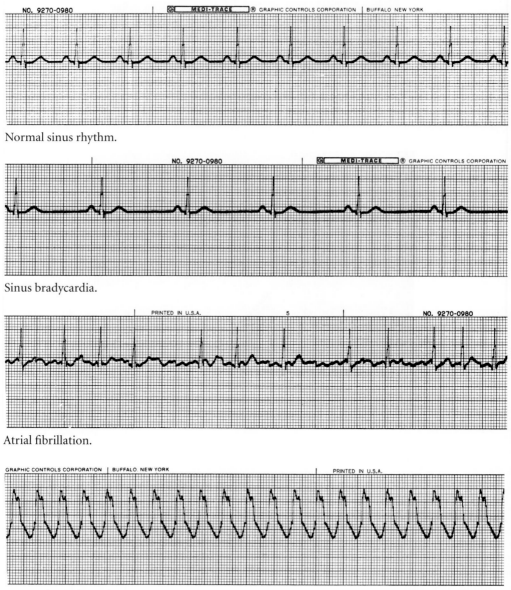

Normal sinus rhythm.

Sinus bradycardia.

Atrial fibrillation.

Ventricular tachycardia.

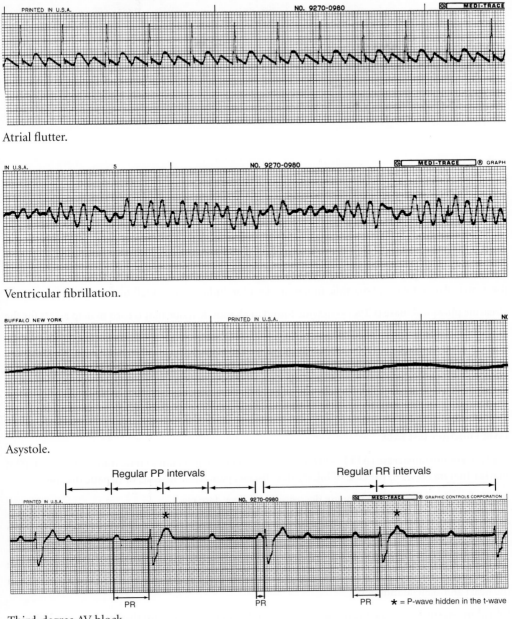

Atrial flutter.

Ventricular fibrillation.

Asystole.

Third-degree AV block.

Reference

1. Dutton AG, Linn-Watson TA, Torres LS. *Torres' Patient Care in Imaging Technology.* 8th ed. Philadelphia, PA: Lippincott Williams & Wilkins; 2013.

Appendix 5
Laboratory Tests

The following information is provided for the student to offer a brief description of the most common laboratory tests performed that are clinically applicable to sonographic practice. Specific ranges are not provided, as these are most often laboratory-specific. Typically, abnormal laboratory findings will be delineated on the laboratory report.

Cardiac Markers (Elevation in the following labs could indicate a myocardial infarction.)

Brain natriuretic peptide—hormone produced by the ventricles of the heart that is used to evaluate for ventricular systolic and diastolic function; elevation indicates heart failure

Creatine phosphokinase (CPK)—enzyme found in all muscle tissue that is used to help assess for the presence of a myocardial infarction

Lactate dehydrogenase (LDH)—found throughout the body but is used to help assess for the presence of a myocardial infarction; elevation indicates possible myocardial infarction; can also be used as a tumor marker

Myoglobin—marker used for muscle damage to the heart

Liver Function Test Labs

Alanine aminotransferase (ALT)—enzyme formerly known as serum pyretic transaminase (SGPT); marker that increases in the case of biliary tree disease, pancreatic disease, or hepatic disease

Albumin—the main plasma protein; decreases with liver damage

Alkaline phosphatase (ALP)—enzyme found in the liver tissue; also found in bone, biliary tract, intestines, kidney, and placenta; elevation indicates biliary obstruction or liver cancer

Aspartate aminotransferase (AST)—formerly known as serum glutamic-oxaloacetic transaminase (SGOT); can be use to indicate liver injury but not as specific compared to ALT; AST is also found in the heart and skeletal muscles

Bilirubin—results from the breakdown of hemoglobin in red blood cells; the liver removes bilirubin and excretes it in the bile; may be described as direct (conjugated) or indirect (unconjugated); elevation indicates liver disease, biliary obstruction, and other systemic disorders and syndromes

Gamma-glutamyl transferase (GGT)—enzyme found in the liver; may be used in conjunction with ALP to differentiate liver verses bone disease

Partial thromboplastin time (PTT)—used to monitor anticoagulation; assessed prior to invasive procedures

Prothrombin—produced by the liver for blood clotting

Prothrombin time (PT)—the amount of time it takes blood to clot when mixed with thromboplastin reagent; assessed prior to invasive procedures

Urobilinogen—urine test used to evaluate for liver dysfunction or biliary obstruction

Lipid Profile Labs

Cholesterol—used to screen for the risk of heart disease

HDL Cholesterol—class of lipoproteins produced by the liver; "good" cholesterol

LDL Cholesterol—class of lipoproteins produced by the liver; "bad" cholesterol

Triglycerides—measures the body's ability to metabolize fat

Thyroid Profile Labs

Calcitonin—hormone produced by the thyroid gland that reduces circulating calcium levels by increasing calcium deposition in the bones; elevation may indicate thyroid cancer, lung cancer, or anemia

Thyroid-stimulating hormone (TSH)—produced by the anterior pituitary gland to regulate the production and release of thyroid hormones; elevation indicates hypothyroidism; decrease indicates hyperthyroidism

Thyroxine (T_4 or free thyroxine)—major hormone produced by the thyroid gland; controls basal metabolic rate; elevation indicates hyperthyroidism; decreased indicated hypothyroidism

Triiodothyronine (T_3)—hormone of the thyroid gland; elevation indicates hyperthyroidism; decrease indicates hypothyroidism

Renal Function Labs

Blood urea nitrogen (BUN)—byproduct of protein metabolism secreted mostly by the kidneys; elevation in most renal diseases but can be the result of dehydration, gastrointestinal bleeding, and congestive heart failure

Creatinine—byproduct of muscle breakdown secreted by the kidneys; increase indicates renal impairment

Specific gravity—measure of the dissolved material in the urine

Obstetrics Labs

Alpha-fetoprotein (AFP)—molecule produced by the developing embryo and fetus; can be used as a tumor marker for some cancers in both male and females; elevated serum maternal levels can indicate fetal open neural tube defects like anencephaly and spina bifida

Dimeric inhibin A (in pregnancy)—hormone produced by the placenta; used as a screening lab for fetal abnormalities

Human chorionic gonadotropin (HCG)—hormone produced by the placenta that indicates pregnancy; can be found in blood or urine; blood is more specific for dating a pregnancy, while urine simply indicates pregnancy; may also be used as a tumor marker for some testicular cancers

MaterniT21 PLUS (LTD)—maternal blood test that is highly effective at detecting Down Syndrome and many other chromosomal abnormalities

Pregnancy-associated plasma protein A (PAPPA)—hormone produced by the placenta; used as a screening lab for pregnancy

Unconjugated estriol (uE3)—hormone produced by the placenta; used as a screening lab for pregnancy

Pancreatic Labs

Amylase—produced by the pancreas; breaks down starch into sugar; elevation indicates pancreatic disorders like pancreatitis and pancreatic cancer; elevates first (before lipase) in cases of pancreatitis

Lipase—produced by the pancreas; breaks down fat; elevation indicates pancreatitis or other pancreatic disorders; more specific for pancreatitis compared to amylase

Other Labs

Bleeding time—assessed by making a 1-mm deep incision and noting the time it takes for bleeding to stop

CA-125—tumor marker elevated in most women with ovarian cancer; often used to monitor cancer after treatment; can be elevated with other disorders as well

Calcium—used to evaluate the parathyroid; elevated levels indicate hyperparathyroidism (often caused by a parathyroid adenoma)

Glucose—used to diagnose and monitor type 1 and 2 diabetes

Hematocrit—also called packed cell volume; the percentage of RBCs in the blood; decreased level could indicate internal hemorrhage (blood loss)

Hemoglobin—main protein in erythrocytes that carries oxygen to the red blood cells and removes carbon dioxide from red blood cells; composed of the pigment of blood, which includes iron and globin (protein)

Platelet count—platelets are cytoplasm fragments that are important in blood coagulation

Potassium—important for the conduction of nerve impulses and the contraction of muscles

Prostate-specific antigen (PSA)—protein made by the prostate gland

Red blood cell (RBC) count—the total number of red blood cells per cubic millimeter of blood

Sodium—critical to body water distribution and overall homeostasis

White blood cell (WBC) count—the total number of WBCs in a cubic millimeter of blood; elevation suggests infection or immune system disorder

Index

Note: Page numbers followed by 't and 'f indicates table and figure respectively.